S0-EJV-202

CANCER
An Introduction

CANCER
An Introduction

WILLIAM A. CREASEY

Department of Pharmacology
University of Pennsylvania
School of Medicine
Philadelphia, Pennsylvania

New York Oxford
OXFORD UNIVERSITY PRESS
1981

Library of Congress Cataloging in Publication Data

Creasey, William A.
Cancer, an introduction.

Bibliography: p.
Includes index.
1. Cancer. I. Title.
RC261.C77 616.99'4 81-3980
ISBN 0-19-502951-8 AACR2
ISBN 0-19-502952-6 (pbk.)

Printing (last digit): 9 8 7 6 5 4 3 2 1

Printed in the United States of America

I would like to thank the authors, journals, and publishers for their permission to reprint the following figures and tables in this text:

Figs. 1-4 and 1-6: J. Rosai and L. V. Ackerman, *Ca—A Cancer Journal for Clinicians*, 29:66 (1979), by permission American Cancer Society, Inc.
Fig. 1-5: S. A. Rosenberg and H. S. Kaplan, *Calif. Med.*, 113:23 (1970)
Fig. 2-1: C. J. Dawe, in *Cancer Medicine*, ed. by J. F. Holland and E. Frei III, Lea & Febiger, 1973
Figs. 2-3, 2-4, and 6-10: R. Süss, V. Kinzel, and J. D. Scribner, *Cancer—Experiments and Concepts*, Springer-Verlag, Heidelberg, 1973
Fig. 3-1: Data reproduced by permission from H. E. Skipper, in *Perspectives in Leukemia*, Vol. 1, Grune & Stratton, Inc., 1968
Fig. 3-3: Data based on reviews by G. G. Steel and L. F. Lamerton, *Br. J. Cancer*, 20:74 (1966) and G. G. Steel, in *Cancer Medicine*, ed. by J. F. Holland and E. Frei III, Lea & Febiger, 1973
Figs. 3-6, 3-7, 3-8, and 3-11: M. L. Mendelsohn, in *The Cell Cycle in Malignancy and Immunity*, J. C. Hampton, chairman, Energy Research and Development Center, 1945
Fig. 3-9: G. G. Steel, *Growth Kinetics of Tumors*, Oxford University Press, 1977
Fig. 3-10: L. F. Lamerton, in *Antineoplastic and Immunosuppressive Agents*, Vol. 1, ed. by A. C. Sartorelli and D. G. Johns, Springer-Verlag, Heidelberg, 1974
Fig. 3-12: E. Stubblefield and S. Murphee, in *Handbook of Experimental Pharmacology*, Vol. 38, Pt. 1, ed. by A. C. Sartorelli and D. G. Johns, Springer-Verlag, Heidelberg, 1974
Fig. 6-2: S. Broder, L. Muul, and T. A. Waldmann, *J. Natl. Cancer Inst.*, 61:5 (1972)
Fig. 6-8: R. H. Harris, T. Page, and N. A. Reiches, in *Origins of Human Cancer*, Book A, ed. by H. H. Hiatt, J. D. Watson, and J. A. Winsten, Cold Spring Harbor Laboratory, 1977
Fig. 6-12: M. Green, K. Fujinaga, M. Piña, and D. C. Thomas, in *Exploitable Molecular Mechanisms and Neoplasia*, Williams & Wilkins, 1969. By permission University of Texas M. D. Anderson Hospital
Fig. 6-13: G. J. Todaro and R. J. Huebner, *Proc. Natl. Acad. Sci. U.S.A.*, 69:1009 (1972)
Fig. 7-1: R. J. Shalek, in *Cancer: A Comprehensive Treatise*, Vol. 6, ed. by F. F. Becker, Plenum Press, 1977
Fig. 7-3: G. W. Barendsen, in *Proceedings of the Conference on Particle Accelerators in Radiation Therapy*, U.S. Atomic Energy Commission, Technical Information Center, 1972
Fig. 7-5: W. K. Sinclair, *Radiation Res.*, 33:620 (1968), by permission Academic Press
Fig. 7-6: M. M. Elkind and C. M. Chang-Liu, *Int. J. Radiation Biol.*, 22:75 (1972), by permission Taylor and Francis, Ltd.
Fig. 7-10: W. R. Bruce, B. E. Meeker, and F. A. Valeriote, *J. Natl. Cancer Inst.*, 37:233 (1966)
Figs. 7-11, 7-15, 7-16, and 7-19: W. A. Creasey, *Comprehensive Therapy*, 1(4) (1975)

Table 1-1: Data derives from E. Silverberg and A. I. Holleb, *Ca—A Cancer Journal for Clinicians,* 23:2 (1975), by permission American Cancer Society, Inc.
Tables 2-1 and 2-3: L. S. Lombard and E. J. Witte, *Cancer Res.*, 19:127 (1959)
Tables 2-6 and 2-8: Data derived from *Ca—A Cancer Journal for Clinicians,* 29(1) (1979), by permission American Cancer Society, Inc.
Table 2-10: H. Seidman, E. Silverberg, and A. Bodden, *Ca—A Cancer Journal for Clinicians,* 28:33 (1978), by permission American Cancer Society, Inc.
Tables 3-1, 3-3, 3-4, and 3-5: G. G. Steel, *Growth Kinetics of Tumors,* Oxford University Press, 1977
Table 3-2: J. Folkman, in *Cancer: A Comprehensive Treatise,* Vol. 3, ed. by F. F. Becker, Plenum Press, 1975
Table 6-1: J. F. Fraumeni, Jr., in *Cancer Medicine,* ed. by J. F. Holland and E. Frei III, Lea & Febiger, 1973
Tables 6-2 and 6-3: F. J. Rauscher and T. E. O'Connor, in *Cancer Medicine,* ed. by J. F. Holland and E. Frei III, Lea & Febiger, 1973
Table 7-1: B. Fisher, in *Cancer: A Comprehensive Treatise,* Vol. 6, ed. by F. F. Becker, Plenum Press, 1977
Tables 7-4 and 7-5: J. F. Fowler and J. Denekamp, in *Cancer: A Comprehensive Treatise,* Vol. 6, ed. by F. F. Becker, Plenum Press, 1977
Table 7-6: Data derived from H. Madoc-Jones and F. Mauro, in *Antineoplastic and Immunosuppressive Agents,* Vol. 1, ed. by A. C. Sartorelli and D. G. Johns, Springer-Verlag, Heidelberg, 1974
Table 7-7: H. E. Skipper, *Cancer Res.*, 31:1173 (1971), by permission Cancer Research, Inc.
Table 7-9: D. A. Karnofsky, *Cancer,* 18:1517 (1965), by permission American Cancer Society, Inc.
Table 7-12: W. B. Pratt and R. W. Ruddon, *The Anticancer Drugs,* Oxford University Press, 1979
Table 7-13: *The Medical Newsletter,* 20:82, 1978
Table 8-1: R. J. Shamberger, and C. E. Willis, *Crit. Rev. Clin. Lab. Sci.*, 2:211 (1971), by permission CRC Press Division, Chemical Rubber Company

This book is dedicated to those patients with whom the author worked, who so willingly gave of themselves to help advance our understanding of cancer and its eventual conquest

Preface

At this time, there is a very intense interest in cancer, a fact reflected in the vast public funding programs for cancer research. This research extends over the whole spectrum of biology, in addition to the traditional medical specialties, and thus involves scientists from a wide range of disciplines. In view of both the public interest, and the variety of disciplines being mobilized for cancer control, it is important that the opportunity to learn about the disease should be available to all. For the most part, the available books on the subject, as would be expected, are either comprehensive volumes aimed at a readership already well versed in medicine or specialized texts dealing with specific areas of medicine or cancer research. There is clearly a need for a broad treatment that has less emphasis on pathology, diagnostic techniques, or details of therapy and more emphasis on cancer biology and trends in research than the traditional medical texts.

While teaching the principles of cancer biology and pharmacology to undergraduate and graduate students, I was made acutely aware of the lack of a suitable introductory text for such students, as well as for non-medical research workers. Medical students would also find such a text useful as a basis for their later, more intensive clinical studies. This book is intended to serve such a need. I have endeavored to bring together in one volume a range of materials on the nature and incidence of cancer, the features of cancer growth and metastasis, the biological interactions between the tumor and the host, the principles of diagnostic approaches, the various factors known or suspected to produce cancer, the forms of treatment, and some of the major directions in cancer research. I have not dealt exhaustively with either the molecular biology of cancer or its clinical aspects; others are better qualified to do this.

I realize that to some extent personal attitudes have determined which topics should be included and which omitted. In this I am reminded of a review of the late Sir Winston Churchill's *History of the English Speaking People*, in which the critic wrote that a more appropriate title would have been *Things that Interest Me in History*. Many, for example, might object to the amount of space given to psychological aspects of cancer etiology, or to an analysis of unproven remedies, but my own feeling is that information on these topics is hard to come by, and its presentation may encourage more definitive studies, whereas the molecular biology of cancer cells or the viral etiology of cancer has been both studied and reviewed extensively. This text will help provide a general basis upon which a sound knowledge of oncology might be built.

I am greatly indebted to Janet Coary for her excellent secretarial assistance.

W.A.C.

University of Pennsylvania
Philadelphia
November 1980

Contents

CANCER
An Introduction

1. The nature of cancer

INTRODUCTION

The term cancer is really a generic name for a group of diseases that share a common type of disordered growth. It originates from the Latin word for crab, itself related to the Greek Καρκινος (*karkinos*) meaning both crab and cancer, from which the term *carcinoma* is derived. Since the original Indo-European root *kar* meant hard, it is evident that the name is suggestive of a hard mass that spreads like the claws of a crab. Galen drew such an analogy nearly two thousand years ago, when he described cancer of the breast with its lateral prolongations of the tumor and the adjacent distended veins (1). Another term applied to cancer is *malignancy,* which refers to the lethal potential of this infiltrative disease and which distinguishes it from *benign tumors;* the latter lack the ability to spread by infiltration and metastasis and thus are not generally life-threatening. However, a benign tumor of the brain, for example, may be deadly, whereas a malignant skin tumor is often curable and thus presents little threat to life. The distinction, then, is certainly not an absolute one. Both these types of growth disorder give rise to tumors, a name that originally meant only a swelling and was thus applied also to inflammatory conditions.

Another term frequently used as a synonym for a cancer is *neoplasm,* although strictly, this only defines a condition as a new growth, that is, a tumor, without specifying whether it is benign or malignant. A number of other growth abnormalities distinguishable from both benign and malignant tumors will be described in the next section. Our immediate purpose is to examine some general concepts and myths about cancer and to introduce some of the topics that will be covered later in this volume.

First we should examine the growth of cancer. There is a widespread conviction that cancer cells proliferate wildly at rates that are quite unlike those of normal tissues. Many, but not all tumors, do indeed exhibit very high growth rates, although it is doubtful if any can match the rate of cellular proliferation in normal bone marrow or intestinal mucosa. In such rapidly proliferating normal tissues, however, the whole process of cell division and replacement is regulated, so that no net accumulation of cells or disruption of tissue structure occurs. This state of dynamic equilibrium contrasts strongly with cancerous growth, in which cell division proceeds without any regard to the need for replacement, and occurs at the expense of normal tissue architecture, which invariably is disrupted in the process. Furthermore, to an extent that varies with the type of tumor, cells may be shed from the main mass and set up new foci of growth—*metastases*—at distant sites.

Another distinctive feature of cancer cells is that they may have lost properties that characterize the cells of their tissue of origin; that is, they are less differentiated. This loss of differentiation includes both morphological and biochemical markers, and may vary from minor deviations, which are barely detectable, to changes so major that the tissue of origin can no longer be identified with certainty. Conversely, cancer cells may acquire metabolic capabilities that are lacking in the parent tissue, such as the ability to elaborate what are known as ectopic hormones. This represents a derepression of gene loci, the activity of which is repressed in the parent cell line, that accompanies loss of differentiation. These distinctive features have been assembled into the concept of tumor progression formulated by Foulds (2). Early tumors are envisaged as being relatively responsive to such host control mechanisms as hormones. Later, as normal features are lost, the responsiveness also disappears, apparently irreversibly, and a stage of independent growth is reached when the tumor spreads freely. Most abnormal growth processes—hyperplasias, benign tumors, and metaplasias—never attain the stage of uncontrolled growth.

The reasons for the most singular characteristic of cancer, its ability to kill those who contract it, are complex. Obstruction of vital functions and disruption of needed organ structure, obvious results of tumor growth, may cause death in those with malignant, or for that matter benign tumors. These, however, are not the most frequent causes of death. Other factors such as malnutrition, cachexia, increased susceptibility to infection, hemorrhage, endocrine disturbances, production of toxins, psychological problems, and the side effects of therapy contribute to the death of a patient.

Recent public pronouncements emphasizing the dangers from environmental carcinogens are based on an assumption that 80 percent or more of human cancer results from exposure to such agents, including dietary items, and is preventable. The claim is based on analysis of worldwide cancer incidence data, in which the lowest figures are taken as the norm (3,4). As we shall see in the next chapter, the death rate from cancer has increased throughout this century (see Figure 2-4). Although much of this increase may be explained by such factors as a fall in mortality from infectious diseases, an altered population with relatively more older people, and better reporting of mortality information, it is likely that there has been a significant increase in the true incidence of cancer. Thus, in the United States, as in other industrialized countries, cancer is now the second major cause of death. In less industrialized societies, lower death rates from malignant disease may reflect shorter life expectancies, the prevalence of infectious diseases, and inadequate data gathering, but it is likely that lower levels of toxic industrial wastes, and other differences affecting life-styles, also contribute. A related epidemiological finding is the wide variation in the incidence of individual types of cancer when different societies are compared. Such variations reflect underlying differences in the spectra of carcinogens to which the populations are exposed, genetic features, infections, diet, amount of stress in daily life, and other personal and cultural factors. Increasing emphasis is now being placed on the epidemiology and etiology of cancer with a view toward reducing the incidence of this disease.

Despite its prevalence, until recently cancer was surrounded by a quite extraordinary secrecy that was intended to protect the patient from knowledge of his or her poor prognosis and to prevent the personal tragedy from becoming public. This was done mainly from consideration for the patient and the family, but also because in the minds of many people a feeling of shame was associated with the disease. The very magnitude of the problem, however, and the slow, but steady progress achieved in treatment, have forced a reevaluation of this secrecy, which usually worked to the detriment of the patient by discouraging early treatment and causing needless anguish. These changed attitudes are typified by the way several prominent victims of cancer have deliberately publicized the nature and treatment of their disease. Such examples serve an educational purpose for

Table 1-1 Incidence of major solid tumors for the U.S. white population per 100,000, and 5-year survival rates for indicated decades.

		Incidence		*Five-year survival in percent*		
Site	*Sex*	1947	1969	1940–49	1950–59	1960–69
Bladder	M	16.3	19.7	41	55	59
	F	7.0	5.2	44	53	58
Breast	F	70.0	72.5	53	60	63
Colon	M	23.4	29.6	29	42	43
	F	25.2	25.0	35	46	46
Lung	M	28.7	67.0	3	7	8
	F	6.5	13.5	8	11	12
Ovary	F	14.7	13.3	25	29	33
Pancreas	M	8.8	10.7	1	1	1
	F	5.6	6.8	2	2	2
Prostate	M	36.4	44.7	37	47	54
Stomach	M	31.4	12.9	9	12	11
	F	17.3	5.8	9	13	14
Uterus	F	60.7	38.1	54	65	65

Data derived from E. Silverberg and A. I. Holleb: Major trends in cancer: 25 year survey. CA-A Cancer Journal for Clinicians 25:2 (1975).

those not aware of the capabilities of current therapy, although harm also may result when recourse to unproven remedies is publicized.

Although significant progress has been made recently toward curing some kinds of cancer, treatment of the more common solid tumors has not dramatically improved cure rates over the period 1940 to 1969 (Table 1-1). This has led many to frustration with orthodox medical therapy and recourse to unconventional treatments. Some of these, which stress dietary supplements, are not unreasonable in themselves, in view of the poor nutritional status of many cancer patients, but others rely on drugs or procedures with no evidence of value or efficacy. Unfortunately, a natural desire to explore any possible cure has all too frequently caused those suffering from cancer to become victims of fraud and deceit.

More research into both prevention and treatment is clearly needed if progress is to be made toward further marked reductions in deaths from cancer. Thus we must redefine goals and develop alternate approaches, since a criticism that has been leveled against current research endeavors is that too many funds have been spent on costly and relatively ineffective human application of therapy. An analogous situation would be one in which polio was still being treated with ever more elaborate and costly supportive devices for maintaining paralyzed victims, while approaches aimed at controlling the virus responsible for the disease were ignored. As will become evident in this book, such an attitude to cancer research is no longer justified, if indeed it ever was, since most researchers are very alert to any new approach, if only to keep up in a very competitive field.

CLASSIFICATION OF TUMORS AND GROWTH DISORDERS

We have introduced a few of the more common terms that relate to growth abnormalities at the beginning of this chapter. Now it is appropriate to discuss these and other terms more comprehensively. As the reader will recall, the tissues derived from the *mesoderm* or middle germ layer in embryonic development are basically *connective and supportive tissues,* whereas *epithelial* organs and the *nervous system* arise from the *endoderm* and *ectoderm.* Tissues of mesodermal origin (*mesenchymal* tissues) account for up to 80 percent of the mass of an animal, including as they do such major structures as bones, tendons, muscles, cartilage, and fat. They also provide a structural basis for epithelial tissues. Apart from various epithelia, parenchymal organs, such as the liver, salivary glands, mammary glands and the nervous system, are primarily of epithelial origin. This distinction between tissue classes is carried over into all forms of abnormal growths. It is interesting that, although normal tissues are predominantly mesenchymal, abnormal growth phenomena, such as tumors, are far more commonly of epithelial origin, indicating that these tissues may have up to 50 times greater incidence of malignant transformation of their cells. This probably reflects the fact that it is the epithelia that are the primary areas of interaction with the environment and its carcinogenic influences.

Several growth disorders do not normally form tumors and thus may be distinguished from malignant and benign neoplasms. In *hyperplasia,* there is excessive proliferation of all the normal cellular elements, which retain an essentially normal appearance, with only a minimal degree of immaturity evident. In Figure 1-1, skin hyperplasia, such as would result from stimulation by a chemical or mechanical irritant, is illustrated schematically. New cell production exceeds cell destruction, with mitoses occurring in the higher layers as well as in the basal layers of the skin. Eventually, increased production of the horny layer, which is sloughed off, increases the rate of cell loss and brings the process back into the original equilibrium state, provided there is not a perpetuation of the stimulus. Psoriasis is in some respects a sustained hyperplasia, with an increased cell turnover

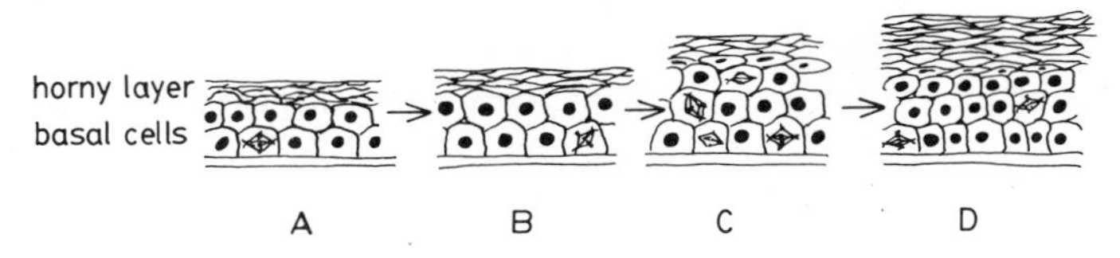

Figure 1-1 Schematic representation of skin hyperplasia. A, normal skin; B, swelling of cells in response to stimulus; C, proliferation of cells at all layers, not only basal layer, as in A; D, production of a thick horny layer, which is sloughed off while cell proliferation diminishes.

such that the time from cell division in the basal layer to appearance of that cell at the outer layer falls from 28 to about 5 days. In *dysplasia*, cell proliferation gives rise to abnormal or atypical cells that may often exhibit features of cancer cells, such as enlarged nuclei with irregular chromatin, but that do not show excessive mitotic activity or invasive growth. *Metaplasia* involves the proliferation of one cell type, which eventually replaces other cell types in the tissue involved. Although these conditions do not usually give rise to tumors directly, there is evidence that some forms of metaplasia, such as squamous cell metaplasia of the uterine cervix, may be obligatory early steps in a progression that can lead to a later malignancy. It is important to note that, in metaplasia, the germ layer of a glandular columnar epithelium may begin to produce flattened or squamous epithelial cells instead of normal cylindrical cells during squamous transformation, but it will not produce other cells, such as mesenchymal connective tissue cells. Thus, continuity of the embryonic germ layer system is preserved. Finally, in *anaplasia*, frankly abnormal cells of malignant appearance may be identified in a tissue, but there are too few cells to have yet established a defined cancerous growth, and this indeed may never occur. There is some confusion regarding this use of the term, but it is the most generally accepted usage. When used with carcinoma, as in *anaplastic carcinoma*, a poorly differentiated cell type, or a tumor that lacks organization, is implied.

In benign tumors of epithelial tissues, connective and vascular cells proliferate along with epithelial cells to form *papillary tumors* (Figure 1-2). A *papilloma*, a protruding peripheral tumor, is composed primarily of epithelial cells with supporting tissues, for no tumor is composed of only one histological cell type. In some cases the actual tumor cells may be of multiple origin, quite apart from the normal supportive elements. This is true of *leiomyofibroma*, for example, in which the tumor cells are of both muscular and connective tissue origin. When the primary proliferating cells originate in glandular epithelium of the parenchymal organs, an *adenoma* results. *Polyps* are stalked tumors, somewhat akin to papillomas in form, that arise from internal mucosal surfaces. Table 1-2 lists a number of the more common benign tumors with their tissues of origin. It should be noted that in most cases the suffix *-oma* denotes a benign tumor, but there are exceptions. *Melanomas* and *lymphomas* are malignant in nature, and should be qualified as malignant, although this is frequently not done. On the other hand, a *granuloma* is really not a neoplasm, but rather a tumor-like lesion of granulation tissue associated with an inflammatory process. Benign tumors do not infiltrate neighboring normal tissues, although pressure exerted by their growth may create some distortions. In general, they remain *in situ,* not crossing the barrier presented by the basal membranes, if they are of epithelial origin, and remaining non-invasive, if of other origins. In effect, the tumor is encapsulated in connective tissue that presents a clear demarcation zone. This is the basis for the frequent finding that benign tumors are mobile, whereas malignant tumors often appear to adhere to their neighboring normal tissues when palpated.

Most benign tumors never progress to become malignancies, but for some time it has been recognized that certain conditions, in themselves benign, show a sufficiently high frequency of becoming malignant to be considered precancerous lesions (5). Some of these are listed in Table 1-2. In *xeroderma pigmentosum,* defects in the DNA repair mechanisms of the affected skin cells are associated with a cutaneous disorder that displays pigmentation and atrophy due to undue sensitivity to ultraviolet light. This leads inevitably to skin cancer, which sometimes is malignant melanoma. Another condition with an inevitable malignant transformation is *Hutchinson's freckle,* a flat pigmented lesion frequently found on the cheek of elderly patients; it should be excised to forstall development of a melanoma. *Von Recklinghausen's disease,* in which a multitude of small tumor nodules

Figure 1-2 Schematic representation of the types of benign epithelial tumors and their progression. A, normal skin; B and C, flat wart and papillary wart; D, papilloma.

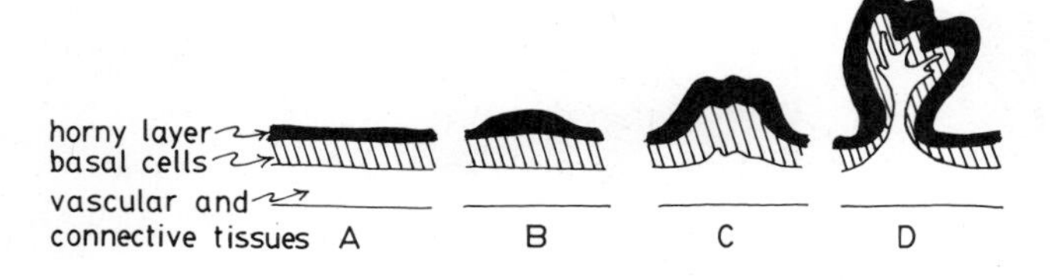

Table 1-2 Nomenclature of the more common types of benign, precancerous, and malignant growth disorders.

Tissue of origin	*Benign*	*Precancerous*	*Malignant*
Primitive	Benign teratoma		Malignant teratoma
Epithelial			
Colonic mucosa	Hyperplastic colonic polyps	Familial polyposis	
	Adenomatous polyps (most)	Villous adenomas	Adenocarcinoma of colon
Glandular	Adenoma		Adenocarcinoma
Liver	Liver cell adenoma		Hepatocarcinoma (hepatoma)
Mucous membrane		Leukoplakia	Epidermoid carcinoma
Nerve cells	Ganglioneuroma		Neuroblastoma
Schwann cells		Von Recklinghausen's neurofibromatosis	Malignant schwannoma
Skin	Papilloma	Xeroderma pigmentosum	Skin (epidermoid) carcinoma
Skin, pigment cells	Nevus (mole)	Hutchinson's freckle	Malignant melanoma
Uterus		Adenomatous hyperplasia	Endometrial adenocarcinoma
		Hydatiform mole	Choriocarcinoma
Mesodermal (*Mesenchymal*)			
Blood vessels, endothelium	Hemangioma		Angiosarcoma
perithelium	Hemangiopericytoma		Malignant hemangiopericytoma
Bone	Osteoma	Paget's disease (rarely)	Osteogenic sarcoma (osteosarcoma)
	Osteochondroma		
Bone marrow, granulocytes			Myeloid leukemias, myelosarcoma
lymphocytes		Fanconi's anemia	Lymphatic leukemias, lymphomas, Hodgkin's disease, lymphosarcoma
Cartilage	Chondroma		Chondrosarcoma
Connective tissue	Fibroma		Fibrosarcoma
	Myxoma		Myxosarcoma
Fat	Lipoma		Liposarcoma
Muscle, smooth	Leiomyoma		Leiomyosarcoma
striated	Rhabdomyoma		Rhabdomyosarcoma
mixed smooth and connective tissue	Leiomyofibroma		Leiomyofibrosarcoma

appear in the skin, has less than a 10 percent incidence of transformation to *malignant schwannoma.* However, excision of such a mass of nodules is not feasible, and in any case malignant disease most commonly arises from more deep-seated nerve tissue. *Familial polyposis* is an autosomal dominant disease in which adenocarcinomas of the colon develop from the *villous adenomas* (i.e., tumors, with villus-like fronds) so frequently that total colectomy is generally the treatment of choice. Most adenomatous polyps, as well as *hyperplastic colonic polyps,* do not give rise to cancer, however. *Leukoplakia,* a hyperplastic condition of mucous membranes, yields keratoses with variable degrees of cellular abnormality that have about a 4 percent incidence of conversion to epidermoid carcinomas. *Actinic* or *solar keratoses* appear on areas of the skin exposed to the sun and most often resemble light-colored nevi. There is a low risk of progression to a relatively indolent epidermoid carcinoma. Dysplasia of the uterine cervix, adenomatous hyperplasia of the endometrium, hydatiform mole, and Paget's disease are other conditions frequently considered precancerous, although, in fact, they have a relatively low incidence of conversion to cancer. For certain other conditions, such as fibrocystic disease of the breast, endemic goiter, cystic endometrial hyperplasia, and osteochondromas of the bone, there is no really convincing evidence that they are precancerous. Finally, a few benign conditions, such as myositis, vaginal polyps, nipple adenomas, nuclear alterations in the endometrial stroma seen in women taking birth control pills, lymphocyte hyperplasia in the lymph nodes of patients with infectious mononucleosis or herpes zoster, and even the sites of insect bites, may present histology resembling malignancies. Such pseudomalignant conditions pose no hazard.

In the nomenclature of malignant tumors (Table 1-2), the term *carcinoma* is used for epithelial tumors and *sarcoma* for mesenchymal tumors. The incidence of carcinomas increases sharply with age, whereas sarcomas, which are more common than carcinomas in younger persons, tend to show a more gradual increase throughout life. *Blastoma* is a suffix indicating that the tumor arises from primitive or embryonic cells, for example, a *nephroblastoma* from immature kidney cells. To these major classes are added qualifiers such as *adeno-* for glandular tumors, *papillary* for tumors that protrude or have villous extensions, *cystic* when the tumor has a cyst-like structure, and *undifferentiated* or *anaplastic* when the tumor really does not resemble normal tissue in its morphology. Some tumors arise from multipotential primitive or embryonic cells and thus may differentiate to varying extents, giving both carcinoma and sarcoma components to the tumor. Examples are the *mixed mesenchymal* tumors of the uterus and the *teratomas* of the gonads. The latter may present a bizarre appearance if they are well differentiated, since they may include such structures as bone, hair, and nails. *Carcinoids* are actively secreting tumors that may cause endocrine disturbances. They were so-named because they were thought to be cancer-like and must be qualified with the term malignant when they are cancerous. A tumor that grows slowly and has little tendency to metastasize is termed *indolent,* whereas rapidly spreading tumors are said to be *aggressive* or highly malignant.

CYTOLOGICAL FEATURES OF MALIGNANT CELLS

Since they are derived from so many different types of normal tissues and because they display a wide range of growth behavior, cancer cells differ markedly in their cytology, yet they do exhibit common characteristics, some of which relate them to embryonic cells (6). Perhaps most noticeable are the large irregular nuclei, often with aggregates of chromatin near the membrane. This may reflect the *polyploidy,* with elevated DNA levels, so frequent in tumors. Most malignant tumors show some chromosomal abnormality, that is *aneuploidy,* which is most often an increased complement of chromosomes, sometimes with visible damage; human diploid solid tumors are rare (7). Within the nuclei, the nucleoli may be larger and more numerous than in normal cells; this could be related to an overall greater rate of RNA synthesis. Mitoses are usually more numerous than in the parent tissue or in benign tumors, and especially in the more rapidly-growing cancers, abnormal mitotic figures such as multipolar mitoses can be seen. These abnormalities probably contribute to the nuclear irregularity (*pleomorphism*) and multinucleation that is also common. The cytoplasm stains more intensely with basophilic dyes, such as methyl green pyronine, because of increased amounts of RNA not associated with the endoplasmic reticulum, and there may be many vacuoles, reflecting increased phagocytotic activity. Electron microscopy has identified such features as an indented, irregular nuclear membrane and more numerous, longer, and thinner microvilli of the cell membrane. These features reflect the demand for more surface area for environmental interactions resulting from greater metabolic activity. Many tumor cells have been shown to have virus-like particles, usually associated with membranous structures, that are relevant to the etiology of cancer. In a few cases, malignancies are identified cytologically by some special feature, such as the Reed-Sternberg cells charac-

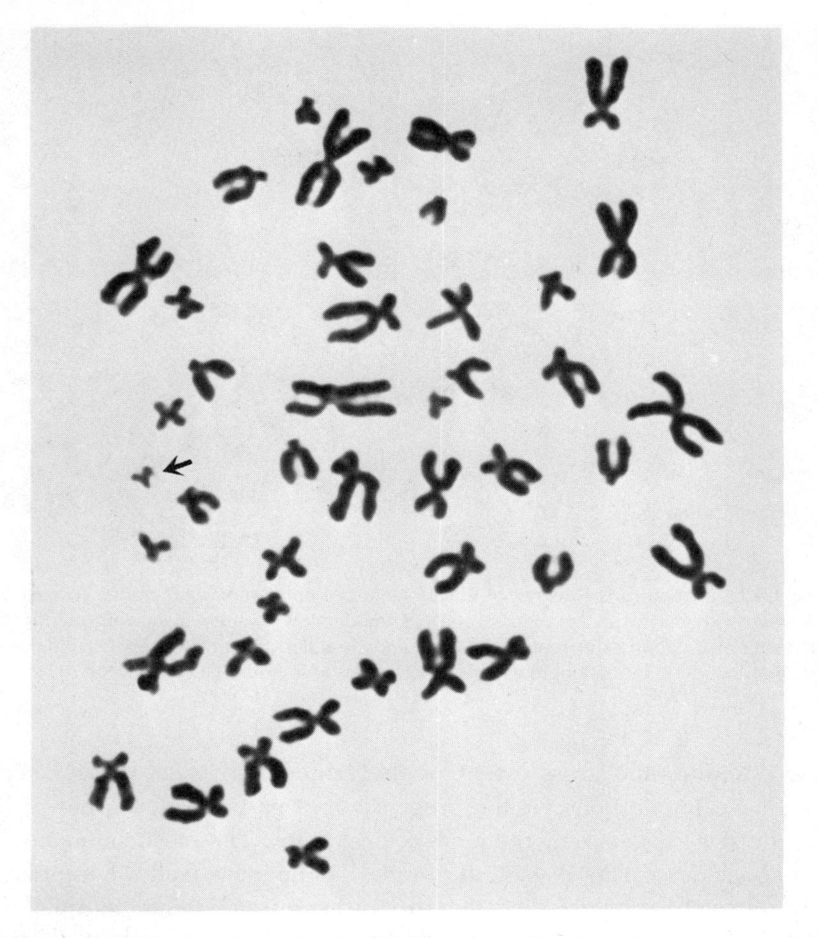

Figure 1-3 Metaphase with 46 chromosomes in the marrow of a male patient with chronic myelocytic leukemia. Arrow points to the Philadelphia chromosome, a characteristic of this disease. Photograph courtesy of A. A. Sandberg.

teristic of Hodgkin's disease or the Philadelphia chromosome often identified in chronic granulocytic (myelocytic) leukemia (Figure 1-3).

GRADES AND STAGES

A malignant tumor is commonly described by grade and stage (8). The grade is based on a microscopic examination of the lesion, whereas the

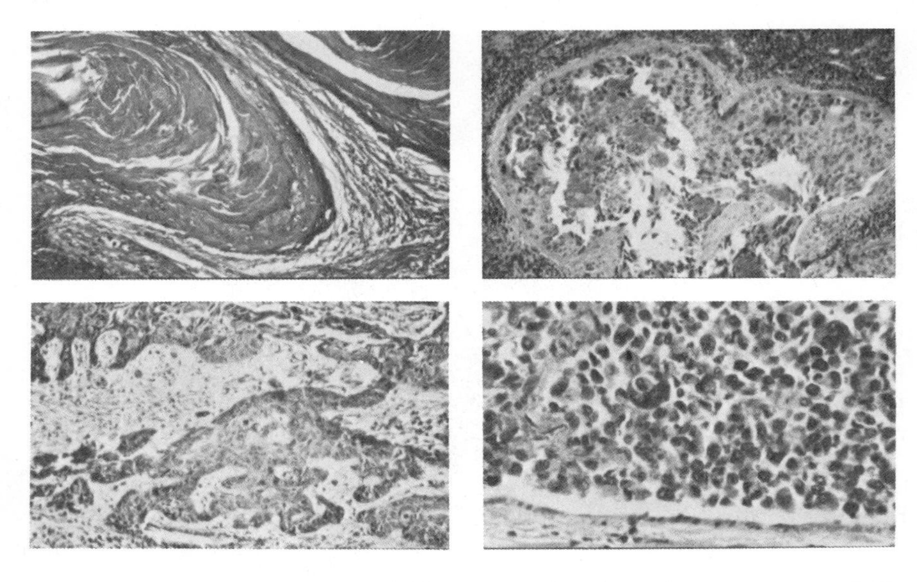

Figure 1-4 Variation in the degree of differentiation of epidermoid carcinoma. A, well differentiated, with masses of keratinized cells; B, moderately differentiated, with identifiable keratinization; C, poorly differentiated, with tumor nodules and no keratin; D, undifferentiated, with no gland formation, mucin secretion, or keratin. Reproduced from Ref. 8.

stage describes the gross extent of the tumor and its metastases. Both terms have implications for the prognosis in a particular case, but of the two, the stage is generally the more critical index. The most common form of grading uses a I to IV system. Grade I tumors are well differentiated, with relatively minimal deviation from the normal tissue morphology. Grades II and III, generally considered moderately and poorly differentiated, respectively, represent intermediate stages in loss of normal structure. Finally, Grade IV tumors are very anaplastic, and there is virtually no resemblance to their tissue of origin. Figure 1-4 shows such a sequence for epidermoid carcinoma. Loss of keratinization is a very notable feature as differentiation is lost. Although, as we have said, grading is usually less significant than staging, there are some tumors in which survival is closely correlated with histological grading. Transitional cell carcinoma of the urinary bladder has a 5-year survival rate of 80 percent for Grade I tumors that falls to 20 percent for Grade III (9). Prostatic carcinomas, chondrosarcomas, and astrocytomas (derived from the astrocytes of the central nervous system) show correlations of this type, but many other tumors do not.

In lymphomas, such as Hodgkin's disease, prognosis is also reflected in a histological classification (Figure 1-5). Lymphocyte predominance, nodular sclerosis, mixed cellularity, and lymphocyte depletion are four histological groups associated with 5-year survivals of 95, 84, 66, and 22 percent, respectively (10).

Staging depends on the extent the tumor has spread, rather than on its histology. The usual system uses numbers I to IV, with additional subclasses appropriate to the tumor under consideration; Stage I represents localized disease, Stage IV widely disseminated disease. In cancer of the uterine cervix, Stage 0 is an intraepithelial tumor; Stage I is strictly confined to the cervix and shows stromal invasion; Stage II extends beyond the cervix, involves no more than the upper two-thirds of the vagina, but does not extend to the pelvic wall; Stage IIIA involves the lower one-third

Figure 1-5 Hodgkin's disease. A, lymphocyte predominance, with mature lymphocytes, some histiocytes and Reed-Sternberg cells (large cells); B, nodular sclerosis, with many atypical histiocytes and Reed-Sternberg cells; C, mixed cellularity, with pleomorphic (varied shapes) cell infiltrate and Reed-Sternberg cells; D, lymphocyte depletion, with numerous malignant histiocytes and Reed-Sternberg cells and only a few lymphocytes. Reproduced from Ref. 14.

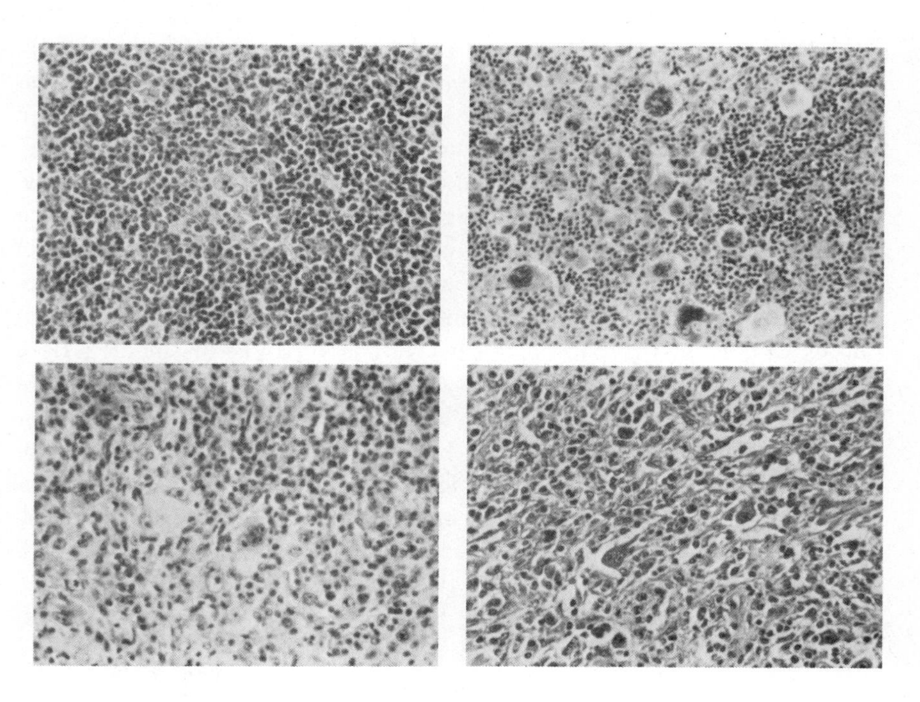

of the vagina, but not the pelvic wall; Stage IIIB involves the pelvic wall; and Stage IV extends beyond the pelvis or involves the mucosa of the bladder or rectum. With current optimal therapy, 5-year survivals are 90, 65, 40, and 10 percent for the four main stages (11). In breast cancer, the criteria for staging are local invasiveness and axillary lymph node involvement (12). Type I are non-invasive tumors of an intraductal type that very rarely show lymph node metastases. Type II are invasive, well-differentiated tumors, generally of circumscribed spread and with a low incidence of lymph node involvement. Most common are Type III, which are ductal or intraductal, but very invasive and with significant metastatic spread. Type IV are undifferentiated tumors that may invade blood vessels and metastasize to both regional lymph node and distant sites. In colorectal cancer, using Duke's system (13), the 5-year survival rate is 90 percent for Stage A, in which disease is restricted to the wall of the bowel; 65 percent for Stage B, in which invasion through the wall has occurred; and only 20 percent for Stage C with regional lymph node involvement. Modifications of the standard I to IV staging system, to reflect the very concrete effect of distribution of specific diseases on prognosis, may be quite complex. In the Stanford classification for Hodgkin's disease (14,15), for example, Stage IA involves a single lymph node region (IA) or a single extralymphatic site (I_EA) and has the same 5-year survival of 90 percent found in the similarly non-symptomatic Stage IIA, which involves two or more lymph nodes on the same side of the diaphragm (IIA) or one or more lymph nodes and a solitary extralymphatic site on the same side of the diaphragm (II_EA). Systemic symptoms (IB, I_EB, IIB, II_EB) lower survival to 75 percent. Splenic involvement (II_SA, II_SB) brings the figure down to 60 percent, which is the same as for IIIA, in which there are positive lymph nodes on both sides of the diaphragm with (III_EA) or without a solitary extralymphatic organ involved. Stage IIIB, in which systemic symptoms are seen, has a survival rate of 40 percent irrespective of extralymphatic (III_EB) or splenic (III_SB) involvement. Stage IV may have 5-year survivals of 0 to 25 percent. In neuroblastoma, a tumor arising in children from primitive nerve cells (neuroblasts), survival is correlated with both the stage of the disease and the age of the child at diagnosis. For Stage I, confined to the structure of origin, 5-year survival ranges from 95 percent at 6 months to 60 percent at 60 months, compared to 80 and 25 percent at the same ages for Stage II with more extensive disease not crossing the midline and with ipsilateral (same side) positive nodes. Corresponding figures for Stage III, with tumor extending beyond the midline and possible bilateral node involvement, are

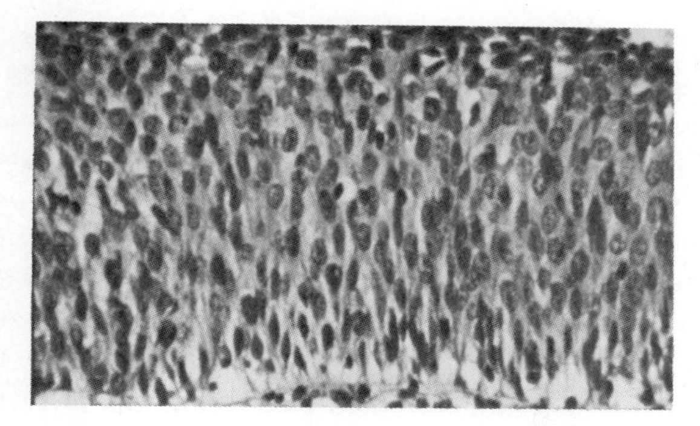

Figure 1-6 Carcinoma of the uterine cervix *in situ*. The disease involves the whole thickness of the epithelium. Reproduced from Ref. 8.

65 and 15 percent. Stage IV, in which there is remote disease of the skeleton, organs, soft tissue, and lymph nodes, has poor survival figures (15 and 2 percent at 6 and 60 months). The unusual IVS category exhibits disseminated disease of the liver, skin or bone marrow, but with a strong trend toward regression and/or maturation of the tumor to a benign ganglioneuroma that leads to a better prognosis (85 and 35 percent survival for the 6- and 60-month-old groups) than for Stage II disease (16). In cancers of epithelial origin, in particular, a very early stage may be distinguished, that of *carcinoma-in situ*. This stage presents cells with all the histological characteristics of malignant cells, but with no invasion or metastasis, the disease being solely intraepithelial. The prognosis when such a lesion is detected is often excellent, for complete excision is easy, since it is highly unlikely that metastatic spread has occurred. Such a carcinoma is shown in Figure 1-6. In contrast to the correlation between stage and prognosis that is so frequently encountered, in certain cancers, such as those of the brain, pancreas, thyroid and esophagus, the extent of spread, whether local or regional has a minimal effect on the outcome.

DIFFERENTIATION, DEDIFFERENTIATION, AND MUTATION

Earlier in this chapter we touched on the concepts of differentiation and dedifferentiation as they relate to cancers and their classification. We shall now return to this topic in more detail, since it is important not only from the point of view of better defining the nature of cancer, but also since alternative therapeutic approaches might arise from exploration of these processes. There has been controversey in the literature over the concept that cancer is the result of genetic mutations and the concept that cancer reflects epigenetic changes concerned with gene expression. Early forms of the mutation theory held that there was "the abnormal mitosis which starts a tumor" (17). This idea has undergone considerable development in response to studies with genetically determined and chemically induced tumors. Evidence that at least two, and probably more steps are needed provides us with a model that has sequential or cumulative mutations (7). For example, in tumors that are clearly genetically determined and inherited, the first step may be a germinal (inherited) mutation carrying a tendency for the disease, which is then manifested through subsequent somatic mutations; in other tumors, a series of somatic mutations may be all that is required. Relatively few human cancers clearly present genetic abnormalities, as we shall see in Chapter 6, and changes are by no means uniform. Many other tumors show no such abnormalities. This, together with the absence of proven unique products of most cancer cells, which would be expected to result from mutations, favors the epigenetic model, in which malignancy is a function of changes related to differentiation. This model has come to be widely accepted (18), although it clearly cannot be applied to all cancer.

Evidence for a primarily epigenetic model comes from several areas. The resemblance between cancer cells and embryonic cells, mentioned earlier, is one such piece of evidence. Tumors may elaborate fetal antigens, which might better be termed transitory cell antigens, that are characteristic of certain periods during cellular differentiation. Thus, hepatomas and embryonal carcinomas may form α-fetoprotein and tumors of the digestive and genitourinary tracts, carcinoembryonic antigens; these substances are formed irrespective of the modality of carcinogenesis (19). In addition, there are such biochemical features as high aerobic glycolysis (20), types of enzyme activity (21), and patterns of isozymes (22) that cancer cells appear to have in common with fetal tissue. Related to this are examples of ectopic or inappropriate hormone synthesis, such as the secretion of gonadotropins by a bronchogenic carcinoma (23), that reflect activation or derepression of a preexisting gene. More striking are the examples of the reversibility of cancer, the ability of cancer cells to differentiate into non-malignant tissue. The nuclei of the Lucke´ adenocarcinoma of frog kidney, when implanted into enucleated ova, may give rise to normal tadpoles (24). Mouse teratocarcinoma (25), mammalian squamous epidermoid carcinoma (26), and human neuroblastoma (27) are among the tumors that have been reported to undergo differentiation to a benign status. Finally, a variety of manipulations with such naturally occurring materials as nerve growth factor and the macrophage and granulocyte inducer, as well as such synthetic compounds as 5-bromo-2′-deoxyuridine and dimethylsulfoxide, can cause tumor cells to revert to the behavioral pattern of normal cells (18). Conversely, nonmalignant T_3 cells in culture may acquire temporarily some features of the malignant transformed strain when they are treated with trypsin, regaining normal behavior spontaneously after some hours (28). These findings are all compatible with a model of the cancer cell in which the primary lesion is in gene expression leading to anomalous differentiation (29). The hope that is held out by this model is that an alternative therapy to the cytotoxic approach with its low specificity and severe side effects is feasible if we can learn to manipulate differentiation and gene expression effectively in a clinical situation.

REFERENCES

1. Galen: *Opera omnia 11:*141, 142.
2. L. Foulds: *Neoplastic Development.* Vol. 1, New York: Academic Press, 1969.
3. J. Higginson and C. S. Muir: Epidemiology. *In Cancer Medicine,* J. F. Holland and E. Frei, III, eds., Philadelphia: Lea & Febiger, 1973, pp. 231–306.
4. Cancer and Environment: Higginson speaks out. Science *205:*1363–1366, 1979.
5. J. Rosai and L. V. Ackerman: The pathology of tumors part I: Precancerous and pseudomalignant lesions. CA-A Cancer Journal for Clinicians *28:*331–342, 1978.
6. E. E. Sproul: Pathogenesis of cancer. *In Cancer Medicine,* J. F. Holland and E. Frei, III, eds., Philadelphia: Lea & Febiger, 1973, pp. 113–124.
7. S. R. Wolman and A. A. Horland: Genetics of Tumor Cells. *In Cancer: A Comprehensive Treatise,* Vol. 3, F. F. Becker, ed., New York: Plenum Press, 1975, pp. 155–198.
8. J. Rosai and L. V. Ackerman: The pathology of tumors part III: Grading, Staging and Classification. CA-A Cancer Journal for Clinicians. *29:*66–77, 1979.
9. F. K. Mostofi: Pathological aspects and spread of carcinoma of the bladder. J. Am. Med. Assoc. *206:*1764–1769, 1968.
10. H. S. Kaplan: Hodgkin's disease and other human malignant lymphomas: advances and prospects. Cancer Res. *36:*3863–3878, 1976.
11. J. F. Fowler and J. Denekamp: Radiation effects on normal tissues. *In Cancer: A Comprehensive Treatise.* Vol. 6, F. F. Becker, ed., New York: Plenum Press, 1977, pp. 139–180.
12. N. T. Kouchoukos, L. V. Ackerman, and H. R. Butcher: Prediction of axillary nodal metastases from the morphology of primary mammary carcinomas. Guide to operative therapy. Cancer *20:*948–960, 1967.
13. C. E. Dukes: Histological grading of rectal cancer. Proc. Roy. Soc. Med. Lond. *30:*371–376, 1937.
14. S. A. Rosenberg and H. S. Kaplan: Hodgkin's disease and other malignant lymphomas. Calif. Med. *113:*23–38, 1970.
15. S. A. Rosenberg: Hodgkin's disease. *In Cancer Medicine,* J. F. Holland and E. Frei, III, eds., Philadelphia: Lea & Febiger, 1973, pp. 1276–1302.

16. C. Pochedly: *Neuroblastoma*, Acton, Mass.: Publishing Science Group, 1976, p. 282.
17. T. Boveri: *Zur Frage der Entstehung maligner Tumoren*, Jena: Fisher, 1914. (English translation: M. Boveri: *The Origin of Malignant Tumors*. Baltimore: Williams and Wilkins, 1929.)
18. A. C. Braun: Differentiation and Dedifferentiation. *In Cancer: A Comprehensive Treatise*, Vol. 3, F. F. Becker, ed., New York: Plenum Press, 1975, pp. 3–20.
19. J. Uriel: Fetal characteristics of cancer. *In Cancer: A Comprehensive Treatise*, Vol. 3, F. F. Becker, ed., New York: Plenum Press, 1975, pp. 21–55.
20. C. A. Villee: The intermediary metabolism of human fetal tissues. Cold Spring Harbor Symp. Quant. Biol. *19:*186–199, 1954.
21. J. P. Greenstein: Enzymes in normal and neoplastic tissues. *In AAAS Research Conference on Cancer*, F. R. Moulton, ed., Washington, D.C.: AAAS, 1945, pp. 191–215.
22. F. Schapiro: Isozymes and cancer. Adv. Cancer Res. *18:*77–153, 1973.
23. C. Faiman, J. A. Colwell, R. J. Ryan, J. M. Hershman, and T. W. Shields: Gonodotropin secretion from a bronchogenic carcinoma: Demonstration by radioimmunoassay. New Eng. J. Med. *277:*1395–1399, 1967.
24. R. G. McKinnell, B. A. Deggins, and D. D. Labat: Transplantation of pluripotential nuclei from triploid frog tumors. Science *165:*394–396, 1969.
25. L. J. Kleinsmith and G. B. Pierce: Multipotentiality of single embryonal carcinoma cells. Cancer Res. *24:*1544–1551, 1964.
26. G. B. Pierce and C. Wallace: Differentiation of malignant to benign cells. Cancer Res. *31:*127–134, 1971.
27. H. Cushing and S. B. Wolbach: The transformation of a malignant paravertebral sympathicoblastoma into a benign ganglioneuroma. Am. J. Pathol. *3:*203–216, 1927.
28. M. M. Burger: Proteolytic enzymes initiating cell division and escape from contact inhibition of growth. Nature *227:*170–171, 1970.
29. C. L. Markert: Neoplasia: A disease of cell differentiation. Cancer Res. *28:*1908–1914, 1968.

SUGGESTED READINGS AND SOURCES

F. F. Becker: *Cancer: A Comprehensive Treatise*. New York: Plenum Press, in six volumes, 1974–1977.

J. F. Holland and E. Frei: *Cancer Medicine*. Philadelphia: Lea & Febiger, 1973.

G. G. Steel: *Growth Kinetics of Tumors*. Oxford: Oxford University Press, 1977.

W. B. Pratt and R. W. Ruddon: *The Anticancer Drugs*. New York: Oxford University Press, 1979.

A. C. Sartorelli and D. G. Johns: *Antineoplastic and Immunosuppressive Agents. Handbook of Experimental Pharmacology* Vol. 38, Berlin: Springer-Verlag, in two parts, 1974–1975.

A. P. Casarett: *Radiation Biology*. Englewood Cliffs, N.J.: Prentice-Hall, 1968.

L. V. Ackerman and J. A. Del Regato: *Cancer: Diagnosis, Treatment and Prognosis*. Saint Louis: C. V. Mosby Company, 1977.

R. Süss, V. Kinzel and J. D. Scribner: *Cancer—Experiments and Concepts*. New York: Springer-Verlag, 1973.

H. C. Pitot: *Fundamentals of Oncology*. New York: Marcel Dekker, 1978.

2. The prevalence of cancer

Cancer is now the second major cause of death in most modern societies. In this chapter, we shall review this situation in more detail in terms of how the pattern of incidence has changed historically, variations in the frequency with which cancer occurs in different societies and locales, and whether the human disease has close counterparts in other species. This information is of interest not only on its own account, but also because it may provide clues to the etiology and prevention of cancer. It is appropriate to begin this survey with a consideration of malignant tumors in various classes of animals and plants.

COMPARATIVE NEOPLASIA

Among the queries posed in 1802 by the Edinburgh Medical Committee of the Society for Investigating the Nature and Cure of Cancer was the following (1):

> It is not at present known whether brute creatures are subject to cancer, though some of their diseases have a very suspicious appearance. . . . This investigation may lead to much philosophical amusement and useful information; particularly it may teach us how far the prevalence or frequency of cancer may depend upon the manners and habits of life. . . .

This query is as valid today as when it was raised nearly 180 years ago, since it goes to the heart of the problem in any discussion of the distribution of cancer among animal and plant species, that is, whether the abnormal growths that have been described are indeed cancerous. In many cases, the reported tumors represent only proliferative responses to injury and disease, responses that may be more marked in lower vertebrates and invertebrates than in mammals because of the frequently greater regenerative powers of lower animals. Once this has been allowed for, it is apparent that all classes of vertebrates may develop cancers and that proliferative disorders presenting analogies to cancer also occur among the more advanced invertebrates. The uncontrolled transplantable neoplasms of plants may also legitimately be considered as cancers. Several excellent reviews of comparative neoplasia in animals (2–4) and plants (5) may be consulted by those wishing to study this area in more detail. In this section we shall outline some of the findings that illustrate the range of neoplastic growths found in the major orders.

Mammals

Although cancer appears to be universal among mammals, there has been much confusion over the classification of tumors and the analogies to human cancers that may exist. Guidelines, such as those developed by the World Health Organization for six species of domestic animals (6), have helped to bring about some uniformity. In surveying the literature, it is immediately apparent that the major tumor types are highly variable in their distribution. For example, lung cancer, which accounts for 22 percent of all male and 8 percent of all female human cancer in the United States (7), was observed in only about 1 percent of cats and dogs at autopsy (8) and in only 19, or 0.1 percent, of the more than 19,000 mammals and birds that died between 1901 and 1963 at the Philadelphia Zoo (9). These findings would be expected if the prime cause of lung cancer were smoking, although inherent interspecies variation cannot be ruled out. Table 2-1 presents summary data for five orders of mammals.

Among non-human primates, proliferative diseases closely resembling human neoplasms have been observed in most families, including prosimians, the marmosets and lemurs (2). About 1 percent of 1,328 primate necropsies at the Philadelphia Zoo uncovered malignancies (10). There is a resemblance to the occurrence of cancer in humans in the types of tumors encountered, lymphomas and brain tumors being rare (11), whereas epithelial tumors are found more often in older animals (12). Experimentally, malignant tumors have been induced in many species of monkey with such

Table 2-1 Frequency of tumors at autopsy in five orders of mammals at the Philadelphia Zoo.

	1901–1934			1935–1955		
Order	*Necropsies*	*Benign (percent)*	*Malignant (percent)*	*Necropsies*	*Benign (percent)*	*Malignant (percent)*
Primates	1,022	0.5	0.7	306	3.6	2.0
Carnivora	801	1.6	3.9	321	11.0	12.0
Artiodactyla	626	0.8	1.1	288	1.7	1.7
Rodentia	461	1.3	3.5	178	0.6	2.2
Marsupialia	422	1.0	2.1	88	1.1	1.1

Both benign and malignant tumors were found more frequently in animals that had been on exhibition longer (averages 104 months in 1901–1934, 143 months in 1935–1955) than the average for all animals (33 months in 1901–1934, 54 months in 1935–1955). Carcinomas (105) outnumbered sarcomas (20) between 1901 and 1955 (Ref. 10).

carcinogens as N-nitrosodiethylamine, and one of the resulting tumors, hepatocarcinoma NCLP-6, has been propagated in culture (13). Another malignant cell line, this time a lymphoid cell (MLC-1), has been induced by Herpesvirus saimiri (14), and C-type virus particles are associated with some primate tumors (15). Finally, granulocytic leukemia has been produced in monkeys by whole-body irradiation (16). The simian cancers that arise spontaneously or by induction behave in the same way as human cancers in terms of metastasis, invasion, lethality to the host, such genetic abnormalities as aneuploidy, and variable degrees of dedifferentiation.

Rodents are the mammalian family in which neoplasia has been most intensively studied outside humans. It is the tumors of mice, and to a lesser extent rats, that serve as the principal screening systems in which modalities for treatment of human cancer are developed and tested. The inbred strains of these animals that have been developed over the past 70 years, which number several hundred, are frequently subject to a high incidence of tumors in a strain-specific manner. In C3H mice, females show almost a 100 percent incidence of mammary tumors, whereas males exhibit almost as high a frequency of hepatomas; these are perhaps the most striking examples. Table 2-2 lists the most frequent spontaneous neoplasma in the major inbred strains of mice. The reviews of Jay (17) and Staats (18) list mouse and rat strains together with their common spontaneous tumors. Transplanted tumors, which are so important in cancer research, will be discussed later in this book when we consider research programs in cancer. When wild mice have been kept and bred in the laboratory, almost one-half of those aged over 25 months were found to have tumors at autopsy. This is a very high incidence compared to that for

Table 2-2 Common spontaneous tumors in major strains of mice.

Strain	*Tumor*	*Incidence*
A	Pulmonary	90%
	Mammary	High in breeding ♀
	Testis	Induced by estrogens
AKR	Leukemia	High incidence
BALB/c	Pulmonary	26–29%
	Mammary	Induced
	Testis	Induced with estrogens
C3H	Mammary	Nearly 100% in ♀
	Hepatomas	85% in ♂
	Subcutaneous sarcomas	3%, most susceptible to carcinogens
C57BL	Pituitary adenoma	Induced by estrogens in nearly all
C58	Leukemia	High incidence
CBA	Subcutaneous sarcomas	High after methylcholanthrene
CE	Adrenal cortical	Following castration
HR	Papillomas	In all mice
	Hemangioendotheliomas	19–33% untreated, up to 76% with carcinogen
DBA	Mammary	High in breeding ♀
SWR	Pulmonary	80%

Data derived from Refs. 2,3,17, and 18.

other mammals. Alveologenic pulmonary tumors, originating from type II cells of the alveoli of the lung, were the most common; this tumor has no true human analogy. Other common tumors encountered were reticulum cell sarcoma, granulosa cell tumors of the ovary, hepatomas (mainly in males), hemangioendotheliomas, and mammary tumors, the latter only in breeding females (19).

Of the major strains of rats, Sprague-Dawley is particularly subject to mammary tumors, Osborne-Mendel to mammary, ovarian, and adrenal cortical tumors, Furth-Wistar to leukemia and pituitary tumors, and Marshall 520 to adrenal medullary tumors (2). Spontaneous leukemias are generally lymphocytic in mice and granulocytic in rats. In both species, the incidence of spontaneous tumors is increased by chemical carcinogens, such as dimethyl [α] benzanthracene, and by irradiation, but other rare tumors, such as hepatomas, may be induced by these modalities. In guinea pigs, papillary adenomas of the bronchi are the most common tumors (46 percent of total neoplasms), with leukemia (7 percent) and mammary adenocarcinoma (6 percent) next common, followed by uterine and gastrointestinal tumors (20). Mastomys (*Praomys natalensis*), a rodent from South

Africa, is of interest because of the high incidence (30 to 70 percent) of carcinoid tumors of the stomach, and renal adenocarcinomas and thymomas are also common (2). The golden or Syrian hamster has been widely used for study of xenografts of human tumors, that is, tumor tissue from humans implanted and growing in the hamster cheek pouches, and for viral induction of tumors.

Among domestic animals, mammary neoplasms are rare in cows, but common in breeding female dogs, where they differ from the human disease in that they usually are of both mesenchymal and epithelial origin and may include bony or cartilaginous elements. Nephroblastomas are common in pigs, but rare in dogs, cats, horses, sheep, and humans (Wilms' tumor). Sheep, cats, and pigs develop melanomas less frequently than do horses or dogs, whereas Hereford cattle are particularly subject to a squamous cell carcinoma of the conjunctiva of the eye, known as cancer eye. The reader is referred to several reviews of the literature for more complete listings (2,3,21–24).

Birds

A certain amount of information is available about the incidence of neoplasms in captive birds in zoos (9,10,22); overall incidence data are given in Table 2-3. Several species have been studied more intensively, namely, the shell parakeet or budgerigar and the chicken, because of its economic importance. The parakeet develops tumors of the kidney and of the pituitary gland rather frequently and is also subject to lipomas and xanthomas of the pectoral subcutaneous tissues (25,26). A monograph has been devoted to tumors found in chickens (27), but in this species most experimental studies have been concerned with the induction of neoplasms by viruses, a subject to which we will return later in this book. The earliest observed neoplastic states in chickens, first defined in 1908, were the erythroblastoses, in which there is excessive proliferation and release into the circulation of immature erythrocytes (28). Subsequently in 1910, Peyton Rous successfully transplanted, using cell-free extracts, a spontaneous sarcoma of the chicken breast (29). In addition, there are chicken leukoses, such as Marek's disease and reticuloendotheliosis, which often take the form of lymphomatous or leukemic proliferative disorders (30,31). Pontén has studied many features of the transplantation of these viral diseases (32–34) and found that, at least in Rous sarcoma, the donor cell line was completely replaced by tumor cells with the sexual karyotype of the recip-

Table 2-3 Frequency of tumors at autopsy in four orders of birds at the Philadelphia Zoo.

	1901–1934			1935–1955		
Order	*Necropsies*	*Benign (percent)*	*Malignant (percent)*	*Necropsies*	*Benign (percent)*	*Malignant (percent)*
Psittaciformes	1,218	0.5	2.0	309	0.6	3.3
Galliformes	660	0.3	1.1	362	0.3	2.8
Anseriformes	601	0	0.8	480	1.0	3.3
Passeriformes	2,977	0.1	0.3	937	0.5	1.2

Both benign and malignant tumors were found more frequently in birds that had been on exhibition longer (averages 59 months in 1901–1934, 93 months in 1935–1955) than the average for all birds (34 months in 1901–1934, 55 months in 1935–1955). A total of 81 carcinomas and 18 sarcomas were reported (Ref. 10).

ient. Thus, increase in the tumor cell population was achieved by recruitment of normal host cells, rather than by proliferation of the donor clone; this is illustrated in Figure 2-1. This type of growth occurring through viral induction of new cells does not seem to fit conventional ideas of neoplasia, yet it is quite possibly involved in the growth of at least some human cancers, although this is difficult to demonstrate. One example that appears to illustrate the process in humans is the recurrence of leukemia with donor karyotype in patients whose leukemia had been treated by bone marrow transplantation (35). A number of mechanisms for transformation apart from viral induction could be involved; these include cell fusion and loss of chromosomes, a fundamental defect in regulation or even immunologically generated damage to donor cells.

Figure 2-1 Clonal growth: as in RPL chicken lymphoma (A), contrasted with the type of recruitment of host cells involved in the proliferation of Rous sarcoma (B). Reproduced from Ref. 2.

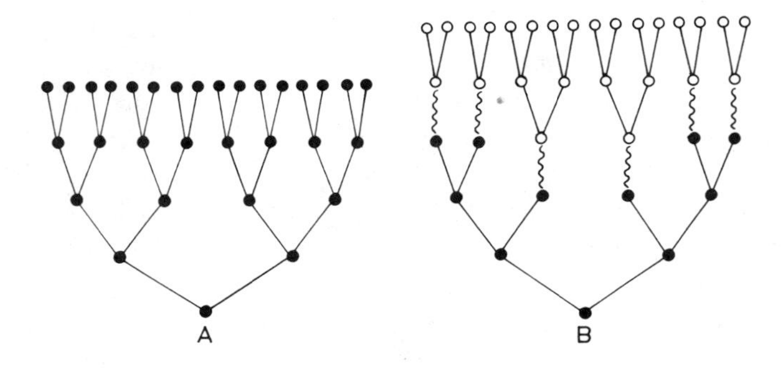

Reptiles

Less is known about cancer in reptiles than in other classes of vertebrates; they are neither of great economic importance nor are they often used as laboratory animals. However, this class is important in that it provides the earliest evidence of growth disorders. This includes fossil remains of what appear to be a hemangioma of a dinosaur vertebra from the Comanchean period and an osteoma of the vertebra of a mosasaur, a giant sea lizard, dating from the Cretaceous period (36). Most anomalous growths that have been described in modern reptiles are benign fibropapillomas or hyperplasias resulting from injury, infection, or infestation by parasites (4). Adenocarcinomas of the kidney and pancreas, malignant melanomas, carcinoma of the bile duct, and ovarian carcinoma have been found in snakes, and squamous cell carcinomas in lizards (37). Hematopoietic neoplasms are rare, but leukemia has been reported in lizards of different families (38). A C-type virus has been associated with sarcomas in the Russell's viper (39). It is interesting that a strain of the chicken Rous sarcoma virus can induce similar tumors in various reptiles (40). There is at present no information about the sensitivity of reptiles to chemical carcinogens.

Amphibians

Amphibians are subject to many neoplasma, of which some are transplantable, including malignant melanoma, neuroepithelioma, and lymphosarcoma (2). Other tumors that are fairly common are the seminomas of the testis in the axolotl and hepatomas and ovarian tumors in the frog (41). However, the best known is the Lucke´ tumor, a renal adenocarcinoma first described in 1905 (42), but later studied intensively by Lucke´ and his collaborators (43). This tumor, which may be present in 2 percent of leopard frogs (*Rana pipiens*), is associated with a herpes virus (44), although there are reports that other viruses are present in the tumor cell nuclei, which may function as helper-viruses in the synthesis of the herpesvirus. But C-type viruses have not been found in amphibians, and these animals also lack papillomas and epidermal neoplasms.

Fish

Of the wide range of neoplastic diseases of fish (45), most occur among the teleosts or bony fishes and very few in cartilaginous fishes. The finding of a variety of tumors in fish raises the question of whether they result from increasing pollution of the waters by such materials as chlorinated hydrocarbons. Chemical carcinogenesis is well known in fish. The rainbow trout (*Salmo gairdneri*) is particularly sensitive to such carcinogens as aflatoxin B, which gives rise to a hepatocarcinoma (4), and dimethylnitrosamine, which can induce both hepatocarcinoma (46) and a nephroblastoma (47). Other tumors, such as the melanomas that are common in platyfish-swordtail hybrids, involve genetic and endocrine factors (48). Although viral particles have been identified in many fish tumors, no infectious tumor-producing agent has been isolated as yet. Among fish we encounter problems in defining neoplasia that reflect the evolutionary distance separating them from mammals. For example, in fish, the thyroid is an ill-defined, nonencapsulated gland, and when thyroid hyperplasia occurs, the tissue invades neighboring structures in much the same way as a malignancy, but no metastasis occurs and the condition is benign.

Primitive vertebrates and invertebrates

A few tumors have been described in lower chordates, including a sarcoma of the sea lamprey, an agnathan fish, and a carcinoid-like tumor of amphioxus, a cephalochordate (2). Among invertebrates, the bivalve molluscs are particularly prone to what are clearly malignant invasive tumors. Such tumors include epitheliomas, sarcomas, leukemia-like diseases, and ganglioneuromas (2,4); herpesvirus has been associated with some of these diseases. Oysters, for example, are found with dense proliferations of enlarged hemocytes (blood cells) that infiltrate other tissues, presenting analogies to leukemia in vertebrates (49). Mussels are subject to what appears to be a diffuse invasive sarcoma (50), with large pigmented binucleate cells having frequent tripolar and tetrapolar mitotic figures. In some areas, such as Yaquina Bay, Oregon, up to 40 percent of the mussels had this disease.

Little work has been done on insects other than fruit flies (*Drosophila*). The melanomas found in this insect appear to be clumps of blood cells with associated deposits of melanin, rather than true tumors (2), although it is possible that an initial leukemic type of neoplasm is subsequently controlled by encapsulation (51). A transplantable, invasive neuroblastoma has also been developed by imaginal disc transplants (52). Imaginal discs, loci of totipotential cells found in insect larvae, are the stem cells from which development of the adult (imago) occurs. In other invertebrates, no systematic search for analogs of cancer has been undertaken, and it is in any case questionable whether they would be recognized as such. An illustration of this point is the mutant giant hydra, described by Lenhoff (53), the cells of which, when transplanted to a normal hydra (*Chlorohydra viridissima*), will totally replace the cells of the latter leaving a complete giant mutant. The whole mutant organism could be regarded, in one sense, as a neoplasm. Sparks has written a review of the many tumors and tumor-like conditions in the lower invertebrates (54), which should be consulted for further examples.

Plants

Plant tumors, specifically crown gall disease, were among the earliest neoplasms to be studied (55). Although the very different structural organization of a plant imposes behavioral and structural differences on a plant neoplasm, as compared with animal cancers, the fundamental characteristic of unrestrained or autonomous growth is common to both types of neoplastic growths. In crown gall disease, a tumor-inducing principle is transmitted by bacteria, the active principle apparently being a virus (56). Autonomous growth is ensured for the tumor cells by derepression of the two systems for elaboration of auxin and of cell division-promoting factors (cytokinins); a variety of other biosynthetic capabilities appear to be depressed at the same time (5). The Kostoff tumors, on the other hand, which arise spontaneously in hybrids within the genus *Nicotiana* (57), represent another type of tumor with a genetic basis. Karyotypes are abnormal in such tumors, but it has been shown that, despite this, normal organization, flowering, and even the setting of fertile seed can occur when the tumor shoots are grafted onto normal parental stems (5). The genetic abnormalities may create a metastable balance between genes that determine growth and those that regulate it (58), so that environmental influences then may determine the direction—toward tumor formation or toward differentiation—in which the metastable state evolves. Plant tumors may offer useful insights into the factors that control tumor growth; in particular, the way cytokinins modulate cyclic nucleotide systems may be very relevant to the basic understanding of differentiation.

HISTORICAL ASPECTS OF HUMAN CANCER

Of necessity, our knowledge of early human tumors is restricted to those involving bone, since that is the only substance usually preserved. Osteomas have been found in femurs from the Neolithic period (59); the reader will recall that these benign tumors have also been found in fossil vertebrae of ancient reptiles. Several cases of osteosarcomas have been reported in the long bones of human mummies, dating from the Vth Dynasty (*c.* 2,700 B.C.) in Egypt (60). A highly vascularized pelvic lesion, also diagnosed as osteosarcoma, and belonging to the Roman period (*c.* A.D. 250), was found in a mummy in Alexandria (61). There is no evidence of cancer in the soft tissues of those few mummies that have been examined in detail. However, it is significant that the Edwin Smith surgical papyrus, composed about 1700 B.C., refers to "bulging tumors of the breast . . . and in any member of a man," for which there is stated to be no treatment (62). Thus, Egyptian physicians appear to have been acquainted with malignant tumors and their unfavorable prognosis.

Much of the medical knowledge of the ancient Greeks is presented in the Hippocratic writings. Cancer was known to the early Greek clinicians, and except for superficial tumors, was not recognized as being treatable. Indeed, one of the aphorisms states that occult cancers should best be left untreated, since the patient will then live longer (63). Although there appeared to be an understanding of the distinction between *phymata* or *oidemata,* which are growths or swellings of an inflammatory nature, and *karkinomata,* which include what we consider to be cancers, caution is needed before assuming such understanding. Lesions described as being *karkinomata* were apparently treated and cured by cauterization, which would argue against their being cancers. There was inevitably some confusion between these types of growths or swellings, since inflammation, benign tumors, and cancers were all ascribed to abnormal fluxes of the four humors, a theory that was to persist until the seventeenth century (64). According to Galen a flux of black bile, unmixed with blood, to any part, could give rise to cancer, which he noted was particularly common in the female breast, for which excision and cauterization were appropriate treatments for superficial disease (65).

It is difficult to determine the relative incidence of tumors of any kind, including malignancies, in ancient societies. They are rare in the Egyptian material (66), the most likely material to yield such evidence because of the practice of mummification. Hard data are sparse or nonexistent over the intervening centuries. We may read that the Empress Theodora, wife of the Byzantine Emperor Justinian, died of cancer in the sixth century, but this tells us nothing of how frequent such occurrences were. Not until the sixteenth century, when parish clerks began to record births and the

(9)

The Diſeaſes, and Caſualties this year being 1632.

Disease	Number
ABortive, and Stilborn	445
Affrighted	1
Aged	628
Ague	43
Apoplex, and Meagrom	17
Bit with a mad dog	1
Bleeding	3
Bloody flux, ſcowring, and flux	348
Bruſed, Iſſues, ſores, and ulcers,	28
Burnt, and Scalded	5
Burſt, and Rupture	9
Cancer, and Wolf	10
Canker	1
Childbed	171
Chriſomes, and Infants	2268
Cold, and Cough	55
Colick, Stone, and Strangury	56
Conſumption	1797
Convulſion	241
Cut of the Stone	5
Dead in the ſtreet, and ſtarved	6
Dropſie, and Swelling	267
Drowned	34
Executed, and preſt to death	18
Falling Sickneſs	7
Fever	1108
Fiſtula	13
Flocks, and ſmall Pox	531
French Pox	12
Gangrene	5
Gout	4
Grief	11
Jaundies	43
Jawfaln	8
Impoſtume	74
Kil'd by ſeveral accidents	46
King's Evil	38
Lethargie	2
Livergrown	87
Lunatique	5
Made away themſelves	15
Meaſles	80
Murthered	7
Over-laid, and ſtarved at nurſe	7
Palſie	25
Piles	1
Plague	8
Planet	13
Pleuriſie, and Spleen	36
Purples, and ſpotted Feaver	38
Quinſie	7
Riſing of the Lights	98
Sciatica	1
Scurvey, and Itch	9
Suddenly	62
Surfet	86
Swine Pox	6
Teeth	470
Thruſh, and Sore mouth	40
Tympany	13
Tiſſick	34
Vomiting	1
Worms	27

Chriſtened	Males—4994	Buried	Males—4932	Whereof, of the Plague 8
	Females-4590		Females—4603	
	In all—9584		In all—9535	

Increaſed in the Burials in the 122 Pariſhes, and at the Peſthouſe this year 993
Decreaſed of the Plague in the 122 Pariſhes, and at the Peſthouſe this year, 266

C 7 In

Figure 2-2 Table reproduced from Graunt's "Natural and Political Observations Mentioned in a following index, and made upon the Bills of Mortality," 1662.

number and causes of deaths, was any numerical indication available. Figure 2-2, a reproduction of such records, was collected by John Graunt in his book "Natural and Political Observations Mentioned in a following Index, and made upon the Bills of Mortality," published in 1662. Assuming that the listed causes are accurate, and discounting some rather obscure descriptions, we find that 64 percent of deaths are ascribable to death during childbirth, infant mortality, and infectious diseases, notably tuberculosis and smallpox. Probable cardiovascular disease—dropsy and sudden death—account for a little more than 3 percent. Only 10 deaths are ascribed to cancer, but if we assume that the "bloody fluxes and aged" categories could contain many cases of cancer mortality, we are left with a figure for this disease of somewhere between 0.1 and 10 percent, with the likely true value near the lower end of this range. Modern data such as those for Germany (Figure 2-3), in which the baseline for cancer mortality was 3.3 percent in 1900, rising to 20.9 percent in 1967, would agree with the above estimate. Thus, it is likely that cancer has accounted for up to 3 percent of deaths during the past few centuries.

Finally, we should turn our attention to the very marked increase in cancer deaths in this century. The Terry Report, covering the period between 1900 and 1960 in the United States, showed a more than sixfold increase in cancer deaths during this time (Figure 2-4). When allowance is made for the doubling of the population that took place over the 60-year period, the calculated incidence is still far short of the actual findings. However, alterations in the age structure of the population, due primarily to a reduction in mortality from infectious diseases, which were formerly very prevalent, mean that 14 percent of the population was over 60 in 1960

Figure 2-3 The rise in cancer deaths in Germany, 1900–1967. Reproduced from Ref. 67.

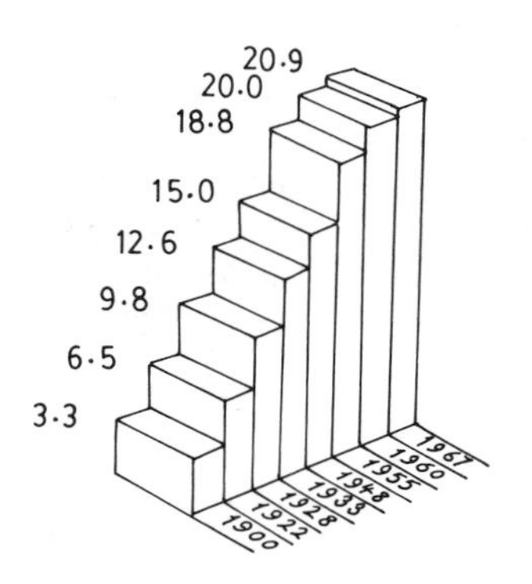

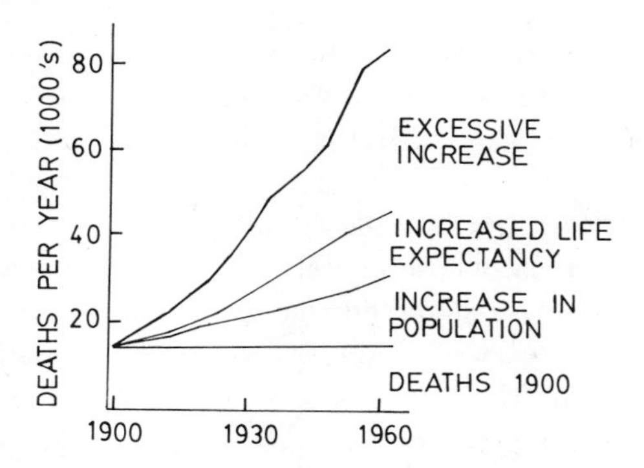

Figure 2-4 Cancer deaths in the United States, 1900–1960, from the "Terry Report." Allowance for increase in life expectancy and increase in population still leaves an excessive increase that requires explanation. Reproduced from Ref. 67.

compared with only 7 percent in 1900. Since cancer, as we shall see later, is far more common in older persons, correction for differences in age structure of the population would significantly increase the expected cancer mortality, although the expected increment is still only about 45 percent of that observed. Some of the excessive increase may be due to more thorough determination and reporting of the causes of death than in the past, perhaps, in part, because far more deaths now occur in hospitals than formerly. The creation of tumor registries has also made statistics more readily available. There remains, however, an unexplained increment that can only reflect increased exposure to carcinogens at the present time.

THE MODERN INCIDENCE OF CANCER

In the United States, cancer accounts for close to 20 percent of all deaths, making it second only to heart disease (Table 2-4). This situation is true of all other industrialized nations, and in fact, in many of them the cancer death rates exceed that for the United States (Table 2-5). In contrast, such countries as El Salvador, Thailand, Honduras, and the Philippines report strikingly low death rates from cancer, even when they are adjusted for age, as in Table 2-5. This could reflect underreporting due to inadequate determination of the cause of death, incomplete data collection, prevalence of other causes of death, such as infectious diseases, or some combination of these. The fact that the lowest rates are found in non-industrialized countries also could be a significant indication of the effect of industrial pollutants in industrialized countries. The data in Table 2-5 also show that the incidence of different forms of cancer varies widely and independently of the overall death rate for cancer. For example, Japan rates number one with respect to stomach cancer, but is in the lower range of death rates for the other listed cancers as well as for the overall average. Scotland heads the list for lung cancer, but has a low incidence of leukemia and of cancer of the uterus. Venezuela, whose overall death rate for cancer is among the lowest of the 44 countries surveyed, has the highest death rate for cancer of the uterus; Costa Rica, Chile, Mauritius, Mexico, Panama, and Romania show a similar pattern. These variations undoubtedly reflect such factors as dietary differences, air pollution, and age at and frequency of childbirth. In Japan, consumption of highly salted foods and rice polished with the aid of materials such as talc has been implicated in stomach cancer; sexual intercourse at an early age and early and frequent childbirth appear to be contributory factors in the development of cancer of the uterine cervix, and thus might be a factor in those countries with high death rates from cancer of the uterus. Although death rates may differ markedly between the sexes, as for example, with cancer of the lung and stomach, the ranking order is generally similar for males and females of each country. In contrast, oral cancers may present marked inconsistencies in ranking, as in the cases of France, Iceland, Italy, Switzerland, and Venezuela. Explanations for this might involve sex differences in smoking and drinking habits, for example. A detailed discussion of international cancer incidences as related to national diets and customs has appeared and should be consulted for further information (68).

If we turn now to figures for cancer death rates within the United States, it is possible to minimize such factors as inadequate determination and reporting of cancer deaths. It is apparent that there are quite marked differences in the prevalence of cancer among the various states (Table 2-6). The low death rate for Utah reflects the high proportion of those inhabitants of the Mormon faith, whose abstemious life-style may lead to a lower incidence of cancer. In contrast, the high rate for Florida reflects the large proportion of elderly retired people, who simply on the basis of their age are more prone to cancer. In the case of Alaska, it could be argued that the opposite is true. Industrial development, particularly with regard to petroleum, has led to a large influx of predominantly younger workers with lower cancer death rates. Looking at the data overall, it is clear that the death rates are greatest for the states on the East Coast, but although these are generally industrialized, and thus more likely to have high levels of environmental carcinogens, this is not true of Maine or New Hampshire,

Table 2-4 Leading causes of death in the United States, 1976.

Cause	Number of deaths	Percent of deaths	Number of deaths: Age 1–14		Age 15–34		Age 35–54		Age 55–74		Age 75+	
			Male	*Female*	*Male*	*Female*	*Male*	*Female*	*Male*	*Female*	*Male*	*Female*
Heart disease	723,729	37.9	305	250	2,506	1,194	45,278	13,613	193,659	99,771	158,257	208,008
Cancer	377,312	19.8	1,457	1,048	3,831	3,457	26,697	28,184	114,742	84,837	58,608	54,324
Cerebrovascular disease (strokes)	188,623	9.9	168	128	836	765	5,075	4,988	30,031	26,930	44,413	75,139
Accidents	100,761	5.3	6,430	3,317	30,394	7,790	13,446	4,519	12,208	6,181	7,018	8,120
Pneumonia/Influenza	61,666	3.2	427	415	775	616	2,446	1,541	9,708	5,509	18,064	20,394
Diabetes	34,508	1.8			386	345	1,654	1,585	6,933	8,694	5,024	9,838
Cirrhosis of liver	31,453	1.6			861	435	8,040	4,109	10,402	5,196		
Arteriosclerosis	29,366	1.5							2,677	2,021	8,961	15,416
Suicide	26,832	1.4	126		7,502	2,309	5,547	2,753	4,920	1,857		
Diseases of infancy	24,809	1.3										
Homicide	19,554	1.0	394	304	8,171	2,133	4,548	1,111				
Emphysema	17,796	0.9					692		7,871	2,180	5,252	
Congenital anomalies	13,002	0.7	917	942	573	428						

Source: Vital statistics of the United States, 1976.

Table 2-5 Cancer death rates in 44 countries world wide (1972–1973).

Country	*All sites*		*Oral*		*Colon & rectum*		*Lung*		*Breast*	*Uterus*	*Skin*		*Stomach*		*Pros-tate*	*Leukemia*	
	Male	*Female*	*Male*	*Female*	*Male*	*Female*	*Male*	*Female*	*Female*	*Female*	*Male*	*Female*	*Male*	*Female*	*Male*	*Male*	*Female*
United States	157.2	106.1	4.6	1.5	18.9	15.1	48.9	10.8	22.4	8.4	2.4	1.4	7.5	3.7	14.4	7.1	4.3
Australia	158.1	100.0	3.9	1.3	20.1	17.4	44.5	6.7	19.9	7.7	4.5	2.6	13.9	7.0	15.7	6.7	4.4
Austria	191.1	124.3	4.0	0.7	23.9	16.8	52.3	6.5	19.2	15.1	2.2	1.7	33.2	17.3	14.3	6.1	4.3
Bulgaria	128.2	81.0	1.6	0.6	8.6	6.9	36.2	6.4	11.2	7.6	1.7	1.1	31.0	18.2	6.3	4.3	3.5
Canada	157.0	109.4	4.5	1.4	21.9	18.2	43.3	8.0	23.9	8.0	1.8	1.3	13.7	6.3	14.2	7.0	4.5
Costa Rica	123.7	111.2	3.0	0.8	4.5	5.1	9.6	4.3	8.3	18.2	1.6	0.7	49.5	30.1	8.0	3.9	4.5
Chile	157.8	133.3	2.5	0.9	7.8	8.0	18.5	4.6	12.2	21.8	1.1	1.1	57.4	30.7	11.5	3.9	3.3
Czechoslovakia	204.1	110.9	3.3	0.7	21.4	14.2	62.9	5.5	8.6	11.7	2.4	1.6	33.5	17.3	10.1	6.5	4.4
Denmark	170.2	132.1	2.1	0.9	23.1	18.5	46.4	9.8	26.3	13.2	2.6	1.9	16.4	8.5	13.4	7.4	4.9
El Salvador	26.7	42.7	0.9	0.3	1.4	1.6	1.8	0.6	1.1	6.5	0.4	0.2	5.6	10.1	1.2	2.9	1.9
England & Wales	184.3	119.6	2.8	1.3	21.7	17.2	73.5	13.4	27.1	8.9	1.6	1.4	17.5	9.6	11.8	5.6	3.7
Finland	182.9	99.1	2.3	0.9	11.4	10.4	64.3	4.1	15.0	7.3	2.8	1.6	27.4	14.1	13.5	7.0	4.8
France	187.0	98.5	13.4	1.0	20.3	13.8	33.6	3.4	17.9	9.7	1.5	1.2	16.6	7.9	14.8	6.8	4.4
Germany, F.R.	178.0	121.2	2.2	0.6	22.4	17.4	46.0	4.7	19.7	11.1	1.8	1.4	28.7	15.1	15.0	6.2	4.4
Greece	124.5	75.3	1.4	0.5	6.0	5.5	35.8	6.0	12.0	6.0	0.9	1.0	13.3	7.8	6.6	6.9	4.3
Hong Kong	170.7	96.8	19.8	7.0	12.9	8.7	41.3	20.0	9.7	9.8	0.7	0.6	16.3	9.1	2.1	3.2	2.4
Honduras	30.6	45.9	0.3	0.1	0.4	0.2	1.5	0.8	0.6	8.4	0.2	0.1	7.0	6.6	0.8	1.6	1.3
Hungary	182.6	125.6	4.6	0.9	19.1	15.5	43.1	8.2	17.5	16.8	2.5	2.0	38.1	18.6	14.7	6.2	4.2
Iceland	114.6	93.8	1.8	2.7	17.4	9.3	11.1	7.4	14.1	5.9	0.7	2.0	31.6	14.9	3.8	4.9	4.7
Ireland	158.0	122.1	4.3	1.8	23.2	19.1	39.1	11.9	23.9	7.7	1.9	1.7	22.8	13.8	13.9	6.2	3.0
Israel	121.5	118.8	1.5	0.8	13.1	12.1	23.1	7.2	25.2	5.3	1.2	1.7	15.7	9.0	7.5	6.2	4.3
Italy	173.3	103.0	6.0	1.0	17.3	12.8	40.9	5.1	18.3	11.2	1.6	1.0	29.3	14.2	10.9	6.9	4.6
Japan	141.2	89.9	1.5	0.6	10.1	8.0	17.7	5.6	4.6	9.8	0.8	0.5	59.6	31.1	2.1	4.1	3.1
Luxembourg	200.7	120.8	6.2	1.4	23.1	17.0	64.5	5.7	21.1	13.9	2.3	0.9	21.6	10.8	13.6	5.0	3.3
Mauritius	80.4	57.4	2.9	0.8	7.6	4.4	15.1	2.2	6.0	16.4	0.0	0.3	16.4	7.1	3.2	2.3	0.8
Mexico	55.2	71.0	1.4	0.6	2.8	3.3	8.1	4.2	5.1	18.8	0.8	0.7	9.7	8.6	5.5	2.5	2.2

Netherlands	186.9	160.2	2.0	0.7	18.4	16.1	67.5	4.0	29.9	10.5	1.7	1.5	22.0	10.7	22.9	12.5	4.3
New Zealand	162.4	114.4	3.1	1.2	25.6	20.8	42.8	10.2	23.5	8.6	4.5	2.2	14.4	6.2	15.8	6.6	4.8
Northern Ireland	159.8	117.1	3.3	2.0	21.8	18.4	50.7	10.1	23.7	9.1	1.3	1.0	20.1	10.7	11.0	6.0	4.0
Norway	133.2	101.4	3.0	0.9	15.8	13.0	19.5	4.1	17.7	8.2	3.0	1.6	20.0	10.0	16.3	6.4	4.3
Panama	75.4	76.1	3.1	1.4	4.3	5.0	11.0	3.1	6.6	17.5	0.3	0.2	13.5	7.6	8.7	3.7	2.4
Philippines	49.8	39.9	4.4	1.9	2.8	2.3	5.2	2.5	4.7	5.0	0.8	0.4	6.0	4.1	1.4	3.0	2.6
Poland	158.3	102.9	4.7	1.0	10.0	8.1	40.8	5.1	12.3	14.2	1.9	1.6	36.7	15.6	8.3	5.5	3.9
Portugal	127.1	91.1	5.3	1.0	14.1	12.9	14.3	3.1	14.3	12.3	2.0	1.6	33.5	19.0	13.0	5.8	4.2
Puerto Rico	119.5	80.3	10.2	2.1	7.2	6.6	14.2	5.9	8.8	12.4	0.9	0.7	19.0	8.1	12.6	5.5	3.3
Romania	126.2	86.2	2.9	1.0	6.7	6.3	27.8	5.4	10.2	17.9	1.6	1.2	30.3	13.6	8.4	4.6	3.2
Scotland	205.0	128.4	2.9	1.3	23.2	19.4	84.1	16.0	27.5	8.4	1.9	1.7	20.8	11.7	12.2	5.3	3.0
Spain	137.4	87.2	3.2	0.6	10.2	9.2	24.4	4.0	11.4	9.0	1.3	0.7	26.2	14.3	11.9	4.3	3.4
Sweden	144.7	111.7	2.7	1.2	18.4	13.9	22.6	5.4	20.2	9.1	2.4	1.6	17.2	9.0	21.1	6.6	4.7
Switzerland	178.8	108.7	6.6	0.9	20.2	12.8	43.8	4.2	23.8	10.7	2.9	1.7	21.2	10.6	19.3	7.1	4.5
Thailand	29.4	19.6	2.2	1.1	1.7	1.2	3.3	1.3	0.4	3.0	0.1	0.0	2.0	0.9	0.2	0.4	0.3
Uruguay	200.6	131.7	5.8	1.1	19.5	19.2	42.6	3.9	24.0	14.7	2.1	1.0	31.4	15.8	17.6	5.8	4.2
Venezuela	116.0	104.0	2.9	2.5	5.0	5.4	14.2	6.8	9.6	25.5	1.5	1.1	29.7	17.7	9.5	4.0	3.0
Yugoslavia	120.4	78.4	3.1	0.7	8.4	7.0	30.1	4.9	10.3	10.6	1.6	1.3	23.0	11.4	7.4	4.3	3.0

Data are age-adjusted rates per 100,000 population.
Source: World Health Statistics Annual 1972–1973.

Table 2-6 Estimated new cancer cases and deaths by state, 1979.

State	*Number of new cases*	*Deaths per 100,000*	*State*	*Number of new cases*	*Deaths per 100,000*
Alabama	13,000	168	Montana	2,300	167
Alaska	500	57	Nebraska	5,300	177
Arizona	7,600	152	Nevada	2,100	141
Arkansas	8,300	195	New Hampshire	3,200	193
California	73,000	169	New Jersey	29,000	206
Colorado	6,500	121	New Mexico	3,000	121
Connecticut	12,000	198	New York	70,000	208
Delaware	2,100	186	North Carolina	17,000	156
District of Columbia	3,100	238	North Dakota	2,000	166
Florida	42,000	250	Ohio	38,000	184
Georgia	15,000	143	Oklahoma	10,000	184
Hawaii	2,100	118	Oregon	8,100	171
Idaho	2,400	145	Pennsylvania	48,000	208
Illinois	40,000	185	Rhode Island	4,100	237
Indiana	18,000	171	South Carolina	8,200	146
Iowa	11,000	194	South Dakota	2,400	187
Kansas	8,100	178	Tennessee	15,000	175
Louisiana	13,000	165	Texas	39,000	151
Maine	4,100	198	Utah	2,500	98
Maryland	15,000	179	Vermont	1,600	172
Massachusetts	23,000	203	Virginia	16,000	157
Michigan	30,000	167	Washington	13,000	174
Minnesota	13,000	164	West Virginia	6,700	190
Mississippi	7,700	160	Wyoming	1,000	129
Missouri	19,000	199	Puerto Rico	6,000	102

Derived from CA Vol. 29, No. 1, 1979.

although they belong to this high cancer risk group. Other factors must be involved, one of which that has been tentatively identified is the level of selenium in soils and crops. Generally, the amounts of selenium found in foodstuff are low in all states of the eastern seaboard as well as the Pacific northwest, whereas in the southwest and west central areas this element is more abundant (69). There is evidence, as we shall see later (p. 234), that selenium is a cancer preventive factor. More detailed statistics have been prepared on the basis of figures from each county (70). This information has shown that the incidence of cancer varies widely within each state, and in many cases this variation has provided evidence of association between particular local industries and cancer. Examples of maps plotted from such data appear in Figure 2-5. Here, for example, areas with high mortality

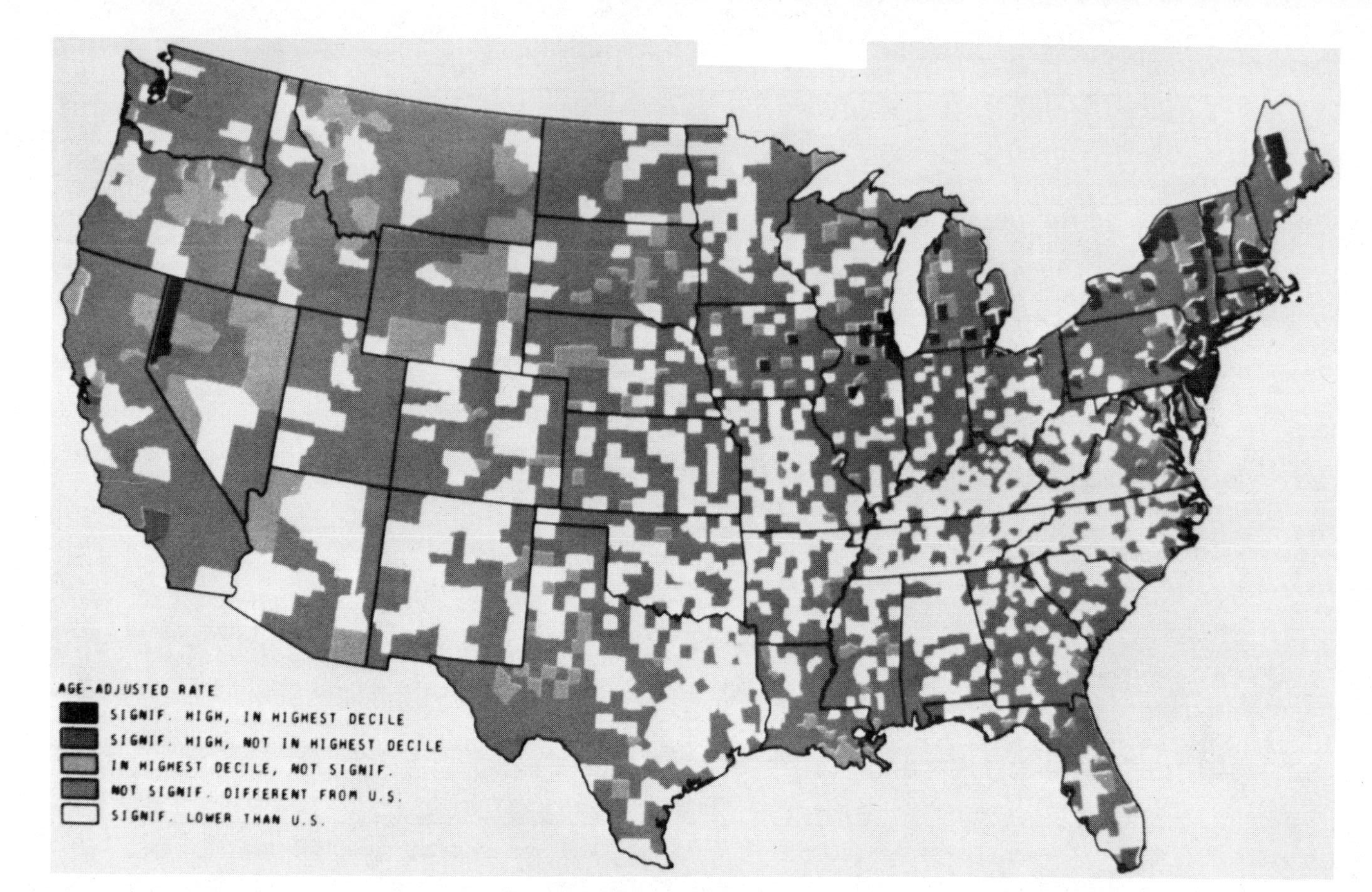

Figure 2-5 The incidence, by county, of bladder cancer in white males in the United States (mainland only), 1950–1969. Note the areas of high frequency, usually associated with concentrations of industry, as in North New Jersey.

Table 2-7 Mortality for the five leading cancer sites for each major age group, United States, 1976.

	Under 15		15–34		35–54		55–74		75 +	
Site	*Male*	*Female*	*Male*	*Female*	*Male*	*Female*	*Male*	*Female*	*Male*	*Female*
Bladder									3,055	
Bone	74	49								
Bone marrow (leukemia)	671	466	738	545	1,059					
Brain & central nervous system	418	335	439	365	1,273					
Breast				535		8,269		16,636		7,678
Colon & rectum					2,445	2,414	13,098	12,250	8,821	11,670
Connective tissue	39	35								
Kidney	45	50								
Lung					10,080	4,276	42,453	12,025	13,200	4,078
Ovary						2,278		5,950		
Pancreas					1,326		6,232			3,521
Prostate							8,640		11,374	
Reticuloendothelial system (Hodgkin's disease)			346	216						
Skin			265							
Stomach							4,629		3,151	
Testis			412							
Uterus				322		2,302		5,591		3,071

Source: Vital statistics of the United States, 1976.

from bladder cancer are clearly located around Northern New Jersey with its concentration of firms in the petrochemical industry. We shall return to this topic later when we discuss chemical carcinogenesis.

The increase in cancer mortality with age is brought out in Table 2-7, which lists deaths attributable to the five leading cancers for each age group; it should be considered in conjunction with the total cancer mortality figures in Table 2-4. It is also evident that the forms of cancer that predominate differ markedly at different ages. The neoplasms of the digestive system, so common in the older age groups, are very rare in children, whereas leukemia and Hodgkin's disease are among the most frequent cancers in younger persons, although they represent only a very small proportion of tumors in the elderly. In children below 15, the overall cancer death rate is only about 5 per 100,000 and many of the tumors, which appear to be of an embryonic origin, represent persistent pockets of incompletely differentiated cells as in neuroblastoma. There is a slight decrease in the cancer death rate for individuals over 75 years of age, both in terms of total numbers and percentage of the total. This has been examined in more detail (71), and it appears that in the United States, the increase in cancer incidence and death slows after 65 and then there is a decline at 90 years of age. In England, this trend occurs after 85, in Sweden after 70.

So far we have been talking primarily of cancer death rates. These do not always reflect closely the actual probability of contracting a disease, because various forms of cancer respond quite differently to therapy, and in some, the cure rate may be higher than in others. Thus, the death rate should always be lower than the figure for incidence of the disease, as is brought out clearly in Table 2-8. Overall, deaths from cancer amount to about 52 percent of the number of new cases, which reflects, but does not directly measure the average curability of cancer. The death rate, expressed as a percentage of the incidence of the disease, ranges from a low of about 11 percent for cancer of the thyroid to a high of 92 percent for patients with bone cancer. A more direct estimate of the success of a given therapy is to determine the 5-year survival rates in groups of patients who have been treated and are without apparent disease. These data are collated in Table 2-9. For most forms of cancer, there is a marked fall in long-term survival when the patient has regional as compared with localized disease at the time of treatment. This points up the value of early diagnosis and treatment of a patient. However, a few diseases have such a poor overall prognosis that the stage of the disease at diagnosis has little or no effect on the outcome. Examples of this are pancreatic and esophageal cancer.

Table 2-8 Estimated new cancer cases and cancer deaths for major sites, 1979.

Site	*Number of new cases (incidence)*	*Number of deaths*	*Deaths (percent of incidence)*
All Sites	765,000	395,000	51.6
Bladder	35,000	10,000	28.6
Bone	1,900	1,750	92.1
Bone marrow (leukemia)	21,500	15,400	71.6
Brain & central nervous system	11,600	9,500	81.9
Breast	106,900	34,500	32.3
Colon & rectum	112,000	51,900	46.3
Esophagus	8,400	7,500	89.3
Kidney	16,200	7,500	46.3
Larynx	10,400	3,500	33.7
Liver	11,600	9,200	79.3
Lung	112,000	97,500	87.1
Ovary	17,000	11,100	65.3
Pancreas	23,000	20,200	87.8
Prostate	64,000	21,000	32.8
Reticuloendothelial system			
(Hodgkin's disease)	6,900	1,900	27.5
(Lymphomas)	7,800	7,100	91.0
(Lymphosarcoma & reticulosarcoma)	15,000	5,200	34.7
(multiple myeloma)	8,800	6,100	69.3
Skin (melanoma)	13,600	5,900	43.4
Small intestine	2,200	700	31.8
Stomach	23,000	14,100	61.3
Thyroid	9,000	1,000	11.1
Uterus	53,000	10,700	20.2

Derived from CA-A Cancer Journal for Clinicians Vol. 29, No. 1, 1979.

Five-year survival is the criterion of "cure" most generally accepted, since the majority of recurrences take place within the first year or two after therapy; by the fifth year relapse rates have leveled off. Some diseases, such as breast cancer and malignant melanoma, however, may recur after more prolonged intervals, so that a 10-year survival figure may be a more meaningful index of successful treatment.

TRENDS IN THE INCIDENCE OF CANCER

Cancer death rate studies over the past forty years or more have helped establish a trend that may be used to forecast rates in the near future. Such data are available for the period 1930–1976 in the United States. Figures 2-6 and 2-7 show these data for females and males, respectively. In the case of males, it is evident that of these eight major forms of cancer, six have shown little net change in death rates between 1950 and 1976. Prior to this period, mortalities from colorectal, prostatic, and pancreatic cancers and leukemia steadily increased. In contrast to these six diseases, stomach cancer showed a continuous steep fall throughout the period, bringing the mortality rate down to about one-quarter of that in 1930. Lung cancer mortality, however, escalated to reach a value close to 18 times the 1930 figure; this rise was the chief contributor to the overall increase in male deaths from cancer. In females, death rates from ovarian, pancreatic, and breast

Table 2-9 Five-year survival rates for period 1965–1969 adjusted for normal life expectancy.

	Percentage 5-Year Survivors			
	Female		*Male*	
Site	*Localized*	*Regional*	*Localized*	*Regional*
Bladder	76	16	71	23
Bone marrow (leukemia)		15		14
Brain & central nervous system	33	37	25	20
Breast	85	56		
Colon & rectum	72	47	71	40
Esophagus	7	10	4	5
Kidney	66	40	70	39
Larynx	75	34	80	38
Lip	89		87	66
Liver	29	5	15	1
Mouth	78	40	64	38
Ovary	78	43		
Pancreas	6	5	5	2
Pharynx	47	29	35	21
Prostate			70	61
Reticuloendothelial system				
(Hodgkin's disease)		57		53
(Lymphosarcoma)		37		34
(Multiple myeloma)		16		17
(Reticulosarcoma)		19		18
Skin (melanoma)	85	41	76	47
Stomach	41	13	39	15
Thyroid	97	87	100	83
Tongue	61	30	55	24
Uterus	83	46		

Derived from Cancer Patient Survival, Report #5, DHEW Publication No. (NIH) 77-992.

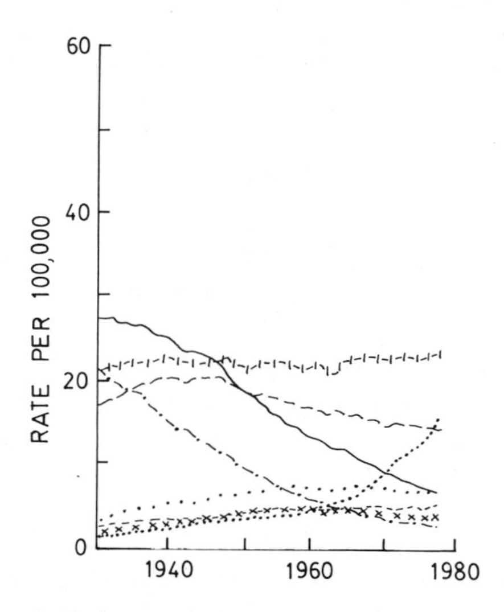

Figure 2-6 Age-adjusted death rates for major sites of cancer in females, United States, 1930–1977: uterus (——); lung (• • •); colon and rectum (— —); stomach (—•—•); ovary (• • •); pancreas (– – –); breast (|—|—|); and bone marrow (leukemia) (× × ×). Data from U.S. National Center for Health Statistics and U.S. Bureau of the Census.

Figure 2-7 Age-adjusted death rates for major sites of cancer in males, United States, 1930–1977: esophagus (——); lung (• • •); colon and rectum (— —); stomach (—•—•); prostate (• • •); pancreas (– – –); bladder (—|—|); and bone marrow (leukemia) (× × ×). Data from U.S. National Center for Health Statistics and U.S. Bureau of the Census.

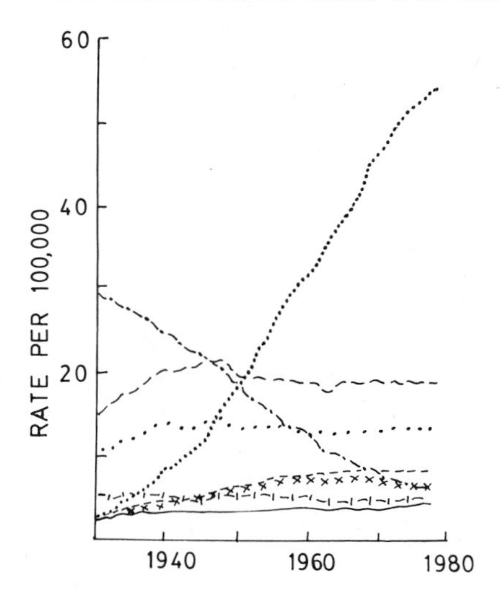

cancer and leukemia remained about the same or increased slowly between 1930 and 1976. Both stomach and uterine cancers showed a continuous steep fall over this time period, whereas colorectal cancer fell slowly after the late 1940's. Death rates for lung cancer, after rising slowly but steadily to double the figure for 1930 in 1960, have escalated thereafter and are now rising faster than in the male population. It is probable that deaths from lung cancer for both males and females will continue to increase, with a likely trend toward similar final values; advances in the treatment of the disease cannot be expected to affect this trend in the near future. Deaths from uterine cancer are unlikely to fall much further because cure rates for early disease are now very high, and most of the population at risk, because of early diagnosis with Papp smears, receive effective treatment while the cancer is still localized. Stomach cancer, on the other hand, is not a particularly curable cancer, and the explanation for its fall lies not in improved therapy, but elsewhere, as for example, in such changes in diet as the consumption of less home-smoked foods. Incidentally, the decline in stomach cancer argues against a major role for dietary or salivary nitrites in cancer induction. The fall in stomach cancer mortality also appears to be leveling off. Leukemias seem to have entered a period of slow decline in terms of mortality rates, which almost certainly reflects the increasing efficacy of modern combination chemotherapy regimens. Deaths from colorectal cancer appear to have dropped off from the peak around 1945, especially in women. Dietary factors such as excess fatty meat, low fiber intake, and lack of vitamin A have been implicated in colorectal cancer. Greater attention to such dietary factors, together with improvements in therapy, may have contributed to this change, and women have generally been more conscious of diet than have men. This trend might be expected to continue.

A final aspect of trends in cancer incidence concerns black Americans (72). In the period from 1950 to 1977, there was a 63 percent increase in cancer mortality in black males compared with 24 percent for white males. Although, to a certain degree, there may have been underreporting of cancer in black males in the past, there has definitely been a real increase, as shown in Figure 2-8. Among the common cancers in which the incidence for blacks exceeds that for whites are those of the esophagus, stomach, prostate, larynx, bladder, and uterus. However, the incidence of breast, ovarian, bladder, and renal cancers is lower among blacks. Available data also suggest that 40 percent more black males than white males are cigarette smokers (72), and smoking is associated with several of the cancers

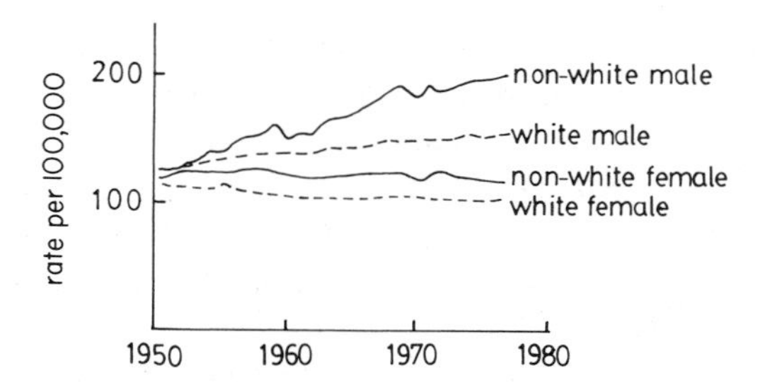

Figure 2-8 Cancer death rates per 100,000, by sex and race, United States, 1950–1977. Derived from National Vital Statistics Division.

more prevalent among blacks. Further etiological study is clearly needed, quite apart from better access to medical care to ensure earlier treatment.

PROBABILITY OF DEVELOPING CANCER

Whereas raw incidence data provide some indication of what might be expected in terms of the probability of an individual developing and dying of cancer, various attempts have been made to arrive at more mathematically sound and numerically precise probabilities (73,74). Although this is not the place for a full consideration, we have reproduced some of the conclusions of Seidman and his collaborators (74). Application of their methodology to available data yielded figures such as those in Table 2-10. In comparison with earlier data, it could be shown that the probability of contracting cancer was increasing in all sex and race groups and that the probability at birth of eventually dying of cancer was greater for males. Problems with these calculations emerge if there is rapid increase (or decrease) in incidence of disease—lung cancer being a case in point—since the assumption of a constant occurrence of disease, made in Seidman's treatment, is not then justified. Readers are referred to the original papers for data on specific forms of cancer.

CONCLUSION

Cancer is widely distributed between species and over time, with growth abnormalities found in modern vertebrates, invertebrates, and plants, as well as in Mesozoic reptiles. Thus, it is evident that the disease is unique neither to humans nor to modern societies. Nevertheless, even with allow-

Table 2-10 Probabilities of developing and dying of cancer within various time periods at different ages, 1970.

	Age and time periods (years)												
	At birth	20			35			50			65		
Group *	*Eventually*	10	20	*Eventually*	10	20	*Eventually*	10	20	*Eventually*	10	20	*Eventually*
Developing cancer													
W.M.	26.3	0.33	0.90	26.87	0.95	3.86	27.15	4.93	13.91	27.12	13.51	22.82	25.04
NW.M.	23.4	0.24	0.82	24.49	1.25	5.00	25.93	6.48	15.55	27.48	14.80	24.00	26.26
W.F.	29.8	0.41	1.53	27.84	1.91	6.08	27.51	5.50	12.64	25.32	9.04	16.76	19.20
NW.F.	25.5	0.48	1.79	22.21	2.11	5.88	22.02	4.94	11.00	20.37	8.27	14.25	16.68
Dying of Cancer													
W.M.	16.9	0.08	0.31	17.21	0.29	1.76	17.23	2.09	7.36	16.69	5.58	11.57	13.47
NW.M.	15.3	0.07	0.36	16.05	0.53	2.89	16.87	3.24	8.87	17.11	6.02	11.45	13.73
W.F.	15.9	0.06	0.35	16.03	0.39	1.91	15.60	1.42	4.64	13.46	2.43	6.63	8.94
NW.F.	13.4	0.08	0.51	13.82	0.56	2.44	13.45	1.70	4.97	11.57	2.72	5.91	8.04

Data reproduced from Ref. 74 with permission of the authors and copyright owners.

* W, white; NW, nonwhite; M, male; F, female.

ances for greater longevity, better recordkeeping, and the control of other diseases, it is evident that the incidence of cancer has increased during the twentieth century. It would appear that about one-half of all cancer is curable at present, but the prognosis varies widely from one tumor to another, with some forms particularly refractory to treatment. There has been a decline in some forms of cancer, which can be expected to continue, but the rise in the incidence of lung cancer has been so marked that it is now responsible for essentially all the recent increment in cancer.

REFERENCES

1. Baillie, Simms, Willan, Sharpe, Home, Pearson, Abernethy, and Denman: Institution for investigating the nature of cancer. Edinburgh Med. Surg. J. *2:*382–389, 1806 (reprinted in Int. J. Cancer *2:*281–285, 1967).
2. C. J. Dawe: Comparative neoplasia. *In Cancer Medicine,* J. F. Holland and E. Frei, eds., Philadelphia: Lea & Febiger, 1973, pp. 193–240.
3. H. L. Stewart: Comparative aspects of certain cancers. *In Cancer: A Comprehensive Treatise,* Vol. 4, F. F. Becker, ed., New York: Plenum Press, 1975, pp. 303–374.
4. D. G. Scarpelli: Neoplasia in poikilotherms. *In Cancer: A Comprehensive Treatise,* Vol. 4, F. F. Becker, ed., New York: Plenum Press, 1975, pp. 375–410.
5. A. C. Braun: Plant tumors. *In Cancer: A Comprehensive Treatise,* Vol. 4, F. F. Becker, ed., New York: Plenum Press, 1975, pp. 411–427.
6. WHO international histological classification of tumors of domestic animals. Bull. World Health Org. *50:*1–142, 1974.
7. Cancer Statistics, 1979. CA-A Cancer Journal for Clinicians *29:*7–21, 1979.
8. H. Stünzi: Zur vergleichenden Pathologie des Lungenkarzinoms beim Haustier. Pathol. Microbiol. *39:*358–363, 1973.
9. H. L. Stewart: Pulmonary cancer and adenomatosis in captive wild mammals and birds from the Philadelphia Zoo. J. Natl. Cancer Inst. *36:*117–138, 1966.
10. L. S. Lombard and E. J. Witte: Frequency and types of tumors in mammals and birds of the Philadelphia Zoological Garden. Cancer Res. *19:*127–141, 1959.
11. C. H. Lingeman, R. E. Reed, and F. M. Garner: Spontaneous hematopoietic neoplasms of nonhuman primates. Review, case report and comparative studies. Natl. Cancer Inst. Monogr. *32:*157–170, 1969.
12. E. Jungherr: Tumors and tumor-like conditions in monkeys. Ann. N.Y. Acad. Sci. *108:*777–792, 1963.
13. C. J. Dawe, J. Whang-Peng, W. D. Morgan, R. W. O'Gara, and M. G. Kelly: Culture of a cell line (NCLP-6) derived from a hepatocarcinoma induced in *Macaca mulatta* by N-nitrosodiethylamine. J. Natl. Cancer Inst. *40:*1167–1193, 1968.
14. A. S. Rabson, G. T. O'Conor, D. E. Lorenz, R. L. Kirschstein, F. Y. Legallais, and T. S. Tralka: Lymphoid cell culture line derived from lymph node of marmoset infected with Herpesvirus saimiri—preliminary report. J. Natl. Cancer Inst. *46:*1099–1109, 1971.
15. G. H. Theilin, D. Gould, M. Fowler, and D. L. Dungworth: C-Type virus in tumor tissue of a woolly monkey (*Lagothrix* spp.) with fibrosarcoma. J. Natl. Cancer Inst. *47:*881–889, 1971.
16. R. Zalusky, J. J. Ghidoni, J. McKinley, T. P. Leffingwell, and G. S. Melville: Leukemia in the Rhesus monkey (*Macaca mulatta*) exposed to whole-body neutron irradiation. Radiat. Res. *25:*410–416, 1965.

17. G. E. Jay: Genetic strains and stocks. *In Methodology in Mammalian Genetics,* W. J. Burdette, ed., San Francisco: Holden-Day, 1963, pp. 83–123.
18. J. Staats: Standardized nomenclature for inbred strains of mice: Fourth listing. Cancer Res. *28:*391–420, 1968.
19. H. B. Andervont and T. B. Dunn: Occurrence of tumors in wild house mice. J. Natl. Cancer Inst. *28:*1153–1163, 1962.
20. H. T. Blunenthal and J. B. Rogers: Spontaneous and induced tumors in the guinea pig. *In The Pathology of Laboratory Animals,* W. E. Ribelin and J. R. McCoy, eds., Springfield, Ill.: Charles C. Thomas, 1965, pp. 183–209.
21. J. E. Moulton: *Tumors in Domestic Animals,* Berkeley: University of California Press, 1961.
22. T. C. Jones: Mammalian and avian models of disease in man. Fed. Proc. *28:*162–169, 1969.
23. R. M. Mulligan: *Neoplasms of the Dog,* Baltimore: Williams & Wilkins Co., 1949.
24. E. A. Cornelius: Animal models: A neglected medical resource. New Eng. J. Med. *281:*934–944, 1969.
25. H. G. Schlumberger: Neoplasia in the parakeet. I. Spontaneous chromophobe pituitary tumors. Cancer Res. *14:*237–245, 1954.
26. H. G. Schlumberger: Neoplasia in the parakeet. IV. A transplantable methylcholanthrene-induced rhabdomyosarcoma. Cancer Res. *19:*954–958, 1959.
27. J. H. Campbell: *Tumors of the Fowl,* London: W. Heinemann, 1969.
28. V. Ellerman and O. Bang: Experimentelle Leukaṁie bei Huhnern. Zentralbe. Bakteriol. Parasitenkd. Abt. *1:* Orig. *46:*595, 1908.
29. P. Rous: A transmissible avian neoplasm (sarcoma of the common fowl). J. Exp. Med. *12:*696–705, 1910.
30. R. M. Dutcher, ed.: *Comparative Leukemia Research 1971,* Basel: S. Karger, 1972.
31. C. F. Helmboldt and T. N. Fredrickson: The avian leukosis complex. Natl. Cancer Inst. Monogr. *32:*29–42, 1969.
32. J. Pontеń: Homologous transfer of Rous sarcoma by cells. J. Natl. Cancer Inst. *29:*1147–1159, 1962.
33. J. Pontеń: Transmission *in vitro* of chicken erythroblastosis by intact cells. J. Cell Comp. Physiol. *60:*209–215, 1962.
34. J. Pontеń: Transplantation of chicken tumor RPL_{12} in homologous hosts. J. Natl. Cancer Inst. *29:*1013–1021, 1962.
35. E. D. Thomas, J. I. Bryant, C. D. Buckner, R. A. Clift, A. Fefer, P. Neiman, R. E. Ramberg, and R. Storb: Leukemic transformation of engrafted human marrow. Transplantation Proc. *IV:*567–570, 1972.
36. R. L. Moodie: *Antiquity of Disease,* Chicago: University of Chicago Press, 1923.
37. H. G. Schlumberger and B. Lucké: Tumors of fishes, amphibians and reptiles. Cancer Res. *8:*657–753, 1948.
38. P. Zwart and J. C. Harshbarger: Hematopoietic neoplasms in lizards: Report of a typical case in *Hydrosaurus amboinensis* and of a probable case in *Varanus salvator.* Int. J. Cancer *9:*548–553, 1972.
39. R. F. Zeigel and H. F. Clark: Histologic and electron microscopic observations on a tumor-bearing viper: Establishment of a "C"-type producing cell line. J. Natl. Cancer Inst. *46:*309–321, 1971.
40. G. J. Svet-Moldavsky, L. Trubcheninova, and L. I. Ravkina: Pathogenicity of the chicken sarcoma virus (Schmidt-Ruppin) for amphibians and reptiles. Nature *214:*300–302, 1967.
41. M. Mizell, ed.: *Biology of Amphibian Tumors.* Basel: Springer-Verlag, 1969.
42. W. M. Smallwood: Adrenal tumors in the kidney of the frog. Anat. Anzeiger *26:*652–658, 1905.

43. B. Lucke: A neoplastic disease in the leopard frog, *Rana pipiens*. Am. J. Cancer *20:*352, 1934.
44. D. W. Fawcett: Electron microscopic observations on intracellular virus-like particles associated with the cells of the Lucke′ renal adenocarcinoma. J. Biophys. Biochem. Cytol. *2:*725–741, 1956.
45. L. E. Mawdesley-Thomas: Neoplasia in fish: a review. *In Current Topics in Comparative Pathology,* Vol. 1, T. C. Cheng ed. New York: Academic Press, 1971, pp. 87–170.
46. L. M. Ashley and J. E. Halver: Dimethylnitrosamine-induced hepatic cell carcinoma in rainbow trout. J. Natl. Cancer Inst. *41:*531–552, 1968.
47. L. M. Ashley: Renal neoplasms of rainbow trout. Bull. Wildlife Dis. Ass. *3:*86, 1967.
48. T. Anders: Tumour formation in platyfish-swordtail hybrids as a problem of gene regulation. Experientia *23:*1–10, 1967.
49. C. A. Farley: Probable neoplastic disease of the hematopoietic system in oysters, *Crassostrea virginica and crassostrea gigas*. Natl. Cancer Inst. Monogr. *31:*541–555, 1969.
50. C. A. Farley: Sarcomatoid proliferative disease in a wild population of blue mussels (*Mytilus edulis*). J. Natl. Cancer Inst. *43:*509–516, 1969.
51. S. Ghelelovitch: Melanotic tumors in *Drosophila melanogaster*. Natl. Cancer Inst. Monogr. *31:*263–275, 1969.
52. E. Gateff and H. A. Schneiderman: Neoplasms in mutant and cultured wild-type tissues of *Drosophila*. Natl. Cancer Inst. Monogr. *31:*365–397, 1969.
53. H. M. Lenhoff, C. Rutherford, and H. D. Heath: Anomalies of growth and form in hydra: polarity, gradients and a neoplasia analog. Natl. Cancer Inst. Monogr. *31:*709–735, 1969.
54. A. K. Sparks: Review of tumors and tumor-like conditions in protozoa, coelenterata, platyhelminthes, annelida, sipunculida, and arthropoda, excluding insects. Natl. Cancer Inst. Monogr. *31:*671–682, 1969.
55. E. F. Smith and C. O. Townsend: A plant-tumor of bacterial origin. Science *25:*671–673, 1907.
56. F. Meins, Jr.: Evidence for the presence of a readily transmissible oncogenic principle in crown gall teratoma cells of tobacco. Differentiation *1:*21–25, 1973.
57. H. H. Smith: Plant genetic tumors. Progr. Exp. Tumor Res. *15:*138–164, 1972.
58. N. Bloch-Shtacher, Z. Rabinowitz, and L. Sachs: Chromosomal mechanism for the induction of reversion in transformed cells. Int. J. Cancer *9:*632–640, 1972.
59. L. Pales: *Paleópathologie et Pathologie Comparative,* Paris: Masson, 1930, p. 263.
60. G. E. Smith and W. R. Dawson: *Egyptian Mummies,* London: Allen & Unwin, 1924, p. 157.
61. M. A. Ruffer and J. G. Willmore: A tumor of the pelvis dating from Roman times (A.D. 250) and found in Egypt. J. Pathol. Bact. *18:*480–484, 1914.
62. J. H. Breasted: *The Edwin Smith Surgical Papyrus,* University of Chicago Press, 1930, p. 405.
63. G. E. R. Lloyd: *Hippocratic Writings,* Harmondsworth, England: Pelican Classics, Penguin Books, 1978, Aphorisms, Section VI, no. 38.
64. L. J. Rather: *The Genesis of Cancer,* Baltimore: Hopkins University Press, 1978.
65. Galen: *Opera omnia* quoted in L. J. Rather op. cit. p. 13.
66. H. E. Sigerist: *A History of Medicine,* Vol. 1, New York: Oxford University Press, 1951, pp. 58–59.
67. R. Suss, V. Kinzel, and J. D. Scribner: *Cancer: Experiments and Concepts.* New York-Heidelberg-Berlin: Springer-Verlag, 1973, pp. 1–3.
68. J. Higginson and C. S. Muir: Epidemiology. *In Cancer Medicine.* J. F. Holland and E. Frei, III, eds., Philadelphia: Lea & Febiger, 1973, pp. 241–306.
69. J. Kubota, W. H. Allaway, D. L. Carter, E. E. Gary, and V. A. Lazar: Selenium in crops

in the United States in relation to selenium-responsive diseases of animals. J. Agr. Food Chem. *15:*448–453, 1967.

70. T. J. Mason, F. W. McKay, R. Hoover, W. J. Bolt, and J. F. Fraumeni: *Atlas of Cancer Mortality for U.S. Counties: 1950–1969*, Pub. (NIH) 75–780, Washington, D.C.: DHEW, 1976.
71. E. A. Lew: Cancer in old age. CA-A Cancer J. for Clinicians *28:*2–6, 1978.
72. L. Garfinkel, C. E. Poindexter, and E. Silverberg: Cancer in black Americans. CA-A Cancer J. for Clinicians *30:*39–44, 1980.
73. M. S. Zdeb: The probability of developing cancer. Am. J. Epidemiol. *106:*6–16, 1977.
74. H. Seidman, E. Silverberg, and A. Bodden: Probabilities of eventually developing and dying of cancer (risk among persons previously undiagnosed with the cancer). CA-A Cancer J. for Clinicians *28:*33–46, 1978.

3. The growth of tumors

In Chapter 1 it was stressed that malignant tumors grow in three ways—enlargement of the original or primary tumor mass, infiltration of tumor cells into neighboring normal tissues, and shedding of cells that then migrate to set up distant metastases; by and large, benign tumors only utilize the first mode of growth. Once established, metastases grow by all three modes, like the parent tumor, but very commonly their growth properties differ markedly from those of the primary tumor, which reflects both the different host environments in which the main tumor and the metastases may be found and the selection of a special subset of the cell population that undoubtedly occurs during metastatic spread.

GROWTH OF TUMOR MASSES

Measurement of tumor size

Growth of human and experimental animal tumors may be assessed both directly and indirectly. Among the direct methods used in experimental systems are excision and weighing of the tumor, vernier caliper measurements of tumor diameters, with or without use of a calibration curve such that linear dimensions can be converted to tumor weight, and finally, determination of the number of tumor cells, usually reserved for ascites tumors growing in the peritoneal cavity. Problems that are encountered include irregular tumor shapes that make estimation of volumes difficult, adherence to tissues such that accurate measurement of linear extension is not possible, and the double thickness of skin and subcutaneous fat. With ascites tumors, the cells in the peritoneal cavity, especially in older tumors, do not represent the total tumor burden, since cancer cells have infiltrated many tissues. In clinical practice, it is customary to take the product of two linear dimensions of a solid tumor, which represents the rectangular area enclosing the tumor, as the criterion of tumor size. This is convenient, since it permits both direct caliper measurements of accessible tumors, rather a rarity, and more importantly, may be used to determine the size of occult tumors only visible on x-ray film. In this latter case, allowance should be made for some degree of magnification of the image that may occur. The method of areas appeared to be free from systematic error when it was applied to rodent neoplasms, giving a two-thirds power relationship to tumor volume, provided there was no major change in the average shape of the tumor. Deviation from the two-thirds power curve occurred with small tumors (< 300 mg), and could be related to a skin thickness of 1.5 mm (1).

Indirect assessments of tumor growth may be based on survival of animals bearing ascitic tumors and on the amounts of special proteins or other tumor-specific products, such as antigens or low molecular weight metabolites. Mouse plasmacytomas and human myelomas and choriocarcinomas secrete specific proteins, whereas human neuroblastomas produce catecholamine metabolites in large quantities. There are varying degrees of correlation between tumor growth or size and the amounts of such tumor products in blood or urine. The incorporation of radioactive precursors has also been used in experimental systems; ^{125}I- or ^{131}I-labeled 5-iodo-2′-deoxyuridine is the tracer that has been used most often, because external monitoring is possible with such a gamma-emitter. Other methods that lend themselves to assessing tumor volumes, but which have not been used extensively for such quantitation, include lymphography, ultrasonic scanning, and xeroradiography and computerized image formation for improved x-ray resolution. Since most patients today receive early rigorous treatment, it is unlikely that much more data will be obtained on the natural growth of human tumors.

Growth curves

Derivation of growth curves may be based on tumor cell number, mass, or volume. In the simplest growth curves, growth rate is a constant fraction of tumor size, leading to a linear increase in the logarithm of tumor volume with time. This is expressed mathematically as

$$V = k \, dV/dt$$

On integration we have

$$V_t = V_o \exp(kt)$$

where V_t is the volume at time t, V_o is the initial volume, and k is the growth constant. In logarithmic form, this becomes

$$\ln V_t = \ln V_0 + kt$$

For doubling of the tumor volume, so $V_t = 2V_0$,

$$\ln V_0 + \ln 2 = \ln V_0 + kt$$
$$kt = 0.693$$

or

$$k = 0.693/T_d$$

where T_d is the *doubling time* of the tumor. This type of *exponential growth* will occur only when there is no nutritional limit to growth, when most of the cell population is capable of division, when there is minimal cell death, or when the proportion of proliferating cells (*growth fraction*) and the specific rate of cell death remain constant. Conditions of this sort may be realized in tissue culture systems and in such transplantable mouse neoplasms as the L1210 leukemia (2), in which exponential growth is approximated over eight logs (Figure 3-1). In humans, lung metastases also may exhibit exponential growth over two orders of magnitude (3).

Most tumors, however, will only follow such an exponential relationship over a limited range, if at all, and the curves describing the logarithm of their growth rates will be convex, reflecting a decrease in the *specific growth rate* (i.e., growth per unit volume) of the tumor with time (4). This decrease results from a declining growth fraction with or without an accompanying increase in the rate of loss of cells from the population through death. Although the specific growth rate falls continuously, tumor size is

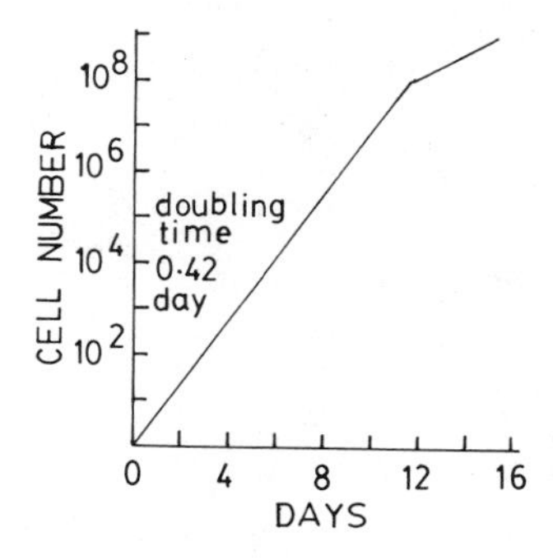

Figure 3-1 Exponential growth of L1210 mouse leukemia after intraperitoneal inoculation of a single clonogenic (i.e., viable, proliferative) cell. Median survival time is the function of the number of cells inoculated, falling from about 15 days after a single cell to about 4 days after 10^7 cells. Derived from Ref. 2.

expanding at a rate that is far greater than linear (Figure 3-2). As a result, the growth rate of the tumor as a whole accelerates to a maximum and then falls off. The total number of dividing cells, which relates directly to growth rate, will also peak at this time (Figure 3-2). A number of different mathematical equations have been proposed to describe this form of tumor growth. To date, it is generally agreed that a *Gompertzian function*, which has a decreasing rate of increase, provides the best fit. Such functions were originally developed for mortality data (5). For growth of tumors, the equation used is of the type

$$V_t = V_0[\exp(1 - e^{-\alpha t}\ A_0/\alpha]$$

where α is the rate constant for exponential decay of the initial specific growth rate A_0. At early times, the function can be reduced to

$$V = V_o \exp(A_o t)$$

and A_o is the growth constant for the limiting exponential and equals ln e or 0.693, divided by the minimum doubling time. At long time intervals $e^{-\alpha t}$ becomes negligible, and the volume V approaches a constant maximum size of $V_o \exp(A_o/\alpha)$. Doubling times increase according to the equation

$$T_d = \frac{\ln 2}{A_o} \exp\ (\alpha t) = \frac{0.693}{A_o} \exp\ (\alpha t)$$

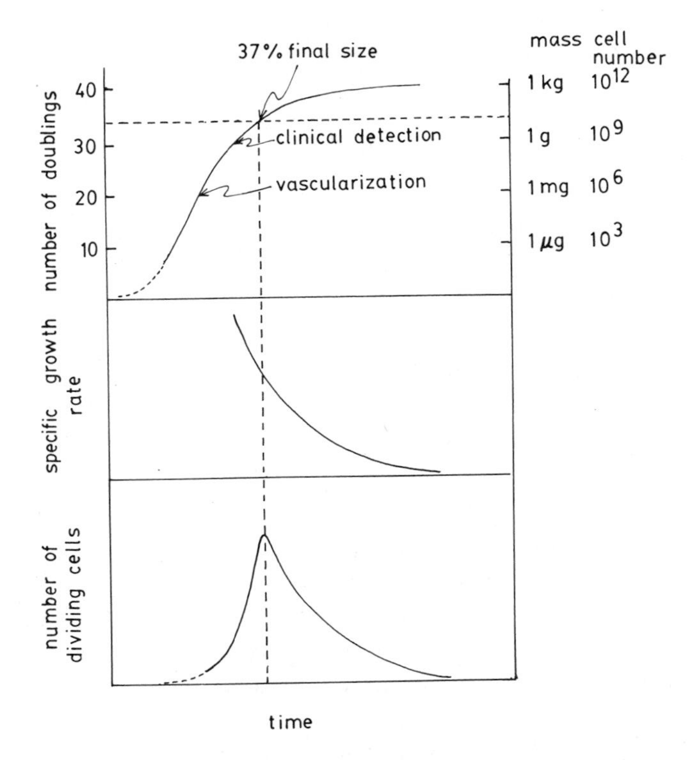

Figure 3-2 Growth of a solid tumor. *Upper curve,* a Gompertzian growth curve shows the points of vascularization, earliest clinical detection, and 37% of final size when rate of increase of tumor mass is maximal; *middle curve* shows continuous decline in the specific growth rate based on unit mass or cell number; *bottom curve,* an arbitrary plot of the number of dividing cells, as a function of both tumor mass and the growth fraction.

Although Gompertz curves are convex on a logarithmic scale, on a linear scale they are sigmoidal, with an inflection point at $1/e$ or 0.368, which corresponds to the point of maximum growth mentioned earlier, when the volume of the tumor will be 0.368 times the volume at the final plateau size. Gompertz curves are a better approximation of tumor growth than simpler functions (6), but they are not universally valid. During the early occult phase of tumor growth, the so-called "*silent interval,*" Gompertz curves yield implausibly short doubling times in many cases. Furthermore, it is questionable whether kinetic calculations derived from these curves are of much applicability in clinical situations (4,7). Theoretical plateau sizes for tumors may frequently be greater than the total body size, which is obviously not a meaningful extrapolation of the data. It is likely that with a massive tumor load, factors such as an inability to maintain an adequate supply of nutrients and oxygen or to remove waste products, together with mounting intratumoral pressure, may markedly increase the rate of cell death and/or suppress cell division and thus greatly reduce actual growth rates below those calculated.

Under some conditions, certain tumors, such as Jensen's rat sarcoma and Krebs ascites tumor of mice, exhibit what is known as *cube-root growth.* Here, a region of the growth curve may show a linear relationship for the increase in tumor diameter with time, that is, the cube root of the volume increases linearly with time. Generally, there is a changeover from exponential growth at low tumor loads. In ascites tumors, the cube root of the cell number is linearly related to time (8).

In this discussion, we have been considering growth of tumors as an orderly process; this is by no means always the case. Empirical clinical observations indicate that tumor growth may often be very irregular. Some metastases may be growing, whereas others may be regressing or remaining dormant. A reduction in the doubling time may defy the logic of Gompertzian functions, but it is entirely compatible with the concept of tumor progression to greater malignancy. Steel has described highly irregular growth curves for experimental tumor systems in rats (8), so the phenomenon is not limited to tumors in humans.

Although the growth rates of rodent tumors have been well studied, information about human tumors is rather fragmentary. This is due both to the difficulty in obtaining reliable measurements of the size of most tumors and to the fact that since nearly all cancer is treated with one or more therapeutic modalities, the innate tumor growth is seldom observed. Steel (4,8) has presented data on human and rodent neoplasms, some of which are reproduced in Figure 3-3 and Table 3-1. It is apparent that very few experimental tumors have growth properties resembling human cancers, and this is undoubtedly a major factor in the often poor therapeutic performance in the clinic of drugs that were very active against experimental tumors. Since, as we shall see later, human cancer cells do not take noticeably longer to divide than do other cells, it is evident that the slower growth rates of many human cancers result from such factors as a lower growth fraction, greater cell loss through necrosis or differentiation, and the operation of endocrine or immunological control mechanisms of the host. Among human tumors, the longer doubling times of carcinomas may stem from the generally greater cell loss in these tumors as compared with

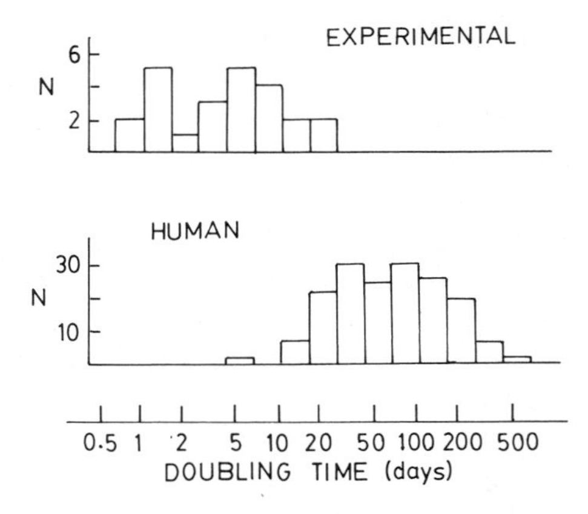

Figure 3-3 Distribution of doubling times for human versus experimental tumors. Reproduced from Ref. 4.

sarcomas. It is also apparent from Table 3-1 that metastatic nodules generally grow faster than primary tumors, a finding we shall return to later.

Tumors are not homogeneous, not only because of the presence of such stromal elements as connective and vascular tissue, but also because of the varied cytology and physiology of the tumor cells themselves. In cancer of the uterine cervix, for example, 41 to 53 percent of the cells in the two outer layers at the periphery are actively dividing, whereas 17 to 20 percent of the interior cells may be capable of division. Necrosis is also a prominent feature of the central region of most large tumor nodules; this situation frequently is the result of poor blood supply. Growth of the nodules involves both outward extension and also an inward migration of cells from the periphery into the interior (9).

Although in general malignant tumors are much less responsive to host growth control mechanisms than normal tissues, there is evidence that such control mechanisms are still operative to some degree. Clinical observation of the highly variable growth rates of essentially similar tumors in different patients, and of different metastases in the same patient, provides general evidence of this. Recently, however, studies with the C755 transplantable mammary carcinoma in mice have indicated that growth of this tumor is affected by antero-posterior and dorso-ventral gradients within the host (10). Growth of the tumors was three to four times more rapid when implantation was anteriorly, rather than posteriorly, with optimal growth in the thoracic region. In anterior and posterior, but not middle regions, there was also a ventro-doral gradient, with anterior middorsal tumor growth markedly greater than the mid-ventral and the reverse situation posteriorly. Since rates of DNA synthesis in damaged epidermis are greater anteriorly than posteriorly (11), tumor yield in response to methyl cholanthrene implants shows a similar anterior preference (12), and similar gradients operate during embryonic development and persist into the adult, it would thus appear that tumors are subject to a preexisting host control system the mechanism of which is unknown. Other control mechanisms that involve endocrine and immunological processes will be discussed later.

Table 3-1 Growth rates of human primary and metastatic tumors.

Tumors	*Number of tumors*	*Doubling time geometric mean (days)*	*95% Confidence limit*
Primary tumors			
Adenocarcinoma, breast	17	95.8	68–134
colon and rectum	19	632.0	426–938
lung	64	148.3	121–181
Sarcoma, bone	6	68.5	
Squamous cell carcinoma, lung	85	84.5	75–95
Undifferentiated, lung	55	79.1	67–93
Lung metastases			
Adenocarcinoma, breast	44	73.7	56–98
colon and rectum	56	94.9	84–107
kidney	14	60.2	37–98
thyroid	16	67.2	44–103
uterus	15	78.2	55–111
Lymphoma	11	26.8	19–39
Melanoma	8	53.5	
Sarcoma, Ewing's	9	17.6	
bone	34	30.2	24–38
fibrosarcoma	28	65.2	46–93
miscellaneous	30	42.9	32–58
Squamous cell carcinoma, bladder	8	70.7	
head and neck	27	56.8	43–75
lung	5	67.2	
Teratoma	80	30.3	25–36
Lymph node metastases			
Carcinoma	9	41.6	
Hodgkin's disease	10	48.6	31–76
Lymphosarcoma	5	19.8	
Reticulum cell sarcoma	12	17.7	12–25
Superficial soft-tissue metastases, breast carcinoma	66	19.4	16–24

Data taken from compilation of Steel (8), Table 1.2

Tumor angiogenesis

The early events in the tumor growth curve of Figure 3-2 that occur prior to detection of the tumor are somewhat obscure. It would appear that the Gompertzian function evolves from an early slow process that represents the initiation of a sigmoid curve. During this phase, limitations are imposed on the growth of the clump of neoplastic cells, and nutritional limitation is the most likely candidate for this role. At this stage, the tumor cells require no special vascular supply because all the cells in the clump have access to diffusing nutrients and oxygen (within 150 μm of a capillary). However, for growth in three dimensions, it should be remembered that whereas the volume, and thus the total number of cells, increases by the third power, surface area will increase by only the second power, and so will the supply of nutrients and elimination of catabolites, which depend directly on area available for diffusion. Thus a discrepancy between demand and supply of nutrients would lead to extensive necrosis in the interior of the tumor as it grows larger. This is seen in many avascular tumor nodules, in which growth appears to be self-limiting, such that they remain below 2 mm in diameter with a cell population of less than 10^6 cells. Although not usually observed clinically, such avascular tumor nodules are very common. Reported examples are the spherical retinoblastoma metastases less than 1 mm in diameter with necrotic centers found in the vitreous humor of the eye (13) and the nodules of carcinoma of the cervix-*in situ*, of which only 33 percent progress to Stage 1 carcinoma, the rest remaining stationary or regressing (14).

Abrupt change in growth characteristics follows the acquisition of a special vascular supply that enters the tumor. When a Brown-Pearce tumor is implanted in the anterior chamber of the guinea pig eye, near the iris vessels, the neoplasm will remain small for 5 or 6 days, at which time it becomes vascularized and increases in volume 16,000-fold over the next 2 weeks (15). As summarized by Folkman, who used chick embryo tumor implants (16), a stable diameter of 0.93 mm was achieved in the avascular state, but within 7 days of vascularization this had increased to 8 mm. The necrotic region of the avascular tumor disappeared 48 hours after vascularization, and capillaries permeated the tumor until it achieved a volume of 1 cm^3. Above this volume, necrosis reappeared as blood vessels were compressed and tissue pressure rose in the tumor. Other changes that accompany vascularization and the abrupt acceleration in growth include the release of tumor antigens into the blood (17), shedding of metastatic cells, and "malignant drift," a progression of the tumor toward a more malignant pattern of behavior (18).

The process by which the tumor stimulates the proliferation of blood vessels is intriguing. Among the early changes that have been observed is a stimulation of thymidine incorporation into the DNA of capillary endothelial cells, determined by autoradiographic studies in which the *labeling index* (i.e., the percentage of nuclei with grain counts from tritiated thymidine) increased from 0.7 to 8 percent (19,20). Bud-like processes develop and may become linked, to form loops through which blood circulates. The sprouting buds often grow in parallel toward the tumor by a process that involves both mitosis of the endothelial cells and their actual migration (21). As measured in normal tissues during wound healing, when angiogenesis occurs, the growth of vessel sprouts averages 0.12 mm/day, and the migration speed of endothelial cells 0.1 mm/day (22), whereas as vessels approach tumors, in such experimental conditions as a corneal tumor implant, mean growth rates as high as 0.61 mm/day have been recorded (23). In contrast to wound healing and inflammatory processes, in which angiogenesis is brief and self-limiting, in tumors a continuous strong stimulus, which is unaffected by such anti-inflammatory agents as hydrocortisone, is produced. Thus, the tumor rapidly elicits an adequate blood supply, but unlike the situation in wounds or in embryonic development, the efficiency of the vascular system deteriorates as the tumor grows. This is the result of an interstitial fluid transfer that may produce a fluid pressure of 8 to 30 cm of water (24), in marked contrast to a pressure of almost zero for neighboring normal tissue; the former leads to compression of blood vessels and necrosis within the tumor (25).

Since stimulation of endothelial cell mitoses and development of new vessels occurred even when the tumor was separated from the vascular bed by a Millipore filter (26), and could take place at distances up to 5 mm from the tumor (27), it is evident that a diffusible humoral factor is responsible. This factor, *tumor angiogenesis factor* (TAF), occurs in both the nucleus and cytoplasm of many human and animal tumors (Table 3-2), as determined by its ability to stimulate development of new vessels when implanted in chick chorioallantoic membranes or rabbit corneas (16). Although not uniquely formed by tumor cells, since the W1-38 cells, which are supposedly normal, secrete it (16), as do spleen and lymph node lymphocytes, macrophages, and thymoctyes (28), TAF is certainly more characteristic of tumors than of other tissues (Table 3-2). Although some progress has been made, TAF has not yet been purified and characterized (29).

Table 3-2 Cells and tissues tested for angiogenesis factor.

Response	*Species*	*Cell type*
Positive	Human	WI-38 embryonic lung
		SVWI-26 (SV40 virus transformed)
		Glioblastoma
		Meningioma
		HeLa (only in suspension culture)
	Mouse	BALB/c 3T3 embryo
		BALBC/c SVT-2 (SV40 virus transformed)
		B16 melanoma
	Rat	Walker 256 carcinoma
Negative	Human	Skin fibroblast
	Mouse	BALBC/c primary embryo
		Placenta
		Liver
		Skeletal muscle
		Myocardium

Tissues and cells were tested by bioassay on chick embryo chorioallantoic membrane. Data from Ref. 16.

It appears in a non-histone nuclear fraction from Walker rat carcinoma 256 cells (30), but is more easily studied in the medium from cell cultures of tumor cells (31). An interesting finding, with potential for future therapeutic approaches, is that angiogenesis is inhibited in the presence of cartilage (23). The active component of the cartilage is in a fraction that is extractable with guanidine hydrochloride, and, by gel electrophoresis, appears to have a molecular weight between 14,400 and 17,800 (32); the same fraction also strongly inhibits proteases. When the nature of this cartilage-TAF interaction, and the nature and function of TAF itself, is better understood, a new therapeutic tool might become available for dealing with metastatic disease.

Cell kinetics

Features of cellular proliferation in normal and tumor cells. The establishment of a tumor blood supply is essential if tumors are to remain viable and attain a clinically evident size. It is now necessary to turn to the kinetics of cellular proliferation to identify features that are characteristic of neoplastic growth. Figure 3-4 outlines the cellular compartments in both normal tissues and tumors. Normal tissues of the renewable type, such as bone marrow, in which cell division is occurring all the time, will have a proliferating compartment and a compartment of similar capability that is not actively proliferating—that is, in the so-called G_0 state. These two compartments include a fraction known as *stem cells,* which are capable of producing a large family of descendants *in situ.* They may be identical with the *clonogenic* cells, which are capable of forming clones *in vitro.* Stem cells, the least differentiated cells in the tissue, are often few in number and may have a relatively slow turnover. Most cell division in the renewable tissues occurs among cells that have been committed to differentiation and a relatively limited number of their descendants. Apart from the bone marrow, this is also true of other tissues, such as the intestinal mucosa. Actively proliferating cells continually pass into a compartment in which differentiation is the major activity. Here the ability to divide is lost as the cells mature. Finally, mature cells are lost from the population through death and migration. In the bone marrow, migration into the peripheral circulation is the predominant fate of the mature cells. This pattern is modified in various normal tissue. In the liver, where cell division is normally minimal, an injury or surgical intervention, such as partial hepatectomy, will recruit cells capable of dividing into the proliferating fraction to replace

Figure 3-4 Cell compartments in normal and tumor populations.

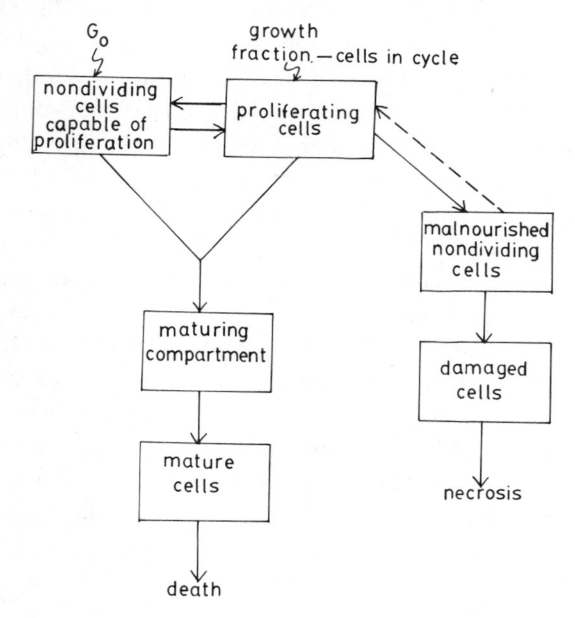

lost cells. Some limited degree of dedifferentiation evidently precedes the initiation of cell division, the biochemical events that occur during this interval have been well studied. Some normal tissue cell populations, the neurons, for example, are committed to differentiation at such an early time in the development of the individual that cell proliferation does not occur through most of the animal's lifetime.

Tumor cells also may follow the same route as normal cells. There may be specific stem cells or a clonogenic fraction that might include several distinct elements, and these cells may differentiate, although the degree of maturation reached is highly variable. In addition, for reasons referred to earlier, an often large fraction of the cells will suffer damage due to deprivation of oxygen and nutrients and to the release of cytotoxic breakdown products by other dead or dying cells (33), and will then die. The rate of cell death within the tumor has a major effect on its response to such treatment as radiation and chemotherapy, during which suppression of mitosis in a population with rapid cell loss will lead to early marked regression of the tumor mass. In a situation of limited cell loss, however, the response of the tumor will be delayed (34). The magnitude of the cell loss factor is seen when actual growth is compared with *potential doubling times* (T_{pot}), derived by isotopic studies of cell division; three- to tenfold discrepancies are not uncommon (8).

All proliferating cells traverse the cell cycle (Figure 3–5). Mitosis, with its subdivisions of prophase, metaphase, anaphase, and telophase, was the first process to have been identified in cell division; it is called *M* phase. All other stages in the recurring cell cycle comprise the intermitotic time (T_i). This is broken down into three periods, the middle period or *S* phase, when DNA is synthesized, and two gap periods that precede (G_1) and follow (G_2) the *S* phase. During the *S* phase, the DNA content of the cells rises until there is twice the normal complement as the cells enter G_2; the original level is restored as a result of mitosis. Data regarding the duration of the cell cycle and its component phases have revealed that tumors and normal tissues differ surprisingly little in their kinetics (35). The means of total cell cycle durations (T_c) may vary from a little over 10 to around 100 hours, with a clustering below 30 hours, but there is no discernible difference between normal tissues and tumors as a class. Furthermore, when we consider the individual phases, there are definite correlations between T_c and the duration of each phase. For G_1 this correlation is expressed as a monotonic curving line (Figure 3–6), whereas for *S* (Figure 3–7), it is a straight line described by the equation $T_s = 4.0 + 0.3\ T_c$ hours. In both

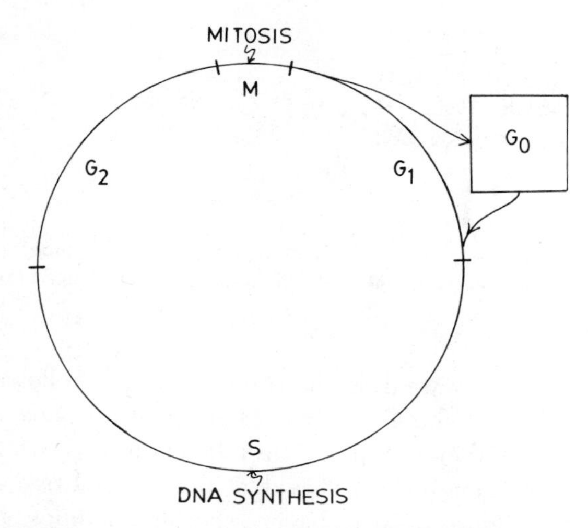

Figure 3-5 The cell cycle: G_0 may or may not differ qualitatively from G_1, depending on the tissue in question; G_1 and G_2, first and second gap phases; *M* mitosis; *S*, phase of scheduled DNA synthesis; G_0, cells capable of proliferating, but not engaged in active division.

Figure 3-6 Mean duration of G_1 phase as a function of total cell-cycle time T_C. Ascites tumors (▲); solid tumors (●); normal tissues (■); cells in culture (▼). Reproduced from Ref. 35.

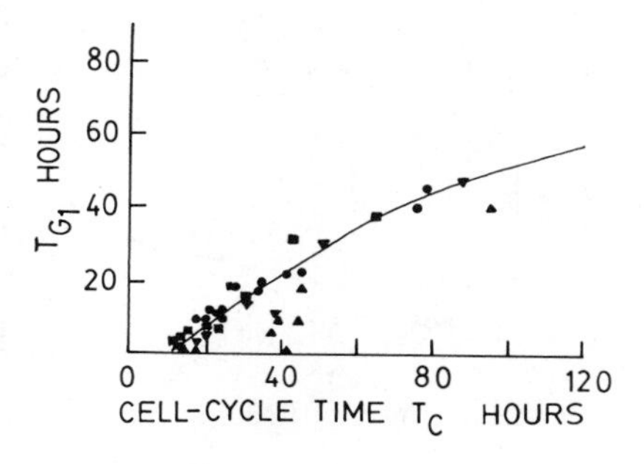

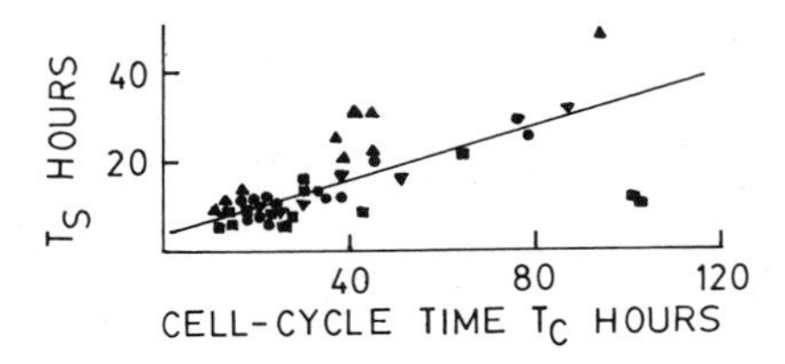

Figure 3-7 Mean duration of S phase as a function of total cell-cycle time T_C. Ascites tumors (▲); solid tumors (●); normal tissues (■); cells in culture (▼). Reproduced from Ref. 35.

cases, ascites tumors deviate from the common pattern followed by normal tissues, solid tumors, and cells in tissue culture, by having relatively abbreviated G_1 and lengthened S phases as a function of T_c. Only in the case of the transit time through G_2 is it evident that normal tissues differ from the other groups (Figure 3–8) in having shorter G_2 times, mostly in the range of 1 to 2 hours. In the mouse this is true, for example, of intestinal epithelium, thymus, spleen, and skin. Ascites tumors and cells in tissue culture show great variation in the lengths of their G_2 phases. Despite this, there appears to be a linear increase in T_{G2}, with increase in T_c. Mitosis itself is a brief event, seldom taking more than 1 hour, except when there are mitotic abnormalities. Tables 3–3 and 3–4 present cytokinetic data for experimental animal and human tumors, respectively. Two points may be noted. First, cell cycle times, as reflected in the values for T_i, are generally longer in human tumors than in experimental systems; this is true of the component phases also. Although this probably only reflects a generally slower cytokinetic system in humans as compared with smaller mammals, it has implications for efforts to develop complex multi-drug and multimodal treatment regimens where the timing of dosages is frequently based on

Figure 3-8 Mean duration of G_2 phase as a function of total cell-cycle time T_C. Ascites tumors (▲); solid tumors (●); cells in culture (▼). Reproduced from Ref. 35.

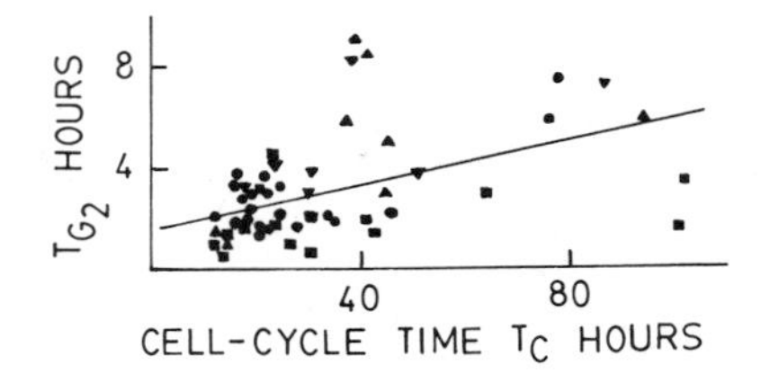

Table 3-3 Cytokinetic data for experimental tumors.

Tumor type	*Host*	T_d	*Medium times (hours)* T_i	G_2	S	G_1	*Growth fraction (percent)*
Primary (autochthonous)							
C3H mammary carcinoma	Mouse	204	25.0	2.5	10.0	14.0	45
Spontaneous AKR lymphoma	Mouse		16.0	1.2	7.6	5.8	
DMBA-induced mammary carcinoma	Rat	340	47.0	1.0	10.0	36.0	35
Polyoma-induced kidney carcinoma	Rat	47	21.0	2.5	7.8	10.8	39
Cheek-pouch tumor	Hamster	295	14.0	1.9	7.8	5.0	69
Anaplastic mammary carcinoma	Dog		50.0	5.2	5.0	48.0	
Early transplants							
C3H carcinoma	Mouse	108	16.0	1.5	6.5	7.8	46
NTI sarcoma	Mouse	118	33.0	3.5	18.1	5.2	24
BICR/A_4 adenocarcinoma	Rat	120	18.0	1.5	10.8	6.0	26
BICR/A_2 fibrosarcoma	Rat	190	53.0	3.5	8.6	39.0	32
Frequently passaged tumors							
Adenocarcinoma 755	Mouse	38	15.0	2.7	5.8	6.8	47
Sarcoma 180	Mouse	33	13.0	2.6	8.6	1.9	63
B16 melanoma	Mouse	72	16.5	1.3	8.3	5.3	85
Lewis lung carcinoma 0.34g	Mouse	53	17.6	1.6	9.6	5.0	92
Lewis lung carcinoma 4.2 g	Mouse	158	26.0	2.5	12.4	7.9	56
L5187 Y lymphoma	Mouse	18	10.0	1.1	6.5	2.7	90
NCTC 2472 fibrosarcoma 0.08g	Mouse	38	17.0	1.7	10.4	4.9	43
NCTC 2472 fibrosarcoma 2g	Mouse	110	15.0	2.0	10.8	2.1	31
BICR/A_3 osteosarcoma	Rat	60	16.0	2.4	8.7	5.2	56
3924 hepatoma	Rat	132	24.0	2.4	7.9	12.7	66
Melanoma	Hamster	74	16.0	1.1	4.8	9.6	42

Reproduced in part from Steel (8), Table 5.1.

cytokinetics (36). Second, in the experimental systems, of which two examples are given (Lewis lung and NCTC 2472), increase in tumor size is accompanied by a very marked increase in the doubling time T_d. Since there is either no change, or a much less pronounced change in the cell cycle parameters, it is evident that the increase in T_d reflects a falling growth fraction and increased cell loss. In human leukemias, the data collated in Table 3–5 give some idea of the cytokinetic features of these cells. There is little comparative data for normal human bone marrow because labeling with radioactive precursors is needed, but Strykmans (37) derived a T_{G2} of about 2 hours and a T_S of 13 to 14 hours from studies with five patients. Thus, T_S appears to be somewhat longer for leukemic myeloblasts than for normal myeloblasts, whereas T_{G2} is about the same in both normal and leukemic marrow and shorter than for most solid tumors.

Table 3-4 Cytokinetic data for human tumors.

Tumor type	Median times (hours) T_i	G_2	S	G_1	Growth fraction (percent)
Epidermal epithelioma	34	5.0	12	14	41
Spindle-cell epithelioma		7.5	10	(38)	82
Basal cell carcinoma		(10.0)	(18)		
Squamous cell carcinoma	52	7.0	18	22	36
Carcinoma of cervix		2.0	(12)		
Melanoma	70	5.0	21	37	20–30
Melanoma	56	8.0	19	20	59
Melanoma	(47)	7.0	14	(19)	70
Carcinoma of breast	(51)	6.0	20	(19)	61
Carcinoma of breast		5.0	14		
Neuroblastoma		3.0	24		
Malignant schwannoma	(39)	5.0	16	(18)	52
Reticulum cell sarcoma	53	5.0	14	32	14
Small cell carcinoma of bronchus		6.0	18		
Villous papilloma of colon		9.0	(12)		
Acites tumors					
Carcinoma of stomach		3.0	19	17	58
Endometrial carcinoma	113	7.0	48	50	25
Lymphosarcoma		(2.5)	(15)		
Ovarian carcinoma		9.0	30		

Reproduced in part from Steel (8), Table 6.3. Data in parenthesis are somewhat doubtful.

Table 3-5 Cytokinetic data for human leukemias.

Type	Median times (hours) T_i	G_2	S	G_1	Growth fraction (percent)
Acute myelocytic	63.9	2.7	18.5	36.9	24
Acute myelocytic and lymphoblastic	67.3	4.1	27.9	32.0	18
Acute lymphoblastic	60.7	4.7	32.7	19.5	25
Acute lymphoblastic	82.0*	2.6	16.8	63.0*	18
Acute myelomonocytic	37.1	2.3	10.9	21.4	61
Plasma cell	57.0	2.1	15.8	37.0	47

Reproduced in part from Steel (8), Tables 6.4 and 6.5.
*These values are mean, not median durations.

Experimental techniques for cytokinetic studies. A number of different techniques have been used to obtain the type of data we have been considering. They include determination of mitotic indices; the use of stathmokinetic agents, drugs that arrest cells in mitosis; continuous or pulse labeling with ^{14}C and/or ^{3}H-labeled thymidine; incorporation of thymidine analogs; cell synchronization; and flow microfluorimetry.

The earliest approach is the determination of the *mitotic index* by microscopic examination of stained preparations. By combining this with the *stathmokinetic technique* of metaphase arrest, in which drugs like colchicine or vinblastine are used, it is possible to calculate the rate of cellular proliferation from the rate at which mitotic figures accumulate (38). If $I_M(0)$ *is the initial mitotic index and* $I_M(t)$ the index at time t after mitotic blocking with a drug, then

$$I_M(t) = I_M(0)\ [1 + t/T_M]$$

where T_M is the duration of mitosis, and thus

$$T_M = I_M(0) \cdot t/[I_M(t) - I_M(0)]$$

During exponential growth, we have

$$T_M = I_M(0) \cdot t/\ln 2\ [I_M(t) - I_M(0)]$$

and if K_p is the rate of cellular proliferation,

$$K_p = I_M/T_M$$

for any tissue. Problems that are encountered with this technique have to do with geometrical artifacts involving the angle at which sections are cut and the tendency to miss small nuclei. Furthermore, the metaphase-arresting agents may be less specific than is generally supposed, and their side effects on the cell may distort its kinetics of division. Although T_M is usually brief, mitotic abnormalities may lengthen the period spent in mitosis (39). Examples of this are the greatly extended prophase (250 minutes) and telophase (110 minutes) in Ehrlich ascites carcinoma and HeLa cells, respectively (8).

Continuous labeling with radioactive thymidine provides information about the growth fraction. Although one might expect a leveling off in the

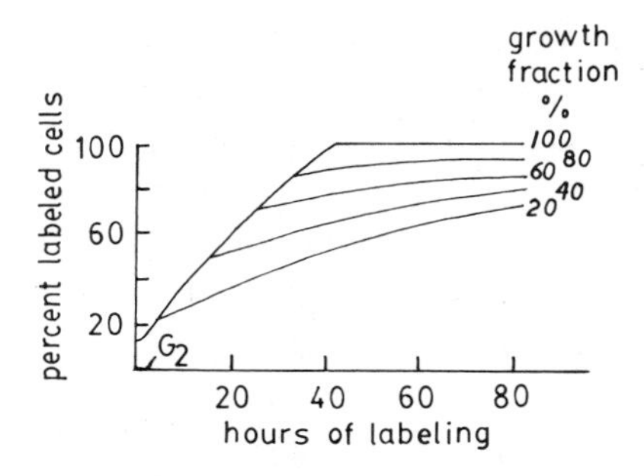

Figure 3-9 Theoretical continuous thymidine-labeled curves for a population in exponential growth without cell loss. Calculation based on 50 hours doubling time, an *S* phase of 8 hours, and a G_2 phase of 2 hours. Reproduced from Ref. 8.

labeling index (LI), the fraction of cells labeled at the appropriate growth fraction, the curves show a discontinuity at this point, with a slow secondary asymtotic approach to 100 percent labeling (Figure 3–9). The labeling index also provides a measure of the potential cell doubling time of the tumor. This is the expected time for doubling of tumor size to occur, based on rates of cell division alone, and it is given by the function

$$T_{pot} = \ln 2/K_p = \ln 2 \cdot t_s/LI$$

It is also related to the cell loss factor ϕ, by the equation

$$\phi = 1 - T_{pot}/T_d$$

where ϕ lies between 0 and 1. As with all techniques that utilize radiolabeled thymidine, autoradiography is the method of choice for determining the extent of incorporation. The fixed, labeled cell preparations are covered with photographic emulsion, set aside in the dark for up to 2 weeks, and then developed. The number of silver grains over the nuclei are then counted during microscopic examination. Since the beta particles from tritium are of lower energy than those from carbon-14, the latter will penetrate further through the emulsion, which must be thicker, before releasing their energy. This permits a measure of discrimination between the isotopes in double-labeling experiments.

Pulse-labeling techniques with thymidine are usually used with the *labeled mitoses* procedure; this is illustrated in Figure 3–10. The intention is to label only those cells in S phase during a relatively short time interval and to follow the kinetics of this synchronized subset of the population. As they progress from S through G_2 and into M phase, labeled mitotic figures appear, reach a peak, and then decline. A second peak should follow, at a time equivalent to T_i after the first peak. The median duration of T_S is usually considered to be equivalent to the width of the labeled mitosis peak at half-height, but as with many of these practices, this decision is essentially empirical. In actual practice, the shapes of the labeled mitoses curves deviate significantly from the theoretical forms (Figure 3–10), and in general, no more than three or perhaps four distinct peaks occur under the best conditions (40). This is the result of the natural broad variation in the duration of the cell cycle phases, which ensures that even completely synchornized cell populations will soon become asynchronous. Double-labeling with tritiated thymidine followed by carbon-14-labeled thymidine, or vice versa, has been used to assess the length of T_S and the G_2 phase, as well as to follow labeled cells through additional cycles (8). In most cases, simple empirical examination and allotment of durations to particular phases on the basis of labeled mitoses curves is not feasible, and recourse to computer simulation based on particular models is necessary, if reliable figures are to be obtained. Steel has discussed this topic (8) and lists references for the major model systems. Among the more extensive treatments are those of Valleron and Frindel (41), Macdonald (42), and Shackney (43). The use of such agents as colcemid, which arrest cells in metaphase, and of such procedures as thermal shock, to induce a degree of synchronization, may simplify the interpretation of labeled mitoses curves, but they may also distort cell kinetics through other actions of the drug, in

Figure 3-10 Thymidine-labeled mitoses curves. A, ideal, B, experimental, for the tail bud of mouse embryo on 12th to 13th day of gestation. Reproduced from Ref. 39A.

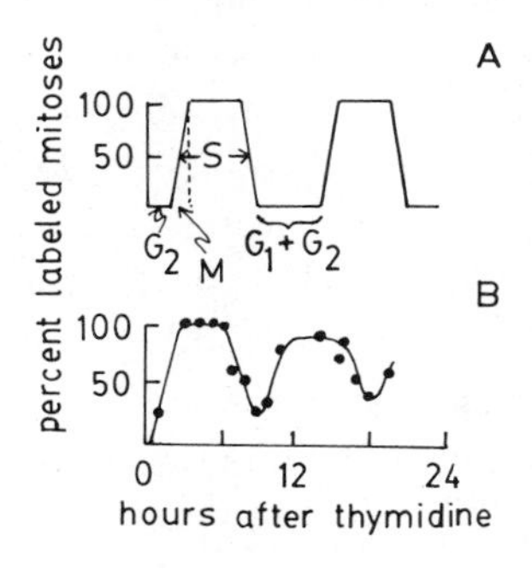

the first instance. There is already concern that beta emissions from incorporated thymidine may cause some intracellular radiation damage.

Labeling with the thymidine analog 5-iodo-2′-deoxyuridine-^{125}I (^{125}IUDR) has been used because reutilization of the isotope and intracellular pool effects are not a problem. The chief virtues of this gamma-ray emitter are that it permits external counting and that it may be used *in vivo*. Study of the cell loss factor is possible with this labeled analog (44).

Finally, flow microfluorimetry has been introduced within recent years to evaluate the cell-cycle distribution of cell populations. Essentially a refinement of earlier methodology that used Feulgen stain of DNA combined with fluorochrome to assess fluorimetrically the amount of DNA, the flow procedure permits the use of smaller numbers of cells. Stained cells are passed through an orifice of the type used in a Coulter counter, excited with a laser beam, and the emission is detected with a photomultiplier. Graphs of the type shown in Figure 3–11 are obtained. The principles and application of this method have been reviewed (45). As with the labeled mitoses technique, mathematical analysis of the data is needed, especially with regard to cells having DNA contents intermediate between those of G_1 and G_2 cells.

Metabolic events occurring during the cell cycle. We have seen that DNA synthesis is a process that takes place specifically during the S phase of the cell cycle. At other times, the only form of DNA synthesis that occurs is the non-scheduled synthesis that represents repair of damaged material (46). Synthesis of RNA, proteins, and lipids occurs continuously throughout the cycle, but at variable rates; late mitosis and early G_1 constitute a period of typically lowered synthetic activity (47). Despite the continuous occurrence of macromolecular synthesis, there are discontinuities in the appearance of specific molecular species. A number of enzymes related to the synthesis of nucleic acids have been assayed and their activities shown to be cell-cycle specific (47). Typical data are shown in Figure 3–12, and it can be seen that the sequence is such as to provide precursors for DNA synthesis as required. Another substance with cell-cycle dependence for its synthesis is tubulin, the microtubule subunit protein and a component of the mitotic spindle, which reaches maximum levels during the late S and the G_2 period (48). Intracellular levels of cyclic nucleotides are known to vary during the cell cycle, with concentrations of cyclic AMP higher, and those of cyclic GMP lower, in non-dividing cells (49). It is a plausible concept that transition between the G_0 and actively proliferating states may be mediated by these changes (50).

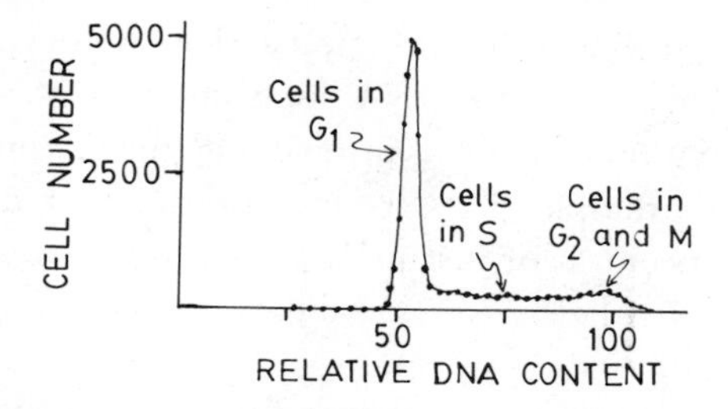

Figure 3-11 Flow microfluorometric analysis curve for the DNA contents of CHO cells growing exponentially in tissue culture; DNA stained with acriflavine Feulgen stain. Reproduced from Ref. 35.

Control of the cell cycle. The mechanisms involved in control of the cell cycle are still obscure. Generally the cycle is, in part, maintained by the necessary sequence of specialized metabolic capabilities discussed above. Thus, DNA synthesis cannot occur until the enzymes that generate the needed precursors are in place, and the mitotic spindle will not form until more tubulin has been formed. However, other control systems are evident within unicellular and multicellular eukaryotes. One of these is the system of internal or primary cilia (51), generally associated with the centrioles, which serve as microtubule organizing centers. These cilia have a 9 + 0 (i.e., no central pair) arrangement of their doublet microtubules instead of the familiar 9 + 2 pattern of motile external cilia. As long ago as 1898, it was suggested that the conversion of the centrioles into ciliated basal bodies was involved in the regulation of mitosis (52), and the sugges-

Figure 3-12 Variation in relative activity of enzymes involved in pyrimidine synthesis during the cell cycle. Ribonucleotide reductase (○——○); thymidine kinase (△– –△); deoxycytidylic deaminase (●– –●); deoxycytidylic kinase (×—×); and thymidylate synthethase (+——+). Reproduced from Ref. 47.

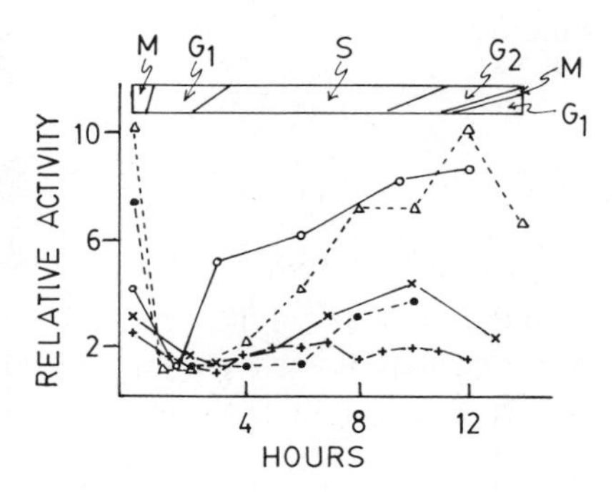

tion has been revived (53). It would appear that the cycle of centriole ciliation and deciliation is tied to DNA replication, a period of deciliation coinciding with initiation of DNA synthesis and reciliation with early G_1 of 3T3 fibroblasts, for example (54). It also appears that duplication of the centriole itself may occur at or just prior to the initiation of DNA synthesis (55). We do not know whether disturbances in centriole function could be involved in carcinogenesis.

A role for cyclic changes in membrane function has also been proposed as a mitotic control mechanism. Changes in the biological properties of cancer cell membranes have been observed, the most notable being the loss of contact inhibition, but in addition, there are changes in the biochemical composition of cultured cell membranes subjected to malignant transformation (56). These changes could undermine a cyclical interaction between structural and functional alterations in the membrane and cell division of the type proposed for normal cells by Burger (57). In a sense, a malignant cell would have the membrane signal for cell division turned on at all times. Another interesting approach to a control mechanism involving the cell membrane is that of Cone (58), which stresses the role of the transmembrane electrical potential difference E_m. This is around -50 to -60 mV in mature interphase (G_1) cells, for example, those of the liver or connective tissue, but declines to about -10 mV when the cells are detached and adapted to proliferation in culture. A similar, or even greater decline occurs on neoplastic transformation; the E_m for a muscle cell falls from -90 mV to -10 mV in myosarcoma cells (59). As monolayer cell cultures approach confluence, that is, with all the cells in contact, the E_m rises from -15 to -55 mV, and cell division ceases, that is, *mitotic contact inhibition* develops. Conversely, high concentrations of sodium ion stimulate mitosis, activate DNA synthesis, and lower the value of E_m; trypsin, which can also stimulate proliferation, has a similar effect on E_m (58).

This latter finding tends to bring together the electrical and biochemical theories of the role of membranes in neoplastic transformation and the control of cell division.

TUMOR INVASION

The second mechanism of tumor growth is invasion, the infiltration of cancer cells into the immediately surrounding normal tissues, which are ultimately destroyed. Infiltration may involve single cells, cell clumps, or large multicellular "tongues." In general, it is clearly limited by the nature of the normal tissue architecture. The thin-walled lymphatics are particularly easily infiltrated, and this is why metastatic disease so often spreads via the lymph. Veins, especially those with thin walls, may also be invaded readily, whereas arteries and arterioles with their thicker walls are rarely subject to infiltration, perhaps because of the barrier created by elastic tissue. Cartilage, elastic, myelinated, and fibrous tissues are relatively resistant to invasion, and in areas where they exist, a tumor will preferentially spread along the fascia planes (i.e., between fibrous bundles) or nerve sheaths. Invasion is a necessary prerequisite for dispersal of tumor cells in the process of metastasis, for it is in this way that the cells gain access to the blood and lymph. It appears that three processes are at work in invasion: release of enzymatic or lytic factors; development of pressure through cellular proliferation; and cellular movement (60). Loss of contact inhibition may play a role in these processes.

Release of enzymatic or lytic factors

Many malignant tumors have been shown to be the source of lytic factors and enzymes, such as proteases, lysosomal hydrolases, collagenolytic activity, and cathepsin B (61–63). These products tend to decrease the efficacy of such normal barriers as fibrous or collagen layers, allowing tumor cells to penetrate what are normally effective barriers to invasion.

Development of pressure

This was invoked earlier as an element in the formation of the inner necrotic cores of tumors. The pressure exerted by the growing mass of tumor cells also may cause pressure atrophy of surrounding normal tissues, as well as act as a sustaining force to produce outward movement of tumor cells.

Cellular movement. Although it was once thought that tumor cells are more motile than normal cells (64), it now appears that most cells are similarly motile *in vitro*. What may differ is that clusters of neoplastic cells lack contact inhibition (65) and will continue to move over each other and to proliferate when normal cells would become quiescent. In addition, the modified membranes of malignant cells also seem to lead to a reduced cohesiveness, so that individual cells or clumps of cells readily separate from the main mass. Most studies of cellular movement have been carried out *in vitro*, but there is little doubt that similar motility is a feature of the cells *in vivo*, having been demonstrated for individual V_2 cancer cells in rabbit tissues, for example (60). Such movement is essentially random and lacks both chemotaxis and contact inhibition (66); but rather like the similar movements of diffusing molecules, it will, in statistical terms, result in a net outward migration from the primary tumor, the region of greatest cellular concentration.

METASTASIS

The production of secondary tumors at sites in the body that are distant from the primary tumor is the basic characteristic defining malignancy. It is these metastases that seem to be the most critical factor in the survival of patients with cancer. We have seen that invasion represents the initial phase of metastasis. In a few cases, such as tumors growing in body cavities, cells may be shed from the primary tumor and lodge at some other point where proliferation is possible, whereas in others, cells may spread by migration along nerve sheaths, for example (67). The bulk of metastatic disease, however, originates by invasion of capillaries, veins, or lymphatics; cells are then carried passively around the body in the blood or lymph until they enter a suitable environment for growth. There seems to be no real evidence for the traditional view that carcinomas spread via the lymphatics and mesenchymal tumors via the blood. Most of the circulating cells in both blood and lymph never give rise to metastases, in part because more than one cell is needed to initiate a metastasis and also because particular cell types are selected from the total population, a subject that will be discussed later.

Vascular and lympatic spread

Some elegant experiments with V2 carcinoma growing in the ear chamber of rabbits have shown that a minimum of three and usually six to ten cells are needed to initiate a metastasis. Another prerequisite is a certain "stickiness," since the cells must adhere firmly to the walls of small venules. Many cells remain dormant or die at this stage, but others initiate a blood clot with fibrin deposition followed by leukocyte infiltration, which tends to disturb the endothelial wall, and allows cancer cells to leave the blood and to enter perivascular connective tissue and neighboring lymphatics (60). A variety of agents may affect the frequency of blood-borne metastases

(Table 3-6). In general, agents that increase leukocyte adhesion or blood coagulability enhance the development of metastases, whereas those that reduce these parameters, or kill cells directly, diminish metastasis. Cytotoxic drugs and radiation, which may damage both normal and cancerous tissues and alter the permeability of small blood vessels, can either enhance or inhibit metastasis, depending on the agent, the dose, and the tumor or tissue in question. Such factors as the size and rate of growth of tumors obviously influence metastatic spread by varying the size of the pool of cells available for invasion and spread. Endogenous host defense mechanisms may even act to the detriment of the host by increasing metastic spread. Thus, lymphocytes and macrophages in the neighborhood of the nascent metastasis release angiogenesis factors that help establish a blood supply for the tumor, whereas platelets secrete a cell growth-stimulating factor. This helps explain the role of blood clotting and leukocyte infiltration in the early stages. The role of the immune response in limiting tumor growth will be discussed in Chapter 5.

Tumor cells may enter the lymphatics either by direct infiltration of the thin-walled vessels or from the blood by way of junctions that are particularly prominent at the venular angles of the neck, but also may occur elsewhere. Once in the lymph, the tumor cells may circulate in the lymph, remain dormant, be eliminated, or form metastases. The lymph nodes present a temporary barrier to the spread of tumor cells because of their complex compartmentalized structure (Figure 3-13). Rather than a smooth

Table 3-6 Factors that affect the frequency of blood-borne metastatic disease.

Increased metastasis	*Decreased metastasis*
Duration and rate of tumor growth	Heparin
Pregnancy	Warfarin or dicumarol
Stress	Fibrinolytic agents (plasmin)
Adrenal steroids	Adrenal steroids
ACTH	Triton WR
Growth hormone	Radiation
Trauma, such as biopsy or massage	Chemotherapeutic drugs
Dead cells	
Hyperlipemia	
Protamine	
Temperature	
Radiation	
Chemotherapeutic drugs	

Data from Ref. 68.

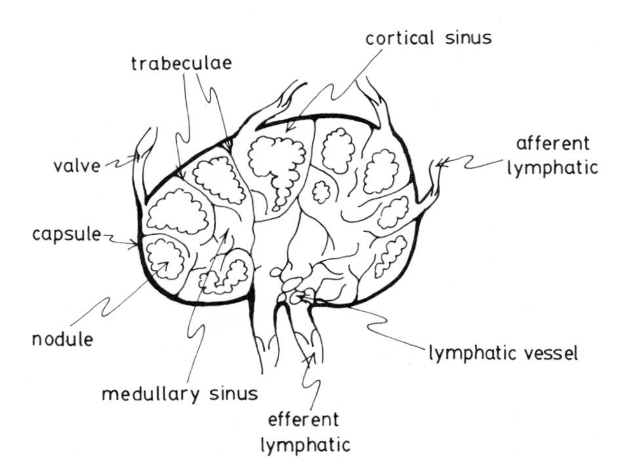

Figure 3-13 Schematic representation of a lymph node.

flow, the passage of lymph through a lymph node is a slow percolation through a series of tortuous sinuses. Lymphocytes appear to squeeze through gaps between the reticuloendothelial cells and to make their way through the ground substance of the parenchyma. Tumor cells may be arrested in this structure, although the node certainly retains less than 100 percent of the cells that reach it, but there is no information about the fate of the cells that are strained off from the lymph (69). Implantation of tumors in experimental animals produces a reactive hyperplasia of the lymph nodes, which can be inhibited by cortisone (70); similar findings have been made in patients with cancer (71). Such reactions could indicate that cellular destruction is taking place within the lymph nodes, but neither the filtration system nor the cellular reaction is likely to control massive loads of tumor cells, although smaller numbers of cells might be destroyed. These considerations, and observations suggesting that manipulation, lymphography, and radiation may enable tumor cells to pass through lymph nodes (60), led Crile to conclude that simple excision or irradiation of lymph nodes might be detrimental to the survival of patients with early cancer, although harmless or even beneficial at later stages (72). This rather controversial concept may be of only limited applicability; for example, it might well be true of breast cancer in which radical mastectomy with extensive dissection of lymph nodes may have little or no advantage over procedures that are at once less radical and better tolerated.

Selectivity in the metastatic process

It is now clear that metastases do not arise by random survival of circulating cells, but rather by a highly selective process that ensures survival of cells with a highly metastatic potential (73). There is a clear individual pattern of metastatic spread for each tumor. Some routes, listed in Table 3-7, give an idea of the degree of individuality that is seen. This specificity may even be seen in an experiment in which a tumor that normally metastasizes to the lung will grow in pieces of subcutaneously implanted lung (75). Membrane components may be involved in this, since fusion of membrane vesicles derived from the F10 subline of B16 melanoma cells, which is highly metastatic, with cells of the F1 line, which produces few pulmonary metastases, led to new cells with metastatic potential intermediate between that of the F1 and F10 lines. The vesicles were incorporated into the plasma membranes of the F1 cells, but persisted there for only 18 to 24 hours, indicating that their role was in facilitating the initial arrest of the cells (73). As we shall see later in this book, spontaneous tumors frequently show no detectable antigenic properties, at least with respect to reactions involving T cells, but the less explored possibility of host protection

Table 3-7 Routes of metastatic spread.

Tumor	*Order of spread* 1	2	3
Bronchial carcinoma	Mediastinal lymph nodes	Pulmonary veins to heart	Brain and liver
Large bowel carcinoma	Mesenteric and para aortic nodes	Portal vein to liver	Lung via vena cava and pulmonary arteries
Prostate, breast, and adrenal tumors	Vertebral vein system to skeleton		
Carcinoma of upper air passages	Cervical lymph nodes	Jugular vein, right heart	Lung
Testicular seminoma	Nodes of external iliac chain	Para-aortic nodes	Thoracic duct and subclavian ~~artery~~ vein to nodes and lung
Ovarian cancers	Spread in peritoneal fluid to viscera		

Derived from Ref. 74.

through natural killer (NK) cells, or armed macrophages, also exists. This represents one other process of selection that might occur during the metastatic process, in addition to others described earlier in this chapter. Finally, we are becoming increasingly aware of just how heterogeneous the cell population of a primary tumor really is (73). This heterogeneity extends to cytology, growth rates, antigenic properties, hormone sensitivity, and metabolic characteristics, and if this list also includes metastatic potential it would be no surprise. We saw in Table 3-1 that growth rates of metastases may be significantly greater than those of primary tumors, and this again is evidence for selectivity, which, moreover, would tend to favor variants with increased malignant capacity, as suggested by Nowell in his concept of clonal evolution (76). The implication for therapy is that efforts must be made to more adequately control the metastatic process. Control or elimination of the primary tumor is of minimal importance, if metastatic disease cannot be checked, and for this, greater attention to the process and availability of meaningful animal models is essential.

CONCLUSION

The overall processes of tumor growth and spread are outlined in Figure 3-14. Malignant tumors grow by the three processes of direct enlargement of the main tumor mass, invasion of adjacent normal tissues, and metastasis to distant regions. In most cases, growth of tumor masses follows, within limits, a type of Gompertzian function with an exponentially decreasing specific rate of growth. Differences between normal and cancer cells in terms of cell cycle kinetics are minimal, and the wide variations that do exist make therapeutic approaches aimed at exploiting such differences difficult. Cell death rates are more critical in determining how fast a tumor will grow than are variations in cell cycle kinetics. During the phase of early tumor growth, an adequate blood supply is assured by elaboration of a tumor angiogenesis factor that stimulates growth of blood vessels into the tumor. Once a blood supply is established, tumors and metastases can exceed the 2- or 3-mm diameter that seems to limit avascular tumors. However, in larger tumors, pressure exerted by growth reduces the efficacy of vascular supply to the inner regions of the cancers, leading to central necrosis.

Invasion and metastasis are selective processes that involve the more agressive elements of the tumor population. Tissue pressure, lack of adhesion between tumor cells, ability to secrete lytic enzymes, formation of

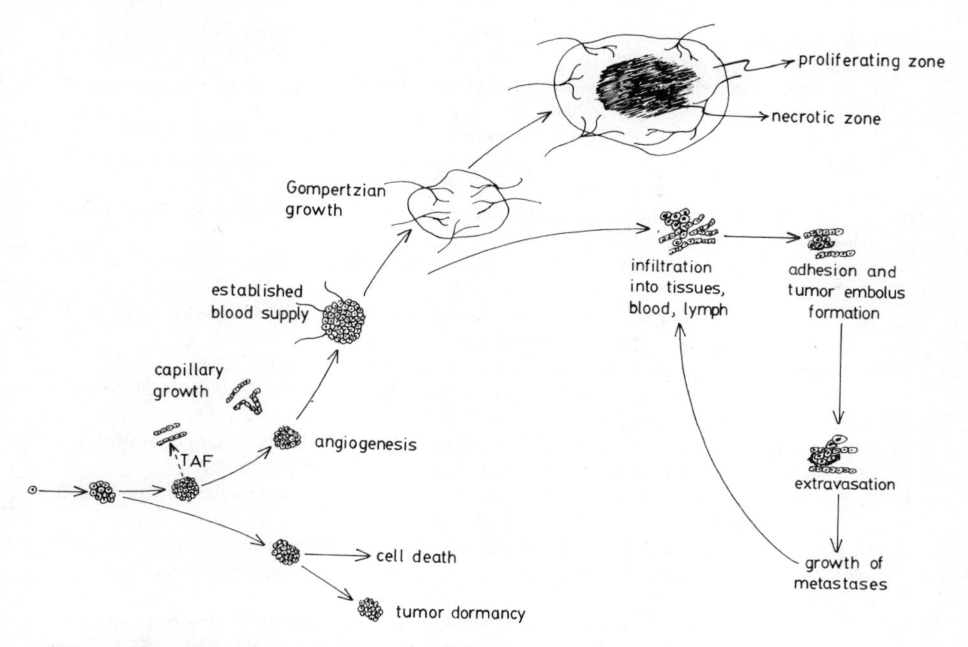

Figure 3-14 Schematic representation of the overall growth of a tumor from a single cell.

blood clots, resistance to host control mechanisms, and ability to proliferate rapidly are among the features associated with various processes in the dissemination of metastases. Thus, the properties of metastatic disease nodules may differ markedly from those of the primary tumor. For this reason, attention to the properties and treatment of metastases is essential if marked improvements in cancer cure rates are to be achieved.

REFERENCES

1. G. G. Steel, K. Adams, and J. C. Barrett: Analysis of the cell population kinetics of transplanted tumors of widely-differing growth rates. Br. J. Cancer *20:* 784–800, 1966.
2. H. E. Skipper: Cellular kinetics associated with "curability" of experimental leukemias. *In Perspectives in Leukemia*, New York: Grune and Stratton, 1968.
3. M. W. Brenner, L. R. Holsti, and Y. Perttala: The study by graphical analysis of the growth of human tumors and metastases of the lung. Brit. J. Cancer *21:*1–13, 1967.
4. G. G. Steel: Cytokinetics of neoplasia. *In Cancer Medicine*, J. F. Holland and E. Frei, eds., Philadelphia: Lea Febiger, 1973, pp. 125–140.
5. B. Gompertz: On the nature of the function expressive of the law of human mortality, and on a new mode of determining the value of life contingencies. Philos. Trans., 1825:513–585.

6. J. A. McCredie, W. R. Inch, J. Kruuv, and T. A. Watson: The rate of tumor growth in animals. Growth *29:*331–347, 1965.
7. L. A. Dethlefsen, J. M. S. Prewitt, and M. L. Mendelsohn: Analysis of tumor growth curves. J. Natl. Cancer Inst. *40:*389–405, 1968.
8. G. G. Steel: *Growth Kinetics of Tumors,* Oxford: Oxford University Press, 1977.
9. J. L. Bennington: Cellular kinetics of invasive squamous carcinoma of the human cervix. Cancer Res. *29:*1082–1088, 1969.
10. R. Auerbach, L. W. Morrissey, and Y. A. Sidky: Gradients in tumor growth. Nature *274:*697–699, 1978.
11. K. Kobayashi: Regional differences in mitotic activity due to injury in mouse skin. Cell Tissue Res. *175:*319–324, 1976.
12. R. T. Prehn and V. Karnik: Differential susceptibility of the axilla and groin of the mouse to chemical oncogenesis. Nature *279:*431–433, 1979.
13. J. Folkman: Tumor angiogenesis factor. Cancer Res. *34:*2109–2113, 1974.
14. O. Petersen: Spontaneous course of cervical precancerous conditions. Am. J. Obstet. Gynecol. *72:*1063–1071, 1956.
15. M. A. Gimbrone, S. B. Leapman, R. S. Cotran, and J. Folkman: Tumor dormancy *in vivo* by prevention of neovascularization. J. Exp. Med. *136:*261–276, 1972.
16. J. Folkman: Tumor angiogenesis. *In Cancer: A Comprehensive Treatise,* F. F. Becker, ed., New York: Plenum Press, Vol. 3, 1975, pp. 355–388.
17. R. Herberman: Cell-mediated immunity to tumor cells. *In Advances in Cancer Research,* Vol. 19, G. Klein and S. Weinhouse, eds., New York: Academic Press, 1974, pp. 207–293.
18. G. Klein and E. Klein: Variation in cell populations of transplanted tumors as indicated by studies on the ascites transformation. Exp. Cell Res. Suppl. *3:*218–229, 1955.
19. T. Cavello, R. Sade, J. Folkman, and R. S. Cotran: Tumor angiogenesis: Rapid induction of endothelial mitoses demonstrated by autoradiography. J. Cell Biol. *54:*408–420, 1972.
20. D. H. Ausprunk and J. Folkman: Migration and proliferation of endothelial cells in preformed and newly-formed blood vessels during tumor angiogenesis. Microvasc. Res. *14:*53–65, 1977.
21. T. J. Ryan: Factors influencing growth of vascular endothelium in the skin. *In The Physiology and Pathophysiology of the Skin.* A Jarret, ed., New York: Academic Press, 1973, pp. 779–805.
22. W. J. Cliff: Kinetics of wound healing in rabbit ear chambers, a time lapse cinemicroscopic study. Quart. J. Exp. Physiol. *50:*79–89, 1965.
23. H. Brem and J. Folkman: Inhibition of tumor angiogenesis mediated by cartilage. J. Exp. Med. *141:*427–439, 1975.
24. T. P. Butler and P. M. Gullino: Bulk transfer of fluid in the interstitial compartment of mammary tumors. Cancer Res. *35:*3084–3088, 1975.
25. R. J. Goldacre and B. Sylvén: On the access of blood-borne dyes to various tumour regions. Brit. J. Cancer *16:*306–322, 1962.
26. M. Greenblatt and P. Shubik: Tumor angiogenesis: Transfilter diffusion studies in the hamster by the transparent chamber technique. J. Natl. Cancer Inst. *41:*111–124, 1968.
27. M. A. Gimbrone, S. Leapman, R. S. Botran, and J. Folkman: Tumor angiogenesis: Iris neovascularization at a distance from experimental intraocular tumors. J. Natl. Cancer Inst. *50:*219–228, 1973.
28. P. M. Gullino: Angiogenesis and oncogenesis. J. Natl. Cancer Inst. *61:*639–643, 1978.
29. J. Folkman and R. Cotran: Relation of vascular proliferation to tumor growth. Int. Rev. Exp. Pathol. *16:*207–248, 1976.

30. D. Tuan, S. Smith, J. Folkman, and E. Merler: Isolation of the non-histone proteins of rat Walker carcinoma 256: Their association with tumor angiogenesis. Biochemistry *12:*3159–3165, 1973.
31. M. Klagsburn, D. Knighton, and J. Folkman: Tumor angiogenesis activity in cells grown in tissue culture. Cancer Res. *36:*110–114, 1976.
32. R. Langer, H. Brem, K. Falterman, M. Klein, and J. Folkman: Isolation of a cartilage factor that inhibits tumor neovascularization. Science *193:*70–72, 1976.
33. B. Sylvén and B. Holmberg: On the structure and biological effects of a newly-discovered cytotoxic polypeptide in tumor fluid. Europ. J. Cancer *1:*199–202, 1965.
34. J. Denekamp: Discussion. In *Time and Dose Relationships in Radiation Biology as Applied to Radiotherapy.* Brookhaven National Laboratory Reports 50203 (C-57), p. 145, 1970.
35. M. L. Mendelsohn: The cell cycle in malignant and normal tissues. *In The Cell Cycle in Malignancy and Immunity.* J. C. Hampton, chairman, Energy Research and Development Administration Technical Information Center, 1975, pp. 293–314.
36. A. C. Sartorelli and W. A. Creasey: Combination chemotherapy. *In Cancer Medicine,* J. F. Holland and E. Frei, eds., Philadelphia: Lea & Febiger, 1973, pp. 707–717.
37. P. Strykmans, E. P. Cronkite, J. Fache, T. M. Fliedner, and J. Ramos: Deoxyribonucleic acid synthesis time of erythropoietic and granulopoietic cells in human beings. Nature *211:*717–720, 1966.
38. P. K. Lala: Studies on tumor cell population kinetics. *In Methods in Cancer Research,* Vol. 6, H. Busch, ed., New York: Academic Press, 1971, pp. 4–93.
39. P. C. Koller: The nucleus of the cancer cell—a historical review. Exp. Cell Res. *31,* Suppl. 9, 3–14, 1963.
39A. L. F. Lamerton: Basic Concepts of cell population kinetics. In A. C. Sartorelli and D. G. Johns, eds. Antineoplastic and Immunosuppressive Agents, vol. I, Berlin–Heidelberg–New York: Springer Verlag, 1974.
40. A. B. Cairnie, L. F. Lamerton, and G. G. Steel: Cell proliferation studies in the intestinal epithelium of the rat. 1. Determination of the kinetic parameters. Exp. Cell Res. *39:*528–538, 1965.
41. A. J. Valleron and E. Frindel: Computer simulation of growing cell populations. Cell Tissue Kinet. *6:*69–79, 1973.
42. P. D. M. Macdonald: Statistical inferences from the fraction labelled mitoses curve. Biometrika *57:*489–503, 1970.
43. S. E. Shackney: A cytokinetic model for heterogeneous mammalian cell populations. Tritiated thymidine studies—the percent labelled mitosis curve. J. Theor. Biol. *44:*49–90, 1974.
44. A. C. Begg and J. F. Fowler: A rapid method for the determination of tumour RBE. Brit. J. Radiol. *47:*154–156, 1974.
45. H. A. Crissman, P. F. Mullaney, and J. A. Steinkamp: Methods and applications of flow systems for analysis and sorting of mammalian cells. *In Methods in Cell Biology,* Vol. 9, D. M. Prescott, ed., New York: Academic Press, 1975, pp. 179–246.
46. M. M. Elkind and J. L. Redpath: Molecular and cellular biology of radiation lethality. *In Cancer: A Comprehensive Treatise,* Vol. 6, F. F. Becker, ed., New York: Plenum Press, 1977, pp. 51–99.
47. E. Stubblefield and S. Murphree: Metabolic events in the regulation of cell reproduction. *In Handbook of Experimental Pharmacology,* Vol. 38 Pt. 1, A. C. Sartorelli and D. G. Johns, eds., Berlin: Springer-Verlag, 1974, pp. 194–204.
48. R. R. Klevecz and G. L. Forrest: Regulation of tubulin through the cell cycle. Ann. N.Y. Acad. Sci. *253:*292–303, 1975.

49. M. Abou-Sabe', ed.: *Cyclic Nucleotides and the Regulation of Cell Growth.* Stroudsburg, Pa.: Dowden, Hutchinson and Ross, 1976.
50. D. L. Friedman: Role of cyclic nucleotides in cell growth and differentiation. Physiol. Rev. *56:*652–708, 1976.
51. S. P. Sorokin: Reconstruction of centriole formation and ciliogenesis in mammalian lungs. J. Cell Sci. *3:*207–230, 1968.
52. L. F. Henneguy: Sur le rapports des cils vibrailles avec les centrosomes. Arch. Anat. Microscop. Morphol. Exp. *1:*481–496, 1898.
53. C. Lloyd: Primitive model for cell cycle control. Nature *280:*631–632, 1979.
54. R. W. Tucker, A. B. Pardee, and K. Fujiwara: Centriole ciliation is related to quiescence and DNA synthesis in 3T3 cells. Cell *17:*527–535, 1979.
55. J. B. Rattner and S. G. Phillips: Independence of centriole formation and DNA synthesis. J. Cell Biol. *57:*359–372, 1973.
56. R. O. Brady, P. H. Fishman, and P. T. Mora: Membrane components and enzymes in virally transformed cells. Fed. Proc. *32:*102–108, 1973.
57. M. M. Burger: Surface changes in transformed cells detected by lectins. Fed. Proc. *32:*91–101, 1973.
58. C. D. Cone, Jr.: Unified theory on the basic mechanism of normal mitotic control and oncogenesis, J. Theor. Biol. *30:*151–181, 1971.
59. K. P. Balitsky and E. P. Shuba: Resting potential of malignant tumour cells. Acta Unio Int. Contra Canc. *20:*1391–1393, 1964.
60. S. Wood, Jr., and P. Sträuli: Tumor invasion and metastasis. *In Cancer Medicine,* J. F. Holland and E. Frei, III, eds., Philadelphia: Lea & Febiger, 1973, pp. 140–151.
61. M. S. Burstone: Histochemical demonstration of proteolytic activity in human neoplasms. J. Natl. Cancer Inst. *16:*1149–1161, 1956.
62. R. Roblin, I. N. Chou, and P. H. Black: Proteolytic enzymes, cell surface changes, and viral transformation. Adv. Cancer Res. *22:*203–260, 1975.
63. B. Sylvén: Metastatic spread of tumors. *Oncology 1970* (Proc. Tenth Intern. Cancer Congr.), Chicago: Year Book Medical Publishers, 1971, Vol. 1, pp. 411–416.
64. L. Florey: General Pathology, 4th ed. Philadelphia: W. B. Saunders Company, 1970.
65. M. Abercrombie: Contact inhibition: The phenomenon and its biological implications. Natl. Cancer Inst. Monogr. *26:*249–273, 1967.
66. S. Wood, Jr., R. R. Baker, and B. Marzocchi: *In vivo* studies of tumor behavior: Locomotion of and interrelationships between normal cells and cancer cells. *In The Proliferation and Spread of Neoplastic Cells,* Baltimore: The Williams & Wilkins Co., 1968, pp. 495–510.
67. R. A. Willis: *The Spread of Tumours in the Human Body,* 3rd ed. London: Butterworths, 1973.
68. S. Wood, Jr., E. D. Holyoke, and J. H. Yardley: Mechanism of metastasis production from blood-borne cancer cells. Canad. Cancer Conf. *4:*167, 1961.
69. P. Sträuli: The barrier function of lymph nodes. A review of experimental studies and their implication for cancer surgery. *In Surgical Oncology,* F. Saegesser and J. Pettavel, eds., Bern: Hans Huber, 1970, pp. 161–176.
70. D. Shepro, L. P. Eidelhoch, and D.I. Patt: Lymph node responses to malignant homo- and heterografts in the hamster. Anat. Rec. *136:*393–405, 1960.
71. U. Fisch: Lymphographische Untersuchungen-über das zervikale Lymph system. Basel: Karger, 1966.
72. G. Crile, Jr.: Rationale of simple mastectomy without radiation for clinical stage I cancer of the breast. Surg. Gynec. Obstet. *120:*975–982, 1965.
73. G. Poste and I. J. Fidler: The pathogenesis of cancer metastasis. Nature *283:*139–146, 1980.

74. J. A. del Regato: Pathways of metastatic spread of malignant tumors. Sem. Oncol. *4*:33–38, 1977.
75. D. L. Kinsey: An experimental study of preferential metastasis. Cancer *13*:674–676, 1960.
76. P. C. Nowell: The clonal evolution of tumor cell populations. Science *194*:23–28, 1976.

4. Host-tumor relationships

As a tumor grows, a point will be reached at which detectable interactions with the host occur. These interactions represent the underlying mechanism of morbidity. Although the perceived changes reflect the growing variety and intensity of actions of the tumor on the host, the relationships operate in both directions, inasmuch as the host exerts some degree of control over tumor growth. Host actions of this sort are described in Chapters 3 and 6 and will, in general, control tumor growth less effectively as it enlarges. Here we are considering the effects of the malignant tumor on the host, restricting ourselves to metabolic derangements, susceptibility to infection, disturbances in appetite, weight loss, pain, psychological disturbances, and other more specific complications associated with cancer. The totality of these effects represents the syndrome of advanced cancer, but for our purposes, it is necessary to isolate the various components in order to understand their roles in bringing about morbidity, and finally death.

CACHEXIA

Progression of neoplastic disease is most commonly associated with symptoms of cachexia (1). This complex syndrome of loss of appetite, weight loss, weakness, pallor, apathy, mental confusion, and depletion or abnormalities of such body components as electrolytes and serum proteins is accompanied by clinical findings of progressive failure of vital functions.

These changes reflect a variety of factors. The direct impingement of the tumor on vital structures and the pressure and destruction of tissues by tumor infiltration would be expected to disrupt normal functions and to obstruct such organs as the esophagus or intestine. In addition, tumors secrete hormones, which produce systemic disorders, as well as other substances of a cytotoxic nature, such as toxohormone or Sylven's octapeptide (2). Toxins also may be released from necrotic regions of both normal and cancerous tissues. A further element that may assume a major role as the tumor burden becomes very large is competition for available nutrients. Finally, there is an overlying psychological component that reflects the patient's response to his or her disease.

Anorexia and depletion of body components

This is one of the commonest findings in patients with advanced cancer (3). It is easy to understand how tumors of the gastrointestinal tract, which produce obstructions that make eating difficult or painful or which prevent passage of food through the intestine, can give rise to anorexia and wasting. In other cases, such as lymphomas (4), infiltration of the gut by tumor cells produces malabsorption. When this occurs in patients with no gastrointestinal involvement, the explanation is more elusive. It has been suggested that lactate, produced in abundance by many tumors, may have an anorectic action, as has been observed experimentally (5). However, there is no proof that such a mechanism is operative clinically. It should be considered, also, that most cachetic patients have advanced disease that has been treated with radiation and anticancer drugs, agents that produce severe side effects including gastrointestinal distress and anorexia (6). An interesting concept that has recently been advanced is that anorexia is a learned food aversion (7). Such learned aversions have been reported among children receiving drugs that induce nausea (8) and consist of aversion to foods consumed during the distressful situation. In rats, aversion to diets eaten during growth of PW-739 transplanted, polyoma virus-induced tumors, developed rapidly, but food consumption rose to the same level as controls when the animals were switched to novel diets (6). Thus, there is likely to be a psychogenic component to the anorexia of cancer, one that is analogous to drug-induced food aversion in children (8) and aversion to vitamin-deficient diets in rats (9). It is probable that such aversions constitute a fundamental protective mechanism for avoiding toxins (10), but in the case of cancer, the response operates to the detriment of the patient. However, these findings do suggest that the appetites of cancer patients could be improved by dietary variety.

Quite apart from anorexia, other processes apparently intervene to deplete the host tissues while the tumor continues to grow. The relative autonomy of an advanced tumor makes it, in many respects, independent of many host control mechanisms, so that in the face of an inadequate dietary intake, which normally prevents growth, the tumor will continue to grow by, in a sense, parasitizing the host tissues. Even in starving animals some tumor growth will occur, for the tumor successfully competes for nutrients with the normal tissues. This aspect can be seen in the hypoglycemia that has frequently been reported in cancer patients since the original finding in 1929 (1). Occasionally, increased glucose utilization directly ascribable to the tumor has been determined (11), whereas in other cases, secretion of insulin or insulin-like substances by the tumor is responsible for the hypoglycemia. However, since tumors may also impair the host's ability to utilize glucose (12), it is obvious that simple competition or insulin secretion are not the only mechanisms responsible for altered carbohydrate demands.

Whatever the mechanisms, the effects of a tumor upon the host are certainly not restricted to glucose metabolism. Depletion of fat reserves is an early result of the presence of a tumor, and may lead to fat contents in muscle samples that are only 50 percent of normal values (1). Possibly more serious, in terms of its contribution to morbidity, is the depletion of body proteins and the appearance of hypoalbuminemia (13). Although it is not possible to distinguish between a generalized loss of protein due to reduced food intake and the more specific effects of the tumor, several findings suggest that the latter may be important. In rats, direct uptake of labeled albumin by tumors has been observed (14); many tumor cells have the pronounced pinocytotic capability needed for this. Abnormal albumin loss could result from damage to the kidneys, and it has been reported that nephrotic syndrome, a kidney disease that appears to have an immunological etiology, is associated with extrarenal cancers (15). Liver catalase is another protein that is depleted by tumor growth (16). In this case, generalized, nonspecific effects on proteins are ruled out, because kidney catalase is much less affected, and the erythrocyte enzyme is not affected.

Treatment of tissue depletion—hyperalimentation. It would seem that some way of increasing food intake should help control cachexia. Although changing diets could help to improve appetite, this obviously will not work in patients who are severely ill, who are undergoing intensive therapy, or who have obstructions of the gastrointestinal tract. Procedures such as the installation of nasogastric tube through which nutrients can be fed may be helpful, but to avoid problems of malabsorption intravenous hyperalimentation has been used as a means of supplying calories and nutrients (17). A catheter is inserted into a jugular vein and threaded through until it is positioned in the mid-superior vena cava. The infused nutrient solutions contain dextrose, protein hydrolysates (amino acids), minerals, and a full complement of vitamins (18). As a result of such infusions, gain in weight, reversal of other cachectic symptoms, such as hypoalbuminemia, greater tolerance to therapy, and improved immune function have been demonstrated (18–20). These improvements may have contributed to a lengthened survival, but hyperalimentation has not been useful in terminally ill patients (18). The major complication has been sepsis because of the indwelling catheter and the excellence of the medium as a growth support for bacteria. Intravenous hyperalimentation has already achieved widespread use, particularly in children (20), because patients feel better, and this should be a major consideration in the treatment of cancer patients, when therapy often seems almost as bad as the disease.

Abnormal retention phenomena

Although depletion of body components is an obvious feature of cachexia, some of the changes that form part of the syndrome and that contribute to morbidity involve abnormal retention of various substances (1). Edema, which may occur due to water retention, is often accompanied by hyponatremia. In fact, the body load of sodium may actually increase, due to the accumulation of fluid, even if the latter has a low sodium content. In many cases, the inappropriate production of antidiuretic hormone is responsible for the changes in sodium balance (21). It is probable that only part of the hyponatremia results from renal mechanisms, since there is evidence of increased intracellular concentrations of sodium in muscle cells (21), representing a possible additional mechanism for depletion of extracellular sodium.

PAIN

Perceived pain represents the product of intensity of peripheral stimulation and the central summation of these stimuli (22); it also probably involves some sort of gate or threshold control mechanism (23). The involvement of several components of this type would explain the wide variations in individual perception of pain, and such variations are accentuated by psychological factors. Early cancers are very seldom associated with pain, and even at later stages, the occurrence and intensity of pain varies considerably. However, there is a widespread conception that the disease is always very painful, so that any pain that occurs is ascribed to cancer, even if it originates from some other condition. This popular expectation may exacerbate the problem by, on the one hand, altering the patient's perception of pain, and on the other, leading physicians not to undertake appropriate specific measures to relieve non-cancer-related discomfort. There are a number of possible sources of pain due to cancer (24).

Obstruction

This is a common source of pain in patients with tumors of the gastrointestinal tract. The pain varies from discomfort and difficulty on eating (esophagus and proximal stomach), through typical ulcer-like symptoms of heartburn (stomach), to acute colicky pain, like that of gallstones (pancreas) or kidney stones (renal obstruction). Usually such pain is intermittent in contrast to the steady, severe pain of peritonitis or occlusion of the mesenteric artery.

Infection and inflammation

Infections may occur more frequently and be more serious in patients with cancer than in the population at large. Lymphomas and leukemias, especially, lower resistance to infection, and impaired immune responses are common in most subjects with advanced cancer. Obstruction of drainage by the tumor mass, ulceration, particularly of tumors on mucosal surfaces, and necrosis of many solid tumors all facilitate the development of infections. Pain then follows as a result of inflammation of the infected region. In other cases, an inflammatory response occurs where tumor infiltration is taking place. Once again the pain may be unrelated to cancer in that an opportunistic infection with such organisms as Herpes zoster or *Pneumocystis carinii* may occur in these debilitated patients. Treatment in all these cases should be directed at the infecting organisms and the inflammatory process, using antibiotics and steroids.

Pressure and tissue destruction

When a tumor is growing in a region such as the brain, where space is limited, the increase in pressure that results displaces normal structures and causes necrosis, processes that lead to pain. In the case of bony metastases, not only may infiltration and pressure create pain, but replacement of bone leads to weakness and results in painful fractures. Intensive radiotherapy may cause necrosis of normal bone, with similar problems.

Referred pain

As with many other painful conditions, pain due to cancer may be referred, so that it is perceived in a region remote from the tumor. This, of course, reflects the particular patterns of regional innervation. For example, advanced cancer of the uterine cervix may be associated with low back pain, whereas biliary tract cancer may lead to pain over the right scapula. Unless tumor growth is unusually rapid, cancers of the viscera often are not notably painful.

Treatment of pain

Surgical measures to deal with severe, unrelenting pain, apart from resection of obstructions, involve such procedures as nerve blocks or cordotomy. Radiation has proven useful in the control of painful bony metastases. The doses used may be lower than those required for effective treatment of a large tumor, since high doses that may cause irreversible damage to normal bone structure may worsen the situation. It is interesting that, as far as drugs are concerned, the study of Moertel, undertaken in ambulatory patients, suggested that aspirin was the best of the nine analgesics examined (25). Aspirin, however, supposedly has more side effects than the almost equally effective acetaminophen (Tylenol), although the latter is known to cause liver damage on occasion. For patients in poorer condition with chronic pain, narcotic analgesics are necessary. Recently, studies have been initiated to evaluate heroin, which has been used elsewhere, notably in Britain, to control severe pain associated with terminal disease. It is not clearly established that heroin is superior to morphine, since both give rise to the same metabolites, but it may be quicker acting. Arguments against the use of heroin, based on its probably greater addictiveness, are irrelevant in terminally ill patients, but undoubtedly widespread availability would create problems for enforcement of drug laws. While on the subject of drugs, it should be stressed that proper preoperative psychological preparation of cancer patients and accompanying emotional support may greatly lessen requirements for medication (26).

Although it is somewhat of a departure from the topic of pain control, the whole question of the care of terminally ill patients deserves discussion. The often dehumanizing nature of both the disease and the methods used to treat it have been stressed by others (27,28). This can add significantly to the psychological distress of the patient and the patient's family. Clearly a greater degree of supportive care is needed, coupled with a willingness to allow the patient to "die with dignity." A model for such care is provided by St. Thomas Hospice in London (29), and there has been much interest in adapting the hospice concept elsewhere. Relief of pain constitutes a major element in such an environment, and in accordance with the significant psychological contribution to perceived pain, understanding and support of staff and family contributes to such relief. In the same vein, the ethics of prolonging life by intensive artificial support procedures has come under much discussion. Selective limitation of the degree of support on the basis of each individual's situation has received widespread agreement. There is no point in maintaining mere basal vital functions in a subject who cannot recover, and attempts to do so can be very troubling to the family, both psychologically and financially. On the other hand, euthanasia is illegal, and the strong moral arguments against it are based on possibilities of flagrant misuse for personal or political ends.

HORMONAL AND OTHER HUMORAL FACTORS

Most important in this category are the ectopic hormones. These are produced by tumors that are non-endocrine in origin and that resemble normal hormones in their action, but that in their production and release are not subject to the usual physiological mechanisms for control that commonly involve feedback pathways. In patients with hormone-producing tumors, not only are there the usual symptoms produced by tumor growth and infiltration, but also symptoms of excessive production of specific hormones may be superimposed. In some cases, the tumor may elaborate multiple hormones (30). The ectopic hormones do show some degree of specificity as regards to the type of tumors that secrete them (31). Secretion of adrenocorticotropic hormone (ACTH) and *melanocyte-stimulating hormone* commonly go hand in hand. Although many varieties of tumors secrete these hormones, oat cell carcinomas of the lungs, pancreatic tumors of non-beta islet cell origin, thymomas, and carcinoids are the most frequent sources. Even large doses of dexamethasone will not reduce ACTH secretion because the feedback pathway of control does not operate in the tumor. The ACTH secreted is similar to the normal hormone (32), whereas the melanocyte-stimulating activity is often found in molecules that differ significantly from the pituitary hormone (33). Obesity, muscle wasting, impaired glucose tolerance, emotional disturbance, hypertension, hypokalemia (low serum potassium) and edema may occur to varying degrees; in women and children, acne and growth of body hair may occur. *Gonadotropins* are most often produced by hepatomas, lung tumors, teratomas, and choriocarcinomas. Luteinizing hormone activity is the major endocrine found, and leads to precocious puberty, as well as gynecomastia, in older men (31). Androgens and estrogens do not suppress gonadotropin levels in the plasma. Carcinomas of the lung are most prone to secrete *antidiuretic hormone,* with resulting low serum sodium and a small output of relatively concentrated urine. Weakness, confusion, gastrointestinal upset, and finally coma and convulsions may occur. Restriction of fluid intake and administration of hypertonic saline is required to deal with the emergency. *Parathyroid hormone* is secreted by a wide range of tumors, with cancers of the lung, pancreas, liver, and colon heading the list. Disturbances in calcium metabolism that occur lead to weakness, nausea, confusion, abnormal cardiac rhythm, coma, and death. *Thyroid-stimulating activity,* leading to a hyperthyroid status, with weight loss, tachycardia, weakness, and excess sweating, is secreted by such trophoblastic tumors (arising from the placenta) as choriocarcinoma and hydatiform mole. *Insulin* may be secreted by bronchial carcinoids and liposarcomas, but it would appear that many more tumors secrete substances with insulin-like activity or that affect carbohydrate metabolism, to produce hypoglycemia (31). As discussed earlier, hypoglycemia may also be the result of competition for glucose. Ectopic *erythropoietin* secretion, giving rise to an elevated hematocrit, has been found in cases of pheochromocytoma, hepatoma, and cerebellar hemangioblastoma (31); the hormone appears identical to the normal molecule secreted by the kidney in response to anemia and anoxia. Bioamines including *serotonin* are excreted by patients with carcinoid tumors.

PSYCHOLOGICAL ASPECTS

We earlier emphasized the role of psychological attitudes on the perception of pain, and it is a common finding of many engaged in the care and treatment of cancer patients that not only pain, but the course of the disease and the success of therapy are also influenced in large measure by these attitudes. Fear of cancer as a major incurable disease has a long history. Once it was associated with feelings of shame or guilt (27,34), perhaps because of the belief that it was the result of some "immoral act," no doubt because of the wasting, disfigurement, and pain that frequently accompanied the disease. Fear remains a potent force, but one that can be modulated or lessened by the concern, honesty, and emotional support of the physician. This is particularly important around the time of the original diagnosis and also before surgery that involves functional loss, such as laryngectomy or mastectomy. There has been a complete reversal of the former pattern of not revealing the diagnosis, so that the appropriate considerations are now concerned with the timing and the extent of the information to be given (28). Within the contexts of the particular disease and the ability of the patient to cope with the information, enough should be provided to prevent feelings of abandonment or helplessness and to encourage realistic hope and a sense of participation in the plan of treatment. Readiness to answer questions honestly, helps to give a sense of alliance with the physician. However, the perceptions of illness by different individuals vary from an adversary to be conquered all the way to an experience to be valued (35), and this will greatly influence the patients' response at all stages of the disease. Kübler-Ross has described six stages of psychological response: denial, anger, depression, bargaining, acceptance, and decathexis—the terminal state (36). However, since a succession of therapeutic attempts may be followed by varying degrees of response, and in many cases, by cures, these stages may not be completed or may be reversed or replayed a number of times (27). Undoubtedly, a major problem for patients with progressive disease that is not curable is the increasing dependence on others and the inability to meet their own needs and those of their families. This may cause a behavioral change in which many patients develop a cooperative, cheerful manner in an effort to ensure the assistance of those they depend on (37). Finally, the attitudes and expectations of the physician regarding cancer, terminal illness and death, may be conveyed to the patient in such a way, albeit unconsciously, as to influence the patient's own feelings and responses (27).

MISCELLANEOUS COMPLICATIONS

There are a variety of other effects of cancer upon the host, all capable of exacerbating the problems presented by the cancer itself.

Neuromuscular disorders

These include weakness, loss of stretch reflexes, atrophy of limb musculature, myositis with chronic inflammatory reactions in the muscle tissue, axonal degeneration with loss of Schwann cells, cerebellar degeneration, and encephalitis (38). Close to 7 percent of cancer patients exhibit these disorders without having any neuromuscular involvement by tumors, and the symptoms are most common (7 to 16 percent) in those with carcinomas of the lung, ovary, or stomach (39). The etiology of these conditions is unknown.

Dermatological complications.

Among these are hyperpigmentation of the skin, erythemas due to vasodilation, localized thrombophlebitis, urticaria, and Paget's disease of the nipple (40).

Skeletal effects

Bony involvement is a prominent feature of cancer. Most familiar is direct involvement by invasion and metastasis of the tumor, but there are also effects produced by the endocrine agents elaborated by many tumors. Such humoral secretions include ACTH, parathyroid hormone, calcitonin, and osteolytic phytosteryl esters (41,42). In many cases these are ectopic hormones, but some are produced by tumors of endocrine origin. Osteoporosis, a generalized fragility of the skeleton, may also occur in patients with advanced cancer and may lead to frequent painful fractures. Hypercalcemia is rather common and results primarily from increased breakdown of bone substance due either to tumor infiltration or to humoral effects on the bone. Prostate and breast cancers and myeloma, in particular, tend to invade the bones. The treatment of choice for bony metastases is radiation; the hypercalcemia is best controlled with hydration, often with the use of a divalent anion such as sulfate or phosphate to complex the calcium.

Hematological effects

Metastatic disease of the marrow arising from carcinomas of the breast, prostate, lung, thyroid, and kidney are relatively common. Neuroblastoma and malignant melanoma also frequently invade the bone marrow (43). This may result in fibrosis of the marrow with anemia, thrombocytopenia, and leukopenia. In other cases there may be thrombocytosis or leukocytosis (increased numbers of platelets and white cells, respectively). Tumors that secrete erythropoietin will stimulate red cell production. Changes in serum proteins frequently occur in cancer patients, as described in the section on cachexia.

Infections

The immunological deficiencies, cachexia, and disturbed marrow function frequently found as cancers progress render patients very susceptible to infection (44). Pneumonias may be associated with pulmonary metastases, and infections can occur in ulcerating lesions of the head and neck, due to necrotic tumor masses and penetration of normal epithelia by tumor. Among the most commonly encountered organisms, and the most serious ones today, are the Gram-negative bacilli *Pseudomonas* and *Serratia,* but increasingly frequent in patients receiving intensive antibiotic therapy are fungal infections by *Candida* and *Aspergillus,* which develop because antibiotics suppress normal flora. Herpes virus infections also are more common in cancer patients. Infections are frequently life-threatening in debilitated patients, and since few antifungal and antiviral drugs are available, there is cause for concern. Attempts to minimize the risk of life-threatening infections in severely immunosuppressed cancer patients include the use of isolation units, such as laminar air flow rooms, where a constant stream of sterile filtered air passes through the room and is recirculated. Entry to the room is made against the air stream, thus preventing passage of organisms to the patient.

CONCLUSION

Tumor growth exerts an increasingly disturbing action on the host. Through infiltration and pressure on normal tissues, release of active endocrine or other secretions, obstruction of vital functions, competition for substrates, pain and discomfort, and a variety of neurological, dermatological, skeletal, and hematological effects, the growth of the tumor weakens the life functions of the host. Psychological responses to the disease are superimposed on these physical changes and may accelerate the downhill course. Although some aspects of the deterioration may be halted by such procedures as intravenous hyperalimentation, other changes are of uncertain etiology and may not be related to such definable syndromes as cachexia. Death may often result from such events as hemorrhage (secondary to thrombocytopenia) or infection.

REFERENCES

1. G. Costa: Cachexia and the systemic effects of tumors. *In Cancer Medicine*, J. F. Holland and E. Frei, III, eds., Philadelphia: Lea & Febiger, 1973, pp. 1035–1044.
2. B. Sylvén and B. Holmberg: On the structure and biological effects of a newly-discovered cytotoxic polypeptide in tumor fluid. Europ. J. Cancer *1:*199–202, 1965.
3. J. C. B. Holland, J. Rowland, and M. Plumb: Psychological aspects of anorexia in cancer patients. Cancer Res. *37:*2425–2428, 1977.
4. B. Ramot: Malabsorption due to lymphomatous disease. Ann. Rev. Med. *22:*19–24, 1971.
5. C. A. Baile, W. M. Zinn, and J. Mayer: Effects of lactate and other metabolites on food intake of monkeys. Am. J. Physiol. *219:*1606–1613, 1970.
6. G. Costa and S. S. Donaldson: Effects of cancer and cancer treatment on the nutrition of the host. New Eng. J. Med. *300:*1471–1474, 1979.
7. I. L. Bernstein and R. A. Sigmundi: Tumor anorexia: A learned food aversion. Science *209:*416–418, 1980.
8. I. L. Bernstein: Learned taste aversions in children receiving chemotherapy. Science *200:*1302–1303, 1978.
9. P. Rozin: Specific aversions as a component of specific hungers. J. Comp. Physiol. Psychol. *64:*237–242, 1967.
10. J. Garcia, W. G. Hankins, and K. W. Rusiniak: Behavioral regulation of the *milieu interne* in man and rat. Science *185:*824–831, 1974.
11. R. W. Carey, T. G. Pretlow, E. A. Ezdinli, and J. F. Holland: Studies on the mechanism of hypoglycemia in a patient with massive leiomosarcoma. Am. J. Med. *40:*458–469, 1966.
12. C. Waterhouse and J. H. Kemperman: Carbohydrate metabolism in subjects with cancer. Cancer Res. *31:*1273–1278, 1971.
13. G. Costa: Cachexia, the metabolic component of neoplastic diseases. Cancer Res. *37:*2327–2335, 1977.
14. H. Bush, E. Fujiwara, and D. C. Firszt: Studies on the metabolism of radioactive albumin in tumor bearing rats. Cancer Res. *21:*371–377, 1961.
15. L. Loughridge and M. G. Lewis: Nephrotic syndrome in malignant disease of non-renal origin. Lancet *1:*256–258, 1971.
16. T. Ohnuma: Hepatic catalase. *In Cancer Medicine*, J. F. Holland and E. Frei, III, eds., Philadelphia: Lea & Febiger, 1973, pp. 1044–1046.
17. S. J. Dudrick, J. M. Long, E. Steiger, and J. E. Rhoads: Intravenous hyperalimentation. Med. Clin. N. Amer. *54:*577–589, 1970.
18. S. J. Dudrick: Intravenous feeding as an aid to nutrition in disease. CA-A Cancer Journal for Clinicians *20:*198–211, 1970.
19. E. M. Copeland: Intravenous hyperalimentation as an adjunct to cancer patient management. CA-A Cancer Journal for Clinicians *28:*322–330, 1978.
20. J. Van Eys: Nutrition and cancer in children. CA-A Cancer Journal for Clinicians *29:*40–45, 1979.
21. K. D. Nolph and R. W. Schrier: Sodium, potassium and water metabolism in the syndrome of inappropriate antidiuretic hormone secretion. Am. J. Med. *49:*534–545, 1970.
22. W. K. Livingston: *Pain Mechanisms*. New York: Macmillan Company, 1943, pp. 62–80.

23. R. Melzack and P. D. Wall: *Pain Mechanisms:* A new theory. Science *150:*971–979, 1965.
24. K. B. Olson: Pain. *In Cancer Medicine,* J. F. Holland and E. Frei, eds., Philadelphia: Lea & Febiger, 1973, pp. 1022–1035.
25. C. G. Moertel, D. L. Ahmann, W. F. Taylor, and N. Schwartan: A comparative evaluation of marketed analgesic drugs. New Eng. J. Med. *286:*813–815, 1972.
26. L. D. Egbert, G. E. Batit, C. E. Welch, and M. K. Bartlett: Reduction of post-operative pain by encouragement and instruction of patients. New Eng. J. Med. *270:*825–827, 1964.
27. J. Holland: Psychologic aspects of cancer. *In Cancer Medicine,* J. F. Holland and E. Frei, III, eds., Philadelphia: Lea & Febiger, 1973, pp. 991–1021.
28. A. D. Weisman and T. P. Hackett: Predilection to death. Psychosom. Med. *23:*232–256, 1961.
29. C. Saunders: The last stages of life. Am. J. Nursing *65:*70–75, March, 1965.
30. W. L. O'Neal, D. M. Kipnis, S. A. Luse, P. E. Lacy, and L. Jarett: Secretion of various endocrine substances by ACTH-secreting tumors-gastrin, melanotropin, norepinephrine, serotonin, parathormone, vasopressin and glucagon. Cancer *21:*1219–1232, 1968.
31. G. W. Liddle and J. H. Ball: Manifestations of cancer mediated by ectopic hormones. *In Cancer Medicine,* J. F. Holland and E. Frei, eds., Philadelphia: Lea & Febiger, 1973, pp. 1046–1057.
32. G. W. Liddle, J. R. Givens, W. E. Nicholson, and D. P. Island: The ectopic ACTH syndrome. Cancer Res. *25:*1057–1061, 1965.
33. M. Shapiro, D. N. Orth, K. Abe, W. E. Nicholson, D. P. Island, and G. W. Liddle: Evidence for the presence of MSH other than α-MSH and β-MSH in tumors of patients with the "ectopic ACTH-MSH syndrome." Clin. Res. *18:*35, 1970.
34. R. D. Abrams and J. E. Finesinger: Guilt reactions in patients with cancer. Cancer *6:*474–482, 1953.
35. Z. J. Lipowski: Physical illness, the individual and the coping process. Psychiatry Med. *1:*91–102, 1970.
36. E. Kübler-Ross: *On Death and Dying.* New York: Macmillan, 1970.
37. R. D. Abrams: The patient with cancer: His changing pattern of communication. New Eng. J. Med. *274:*317–322, 1966.
38. E. P. Richardson, Jr.: Neurologic effects of cancer. *In Cancer Medicine,* J. F. Holland and E. Frei, III, eds., Philadelphia: Lea & Febiger, 1973, pp. 1057–1067.
39. P. B. Croft and M. Wilkinson: The incidence of carcinomatous neuromyopathy in patients with various kinds of carcinoma. Brain *88:*427–434, 1965.
40. W. L. Dobes, Jr., and R. R. Kierland: Dermatologic effects of cancer. *In Cancer Medicine,* J. F. Holland and E. Frei, III, eds., Philadelphia: Lea & Febiger, 1973, pp. 1067–1074.
41. B. F. Bower and G. S. Gordan: Hormonal effects of nonendocrine tumors. Ann. Rev. Med. *16:*83–118, 1965.
42. G. S. Gordan, B. S. Roof, and A. Haldan: Skeletal effects of cancers and their management. *In Cancer Medicine,* J. F. Holland and E. Frei, III, eds., Philadelphia: Lea & Febiger, 1973, pp. 1075–1083.
43. W. B. Kremer and J. Laszlo: Hematologic effects of cancer. *In Cancer Medicine,* J. F. Holland and E. Frei, III, eds., Philadelphia: Lea & Febiger, 1973, pp. 1085–1099.
44. G. P. Bodey: Infections in patients with cancer. *In Cancer Medicine,* J. F. Holland and E. Frei, III, eds., Philadelphia: Lea & Febiger, 1973, pp. 1135–1165.

5. Detection and diagnosis

In Chapter 4 we discussed briefly the effects of a tumor on the host, outlining a variety of problems commonly associated with more advanced cancer. These effects on the host constitute diagnostic signs of the disease. Although many patients do have advanced disease when they are seen initially in the clinic, and thus may exhibit these overt, unmistakable symptoms, most present with less advanced or even asymptomatic cancer. The latter frequently may be diagnosed only when the patient is being examined for some other condition. Since, as we saw in Chapter 1, small and asymptomatic tumors tend to be more curable than larger cancers, it is clearly vital that the disease be diagnosed at as early a stage as possible. Not only is the tumor then more amenable to therapy, but the patient is likely to be in comparatively good health and better able to tolerate rigorous treatment than a patient who is debilitated. Unfortunately, ideals of early detection are not always realized. Current diagnostic techniques are unable to detect most forms of cancer when the tumor volume is less than about 1 cm^3, by which stage metastasis may already have occurred. To compound the problem, a large section of the population, especially the poorer section, have no routine physical examinations and resort to a doctor only when a serious problem exists. These factors emphasize the need for improvements in both diagnostic techniques and the medical sophistication of the lay population. In addition to merely detecting the presence of a cancer, accurate diagnosis establishes the cytological type and stage of the disease, basic parameters that are essential in making rational therapeutic decisions.

In this chapter, we will outline the types of test used to diagnose cancer, pointing out their limitations as well as their advantages. In keeping with the fact that the larger proportion of cancers are diagnosed as a result of patients visiting a physician because of some symptom that causes concern, we shall begin with a brief consideration of self-examination.

SELF-EXAMINATION

The effective use of self-examination depends upon public information as to its need and the methods to be used. Two major objectives exist in this public effort, the first to persuade people to seek medical help when certain warning signs appear, the second to persuade them to take part in special screening programs even when they have no obvious health problem. It is interesting that studies made in Britain, Canada, and the United States all suggested that large-scale public educational programs, using pamphlets, posters, books, or films, are less effective than person-to-person communication and television in reaching and influencing people, particularly those in less advantaged socioeconomic groups, precisely the ones most at risk (1,2). The role of the physician as an informed individual who can relate to the patient on a one-to-one basis is particularly important in terms of ability to persuade people to enter screening programs, for example, although doctors are not always well prepared for this (3). Among organizations involved in public education about cancer, the American Cancer Society has been prominent, and its efforts are typified by the widely publicized "seven warning signals":

Change in bowel or bladder habits
A sore that does not heal
Unusual bleeding or discharge
Thickening or lump in breast or elsewhere
Indigestion or difficulty in swallowing
Obvious change in wart or mole
Nagging cough or hoarseness

Among the self-examination procedures that can be taught are breast examination, a guaiac test for blood in the stools, an irrigation test for cervical cancer, and sputum collection (4). In the latter three examples, samples are mailed to a laboratory or a physician's office for the actual diagnostic workup. The self-examination involves the obtaining of specimens, which often may be much less embarrassing to patients than when a physician obtains them.

Although self-examination is clearly important for its role in encouraging patients to seek early medical help, the degree of adherence to recommended procedure and frequency may be so low that its full advantage may not be realized in practice. Such methods as irrigation for cervical cancer are clearly less adequate than the Pap smear carried out by trained personnel, but where the alternative is no examination, irrigation is preferable.

SURGICAL DIAGNOSIS

Surgical intervention followed by cytological study of the specimens that are collected is the major procedure for detection and diagnosis of cancer. Two approaches exist, biopsy and laparotomy. The form of biopsy that is preferable is excision biopsy, in which the lesion and surrounding normal tissue are removed. For very large tumor masses, only a portion may be excised for examination, but the specimen must be removed in such a way as to cause minimal injury and dissemination of cells (5). Once obtained, the specimen is studied cytologically. In many cases, a patient may remain on the operating table while frozen sections of the biopsy material is examined. It should be noted that so-called frozen sections are less satisfactory than conventional stained sections, and it may be necessary to wait for the results of the latter if there is doubt over the diagnosis. In the case of many soft-tissue tumors, it may be that a delay of 5 days or more between biopsy and surgical removal of the tumor is needed to enable residual tumor cells in the area of excision to become immobilized by biopsy-induced fibrosis.

In needle biopsy, the needle is positioned so that on penetrating the tissues it cuts out a small round section. A needle and syringe is used for aspiration biopsy, in which interstitial fluid and cells are drawn back into the syringe. Needle biopsies do not involve the need for cutting or suturing in all cases and can thus be used with minimal distress to the patient. The method is applicable to all sites within reach of the usual 20-cm needle.

The major problem with all forms of surgical biopsy is the danger of spreading cancer cells along the track of the needle or the line of sutures. Penetration of a highly vascularized organ could also lead to serious internal bleeding. Also, an adequate number of samples should be collected, since, especially with needle biopsies, the chance of false negatives is high.

Laparotomy, an exploratory opening of the abdominal cavity, has long been used when symptoms suggest the presence of a tumor, but no radiological procedure can demonstrate it. Such surgery serves both to obtain samples and to visualize the extent and location of the tumor. In some cases, particularly with the lymphomas, laparotomy is valuable in the staging of the disease, which, as we saw in Chapter 1, is very critical for prognosis. In these patients, exploratory laparotomy is combined with removal of the spleen, which contributes both to proper diagnosis and to therapy of the lymphoma. A procedure often carried out during laparotomy is to affix radiopaque clips so that the involved region can be accurately defined when portals for radiation therapy are being mapped out. Another advantage of laparotomy is that biopsy specimens can be collected from regions that clearly look abnormal; needle biopsies undertaken without opening the body cavity may miss such regions and thus give false negatives. However, any major resection of this type entails the traumas of anesthesia, surgery, and recovery, as well as the risk of infection or dissemination of tumor cells.

CYTOLOGICAL DIAGNOSIS

In the section on surgical detection of cancer, it was stated that samples obtained by those methods are examined cytologically; this is also true of specimens obtained by non-surgical procedures. Although cytological diagnosis of cancer has been used for more than a century, the modern development and widespread use of this approach is tied to the studies of Papanicolaou (6). His work on cancer of the uterine cervix served as a model for application to many other tumor sites and established the value of *exfoliative cytology*, the examination of cells shed from such accessible sites within the body as the female genital tract, the respiratory pathways, and the urinary and gastrointestinal tracts.

Technical details of cytological diagnosis may be found elsewhere (7). Freshly collected specimens or those fixed in alcohol immediately after collection are best, as deterioration of the specimen may mask many of the abnormalities diagnostic of cancer. For the study of cells, smears are most satisfactory, with embedding in paraffin of sediments centrifuged down from fluids a less preferred method. In studying cells from the female genital tract, cervical smears, vaginal or endometrial aspirates obtained with appropriate pipettes, and material collected during curettage are the types of specimen usually obtained. Sputum coughed up from the bronchial tree can be used in preliminary screening for disease of the respiratory tract. However, sputum collection has been supplemented by the use of bronchial brushing (this serves to remove surface cells) and thin-needle aspiration. For urinary tract examination, separation of sediment from the urine, scraping from the urethral wall, aspiration of prostatic fluid, and bladder washing carried out during cystoscopy are the usual procedures. During examination of the gastrointestinal tract, specimens may be obtained by scrape smears of visible lesions, for the mouth; lavages with saline, use of a Levin tube, or collection with a fibergastroscope equipped with a saline jet stream and an aspirator for disease of the esophagus and stomach; saline lavages for the colon; and needle biopsy for the liver. For effusions, sediment from fluids that accumulate in body cavities, as well as spinal fluid, is examined after fixation. Nipple secretions may be so examined (8). Cytological techniques have also been applied to other sites, such as the skin, ears, eyes, and larynx, with varying degrees of success (8).

Once collected, fixed, and stained, cancer cells are identified by their special features (see Chapter 1). They include abnormal nuclei, enlarged nucleoli, altered staining properties, lower mutual adhesiveness, increased numbers of mitotic figures with more frequent abnormal figures, occasional chromosomal abnormalities, such as the Philadelphia chromosome, and the presence of special "signal" cells, such as the Reed-Sternberg cell. Changes in cell type indicative of metaplasia or infections often may be seen. However, a considerable element that is subjective and dependent on the experience of the pathologist goes into the diagnosis, especially in borderline cases. Occasionally, therapeutic modalities used in a patient may modify the appearance of cytological specimens collected from a region that has no disease. Thus, cells collected from the uterine cervix or even from the bronchial tree of patients receiving the alkylating agent busulfan for myelogenous leukemia may show abnormalities resembling cancer (9). Similar changes may result from other drugs and from radiation.

RADIOLOGICAL TESTS

A range of diagnostic techniques may be loosely grouped together as radiological, even if certain of them, such as thermography, make no use of ionizing radiation. The use of x-rays for both diagnosis and therapy followed within months of their discovery by Roentgen in 1896. Over the intervening years, an impressive array of procedures have been developed and represent major tools in the diagnosis and evaluation of most cancers. For more comprehensive descriptions the reader is referred to other texts (10,11), the sources of the present outline.

Conventional x-rays

Conventional x-ray examination is one of the most generally useful techniques for diagnosing and staging cancer. In its simplest form, it is exemplified by the chest x-ray, which is, with sputum cytology, the major method of diagnosing lung cancer. For this purpose x-rays between 70 and 150 kVp are needed, and postero-anterior and lateral films are obtained. Comparison with previous films is always preferable because of the information provided about growth rates. Primary lung tumors are usually not visible until they are about 1 cm in diameter. Lesions that do not change over a 2-year period or which take more than 16 months to double in size are unlikely to be malignant. Those that double in size in less than one month are also probably not malignant, although metastatic osteosarcomas, testicular tumors, and choriocarcinomas often grow extremely rapidly. The type of tumor is also suggested by its effects on the bronchi, as visualized in selective bronchograms.

For tumors of the gastrointestinal tract, it is necessary to administer a radiopaque material, usually containing barium, which outlines the inner contours of the parts of the tract. Sequential x-ray films of the passage of the barium swallow can reveal points of constriction, or other abnormalities along the tract, that result from the presence of a tumor. Malignancies on the outer wall of the gut will not be visualized unless their growth distorts the inner cavity; early pancreatic cancers are similarly difficult to diagnose.

Angiography

As they grow, tumors will distort the preexisting vascular supply, and through angiogenesis, direct new supply vessels toward the neoplastic tissues. By the injection of water-soluble radiopaque material, x-ray films may be made of the blood supply to establish whether there is a disturbance that could be attributed to a tumor. Angiography is usually used as an additional procedure to confirm a tentative diagnosis made by some other method. In such diseases as pancreatic carcinoma, in which other methods may not be applicable, angiography is a primary diagnostic tool. Similar in principle to angiography, in *percutaneous transhepatic cholangiography* the smaller bile ducts are punctured blindly with a needle, the bile is aspirated, and radiopaque dye is injected to allow the biliary tree to be visualized. In lymphangiography, drainage of radiopaque dye is observed in the lymphatic system.

Pneumoencephalography

Displacement of cerebrospinal fluid with a gas, such as air, helps to outline the subarachnoid space and the ventricular system when x-rays are taken, giving better definition of tumors.

Intravenous urography

This involves injection of radiopaque dye into the peripheral circulation, and observation of the progress of the dye into the urinary system. It has been used most often in the workup of children with Wilms' tumor and in bladder cancer.

Radionuclide scanning

In contrast to methods that involve radiopaque materials and external radiation, radionuclides may be administered and this internal radiation scanned from outside. One such radionuclide preparation is technitium-99m pertechnetate, perhaps the most widely used material currently. In brain tumors, for example, the tumor engenders a breakdown of the local blood-brain barrier, or increased local vascularity, and in some cases may take up the isotope, which gives rise to a region of higher density on a scan than the normal brain. Among other radionuclides are iodine-131 or iodine-125, which because of their selective uptake by the thyroid may be used in scans of this organ. Selectivity of uptake and tissue penetration and the emission of gamma rays that can be detected externally are necessary criteria for choice of radioisotope. Radionuclide scans have a fairly high frequency of false negatives, although probably less than angiography has. For tumors such as glioblastomas and meningiomas (brain tumors), however, radionuclide scans may be effective in diagnosing around 95 percent of the cases, but metastatic disease and astrocytomas are much less easily detected (around 70 percent). Apart from the two isotopes mentioned, gallium-67 as the citrate has found increasing use, particularly for such conditions as Hodgkin's disease. Other salts and complexes of technetium are also used quite frequently.

Computerized axial tomography (CAT scans)

This comparatively new technique, which has been of special value for brain tumors, depends on the fact that different tissues absorb x-rays to varying extents. Although many of the differences may be minor, computerization maximizes them. A narrow beam of x-rays is directed at a patient's head, or other parts of the body, but instead of remaining stationary, the source is rotated slowly about the part in synchrony with very sensitive detectors. Data are processed by computer and pictures generated on a cathode ray tube; these are photographed. Each picture represents a slice through the part x-rayed. In the brain, ventricular spaces appear black or dark gray as does air or fatty tissue, neurons are light gray, and bone and choroid plexuses appear white, as do calcified lesions and clotted blood. Injection of radiopaque dyes may increase the contrast of CAT scans, so that less well-defined lesions can be identified. To a large extent the CAT scan is displacing the use of radionuclide scans for brain tumors in the large hospitals possessing the necessary equipment, and is being adapted for other tumor sites.

Mammography, xeroradiography, and thermography

These techniques have been widely used in the diagnosis of breast cancer. In mammography, the x-ray unit uses a molybdenum target tube and filter, which provide low energy photons that give good contrast of the breast structures and low radiation doses. With age there is increasing replacement of breast tissue with fat, which offers a radiolucent background. Benign tumors frequently show well-defined borders and are rather homogeneous, whereas malignancies are usually poorly defined with infiltrations into neighboring tissues and variable radiographic density within the tumor. Some malignant lesions show fine sand-like calcifications. Other changes include deposition of fibrous tissue, which disturbs the symmetry of the breast and may shorten Cooper's ligaments, the major supportive element in the organ, leading to skin and nipple retraction.

With xeroradiography, films are not used, but instead x-rays from a tungsten target impinge on an electrostatically charged aluminum plate covered with the semi-conductor selenium. Charges leak from the plate in proportion to the amount of x-rays falling on it. The electrostatic image is visualized by applying an oppositely charged blue powder, and this image is then transferred to paper and sealed in plastic. The image has superior detail, especially in regard to edges and boundaries of anatomical structures, but large soft tissue regions give less contrasting images than they do in conventional films.

Thermography entails no radiation, and thus offers advantages over even low-dose mammography. The temperature of the skin near a tumor is generally higher than that in other areas, and in addition, because of the insulating nature of fatty tissue, heat can only be carried away from underlying tumors by venous blood flow that leads to the subareolar venous plexus. "Hot spots" in the skin and excessive heat carried by blood into the superficial veins can be identified by appropriate infrared scanners. The infrared emission from the breast is detected with a sensitivity around 0.1 to 0.2°C. When the superficial vascular patterns are visualized in the normal breast, they may vary from a virtually avascular to a diffuse, but highly vascularized pattern. Unilateral exaggeration of the pattern, areas of localized elevated heat emission from the skin, and abnormal emission from the areola are the usual findings associated with breast tumors. Apart from the malignancies, many benign tumors, especially fibroadenomas, increase heat emission.

Ultrasonography

Narrow beams of ultrasound may be used for purposes of scanning for tumors in such solid, soft-tissue organs as the liver, spleen, pancreas, and kidneys. The sound is reflected from tissue interfaces, much as in the well-known sonar system used by ships. These reflections are detected and visualized as a cross-sectional image. Many tissues, such as the liver, are free of internal echoes, but a tumor within the organ can often be identified by its scattered echoes. Solid malignant tumors may be distinguished from cysts, but not from benign tumors or granulomas. This technique cannot be used for hollow, gas-filled organs, such as the intestines, since gas within the organ scatters the ultrasound.

DIRECT INSPECTION OF LESIONS

Instrumentation now exists to examine tumors on the walls of most hollow body structures. This approach has been used since the early nineteenth century, but semirigid instruments prevented its widespread application. Beginning in 1958, flexible fiberoptic techniques became available and were immediately applied to medical instrumentation, leading to a quantum jump in the usefulness of this procedure (12). The fiberoptics permit illumination and viewing around curves and can detect lesions too small to be seen on x-rays. Complete, detailed examination of a wide area is possible, for example, 95 to 100 percent of the stomach can be studied by gastroscopy. Proctosigmoidoscopy, in which the rectum and up to 25 cm of the distal colon can be examined, has been recommended as a routine biennial examination for those over 40 because of the high incidence of colorectal cancer in this population; similar instruments are used to examine the bronchi (bronchoscopy) and the bladder (cystoscopy). The chief risk of such procedures is from perforation of the walls of the organ, an emergency to be met with antibiotics and surgical repair. Laparoscopy, in which the fiberoptic endoscope is passed into the peritoneal cavity through an abdominal incision, is a modification of this type of procedure that permits detection of metastases on the outer surfaces of the viscera and the walls of the peritoneum.

BIOCHEMICAL DIAGNOSTIC TESTS

A wide variety of biochemical tests are used to help in the diagnosis of cancer (13,14). Some of these are rather general tests, whereas others are specific for certain diseases; all involve sampling of blood or urine.

General tests

Lactic dehydrogenase is elevated in the plasma of about 40 percent of cancer patients, but more pronounced in a greater proportion is a shift toward isozymes that do not migrate far from the cathode during electrophoresis and which are more effective catalysts under anerobic conditions. This may relate to Warburg's theory of greater anerobic metabolism in tumors (15). *Aldolase* isozymes show differential ability to catalyze the breakdown of fructose-6-diphosphate (FDP) and fructose-1-phosphate (FIP). In tumors, and in the plasma from many cancer patients, the ratio of activities with FDP to those with FIP rises. Among trace elements, serum levels of *zinc* appear to be lower ($< 100\ \mu g/ml$) in cancer patients than in controls (75 to 125 $\mu g/ml$), whereas serum *copper* is elevated (13). Metastatic bone disease frequently leads to elevated *calcium* levels. We described *hypoalbuminemia* in Chapter 4, but in addition, plasma α_1 and α_2 globulins may be elevated, and abnormal globulins appear. These abnormal globulins and fetal proteins may sometimes be used as indices of response of the tumor to treatment.

Specific tests

Carcinoma of the prostate is associated, in 75 percent of patients, with elevated serum *acid phosphatase*. It may also be elevated in such other diseases as osteogenic sarcoma, breast carcinoma, and chronic granulocytic leukemia. *Amylase* in the serum is elevated in about one-quarter of patients with carcinoma of the pancreas. *Alkaline phosphatase* is frequently found at higher levels in the serum of patients with primary liver and bone cancer, and a placental type isozyme occurs more commonly in patients with cancer. This enzyme comes from the tumor itself. Alkaline phosphatase is also a reliable indicator of metastatic liver disease. Excretion of *catecholamine metabolites*, particularly 3-methoxy-4-hydroxymandelic acid (vanillylmandelic acid; VMA), in greater than normal amounts is characteristic of nearly all children with neuroblastoma (16).

IMMUNOLOGICAL DIAGNOSIS

Two types of immunological tests may show change in cancer patients (17). In many cases, there is a relatively nonspecific drop in immune competence, visualized by such procedures as inability to react to vaccines and failure to reject skin grafts. Apart from this, a variety of tumor-associated antigens are found in the serum. They include carcinoembryonic antigen of the digestive tract, α-fetoprotein, placental alkaline phosphatase, α_2-H-ferroprotein, fetal sulfoglycoprotein antigen, and T-globulin.

CONCLUSION

Although advanced cancer may present distinct symptoms, for most patients a battery of tests must be used to establish not only the presence of a cancer, but its stage and type, criteria that are vital predictors of response. Such tests include biopsy, cytological examination, a number of radiographical procedures, direct examination with fiberoptic equipment, and biochemical and immunological studies. A necessary component of cancer diagnosis, however, is willingness of the population to take part in screening programs and to visit physicians promptly when symptoms occur.

REFERENCES

1. J. Wakefield: *Cancer and Public Education*. London: Pitman Medical Publishers, 1963.
2. C. D. Sansom, J. Wakefield, and K. M. Pinnock: Choice or chance? How women come to have a cytotest done by their family doctors. Int. J. Health Educ. *14:*127–138, 1971.
3. International Union against Cancer Monograph Series, Vol. 4: *Cancer Detection*. Berlin-Heidelberg-New York: Springer-Verlag, 1974.
4. A. I. Holleb: Self-examination in the asymptomatic patient. *In Cancer Mdicine*. J. F. Holland and E. Frei, III, eds., Philadelphia: Lea & Febiger, 1973, pp. 315–320.
5. A. S. Ketcham: Modern trends in the prevention of cancer recurrence. *In Current Problems in Surgery: Surgical Oncology*. Bern: H. Huber, Publ., 1970.
6. G. N. Papanicolaou: *Atlas of Exfoliative Cytology*. Cambridge: Harvard University Press, 1954; Supplement I, 1956; Supplement II, 1960.
7. L. G. Koss: *Diagnostic Cytology and Its Histopathologic Bases*. Philadelphia: J. B. Lippincott, 1968.
8. L. G. Koss: Cytologic diagnosis of cancer. *In Cancer Medicine*, J. F. Holland and E. Frei, III., eds. Philadelphia: Lea & Febiger, 1973, pp. 320–335.
9. M. L. Feingold and L. G. Koss: Effects of long-term administration of busulfan. Arch. Int. Mad. *124:*66–71, 1969.
10. J. F. Holland, and E. Frei, III., eds. *Cancer Medicine*. Philadelphia: Lea & Febiger, 1973, pp. 391–488.
11. R. J. Steckel and A. R. Kagan: *Diagnosis and Staging of Cancer: A Radiologic Approach*. Philadelphia-London-Toronto: W. B. Saunders, 1976.
12. B. F. Overholt: Gastrointestinal endoscopy. *In Cancer Medicine*, J. F. Holland and E. Frei, III, eds. Philadelphia: Lea & Febiger, 1973, pp. 378–382.
13. G. Raynoso: Biochemical tests in cancer diagnosis. *In Cancer Medicine*, J. F. Holland and E. Frei, III, eds. Philadelphia: Lea & Febiger, 1973, pp. 335–348.
14. J. H. Wilkinson: Clinical applications of isoenzymes. Clin. Chem. *16:*733–739, 1970.
15. O. Warburg and S. Minami: Versuche an uberlebenden Carcinomgewebe. Klin. Wochenschr. *2:*776–777, 1923.
16. S. E. Gitlow, L. B. Dziedzic, and S. W. Dziedzic: Catecholamine metabolism in neuroblastoma. *In Neuroblastoma*. C. Pochedly, ed. Acton, Mass.: Publishing Sciences Group, 1976, pp. 115–154.
17. P. Gold: Immunologic diagnostic techniques. *In Cancer Medicine*, J. F. Holland and E. Frei, III, eds. Philadelphia: Lea & Febiger, 1973. pp. 349–356.

6. The etiology of cancer

The cause of cancer is a topic that has excited speculation since the days of Galen. In earlier chapters we considered the implications that could be drawn from cancer epidemiology and alluded to such agents as viruses, chemical carcinogens, radiation, and dietary factors that appear to be involved in the development of cancer, and it is now appropriate to consider them in more detail. These agents may be grouped into two categories. In the first category we have those that are basically endogenous to the host, such as genetic predisposition, psychological makeup, immune competence, and endocrine or metabolic factors. To these innate factors must be added a second category: assaults of external origin, such as chemical carcinogens, radiation, sunlight, and viruses or other infectious agents.

For both etiological categories there probably exists a similar underlying sequence of events involving the interaction of two or more factors of those listed. It is well established that more than one step is needed to transform a normal cell into a cancerous one. This is compatible with the action of chemicals that induce cancer in experimental animals and with clinical observations of human cancers, such as carcinoma of the uterine cervix with its long latent phase during which stages of metaplasia and dysplasia finally give way to carcinoma-*in situ*. Also in agreement with this is the concept of tumor progression to greater malignancy as manifested during the growth of a cancer. This multistage theory of carcinogenesis was proposed first by Nordling (1) to explain the fact that in many forms of human cancer the logarithm of the death rate increases in direct proportion to the logarithm of age. If only one event were necessary to transform a normal cell into a cancer cell, there would be no such time dependency, since the event would be expected to occur randomly throughout life. In contrast, the accumulation of a series of random events is, of necessity, time-related. Subsequently, the theory was modified mathematically to take into account the importance of the order in which the events occur (2) and observable departures from expected cancer death rates (3). In this discussion we shall outline the factors that have been implicated in the development of cancer, beginning with those classified within the endogenous category.

GENETIC FACTORS IN CANCER DEVELOPMENT

The fact that a cancer cell is able to pass on its characteristic features to a large progeny as the tumor grows, suggests that the initial events underlying malignant transformation include inheritable genetic changes. However, without additional study, it is impossible to determine the type of inherited change involved. Three major possibilities present themselves: genetic mutation in the germ cells such that the initial change is inherited in a Mendelian pattern; somatic mutation in which the primary events originate in tissue cells during the life-span of the individual who contracts cancer; and epigenetic changes that permanently alter gene expression.

Hereditary neoplasms

A number of cancers and preneoplastic states appear as inherited traits. Some of these conditions represent the sole expression of a genetic defect, but in many cases cancer, or a precancerous condition, is part of an overall syndrome that includes other abnormalities. The pattern of genetic transmission is commonly one of autosomal dominant inheritance, and since the defective gene is usually expressed in the heterozygous state, about one-half of the children of an affected subject will have the disease. However, the defect does not always find expression; it is then *incompletely penetrant,* with the penetrance expressed in percent, and as a result, persons without clinical symptoms may transmit the condition. These clearly inherited syndromes tend to be rather rare, to arise in life earlier than nonhereditary cancers, and to show multiple sites of origin within a tissue (4). To illustrate with a few examples we might cite retinoblastoma, an embryonic eye tumor with an incidence of 1:20,000 live births that is often associated with partial deletion of a D chromosome. Since the penetrance for this disease is between 80 and 90 percent, persons with no apparent defect can transmit the tumor to their offspring. About 5 to 10 percent of all cases involve familial occurrence with a higher incidence of bilateral tumors than in a non-familial or sporadic pattern (5). Nevoid basal cell skin cancers are part of an overall syndrome that includes such developmental defects as jaw cysts, skeletal abnormalities, calcification of soft tissues, and skin pits on the feet, as well as increased risk of medulloblastoma and ovarian fibromas. Although these tumors generally develop in childhood, a few may appear up to age 40, an age when the incidence of non-hereditary cancer is rising (6). Rather more common is polyposis coli, a condition with adenomatous polyps of the colon and rectum that in almost all cases give rise to carcinomas (7). The frequency of this disorder is around 1:8,000 live births and the penetrance is close to 80 percent. Gardner's syndrome, which includes osteomas, fibromas, and lipomas, in addition to intestinal polyps, may be a variant of polyposis coli (8). Table 6-1 lists some of the better known or more definitely genetically ascribed neoplastic conditions.

In addition to the neoplasms, a variety of preneoplastic states are hereditary. The *hamartomas* are malformations characterized by excessive localized tissue growth, which occasionally show neoplastic changes. Von Recklinghausen's disease, which was described earlier, is the best known of

Table 6-1 Some hereditary neoplasms and preneoplastic states.

Neoplasms	*Preneoplastic states*
Chemodectomas	*Hamartomatous lesions*
Gardner's syndrome	Multiple exostoses
Multiple endocrine adenomatosis	Tuberous sclerosis
Nevoid basal cell carcinoma	von Recklinghausen's neurofibromatosis
Pheochromocytoma	*Genodermatoses*
Polyposis coli	Albinism
Retinoblastoma	Dyskeratosis congenita
Trichoepithelioma	Werner's syndrome
Tylosis with esophageal cancer	Xeroderma pigmentosum
	Bloom's syndrome
	Fanconi's syndrome
	Immune deficiency
	Ataxia-telangiectasia
	Late-onset immunological deficiency
	X-linked agammaglobulinemia

Data derived from Table 1-2-1, Ref. 9.

these syndromes. Harmartomas show autosomal dominant inheritance. In contrast, the *genodermatoses*, of which xeroderma pigmentosum (10) is the most studied example, are usually autosomal recessive. Genodermatoses are genetic skin disorders, and such environmental factors as exposure to ultraviolet radiation, although they do not affect the underlying disorder, do increase the frequency of conversion to malignancies. Leukemias show a much higher incidence in individuals with certain genetic abnormalities (11). Other conditions are Bloom's syndrome, which exhibits photosensitive facial erythema; Fanconi's syndrome, which is an aplastic anemia accompanied by developmental abnormalities; and ataxia-telangiectasia, which involves cerebellar ataxia, telangiectasia (skin spots due to dilation of capillaries), and recurrent infections due to immune deficiency. These conditions may entail a 10 or 12 percent incidence of leukemia. All appear to involve chromosomal fragility with increased breakdown and recombination (12), and there is evidence of a deficiency in DNA repair mechanisms (13), as there is in xeroderma pigmentosum. It is of interest that chromosome abnormalities occur also in noninherited syndromes associated with leukemia. In Down's syndrome, an extra chromosome is produced during meiosis around the time of conception, and there is a 30-fold greater risk of contracting leukemia; the Philadelphia chromosome is associated with chronic myelogenous leukemia. Although the risk of acute lymphocytic leukemia is elevated in patients with ataxia-telangiectasia, this and other immune deficiency diseases are more characteristically associated with lymphorecticular tumors (14).

Turning from the rather uncommon conditions in which a tendency to develop cancer is clearly hereditary, we encounter a more nebulous group in which Mendelian inheritance is not involved, but in which there is a genetic predisposition to cancer. These conditions may be spoken of as *familial cancer* and have been uncovered empirically in the course of large statistical surveys. A major problem in establishing that such susceptibility is genetic is that environmental factors are usually difficult to rule out. It is in this area that study of twins may be most helpful. Comparison of identical twins has shown that for childhood leukemia there is about 20 percent correlation of incidence in the siblings, whereas fraternal twins showed no concordance (15). Similar suggestive evidence was obtained in Japan where the parents of sibling-pairs contracting leukemia had a high rate of consanguinity through cousin marriages (16). In adults, there may be as much as a threefold increase in risk among close relatives of subjects who develop carcinomas of the breast, stomach, prostate, colon, and lung (17); and childhood brain tumors and soft-tissue sarcomas may occur four times as frequently in the siblings of children with these tumors than in the population at large (15). These latter tumors would be expected to be less associated with environmental factors than would carcinomas, and hence afford a better opportunity to observe genetic effects. The genetic basis of breast cancer has recently been substantiated in more detail (18), although for this disease the appearance of virus particles in milk from women belonging to families with a history of the tumor does provide an alternative etiology (19). This viral aspect will be discussed later in the chapter. Although familial cancer is usually taken to refer to one particular site, examples of "cancer families" include also those with tumors at various sites, but of the same type, such as adenocarcinomas (17,20), and the increased incidence of rhabdomyosarcoma in children from families with high rates of cancer, particularly breast cancer (21). Many other examples of this phenomenon have been described (9). Finally, on a wider scale, the association of certain types of cancer with certain races and particular genetic groups have been observed. In the first example, Japanese families experienced a rise in the prevalance of colon cancer after migrating to the United States, which exhibits a high incidence of this disease, whereas rates for breast cancer remained at the low Japanese level in the first- and second-generation migrants (22), as would be expected for genetic determination. The second example is the association between blood group A and a higher incidence of stomach cancer (23).

Somatic mutations

An alternative genetic basis for permanent malignant change is a mutational event in a normal tissue cell, a so-called somatic mutation in contrast to mutations in the germ cells. From the early concept of a single event, as suggested by Boveri in 1914 (24), the theory has progressed through a two-stage initiation and promotion model (25) to a multistep process that involves somatic mutations and changes in gene expression. In such a modified theory, somatic mutations serve mainly to increase genetic variability so that cells with properties advantageous for their uncontrolled growth may be more readily selected (26). As we have seen in Chapter 2, the incidence of cancer increases with age, which is compatible with accumulation of mutational changes. Cultures of human cells from older individuals, as well as aging cultures of normal human cells, may show such aneuploid changes as loss of the second sex chromosome (27), increase in chromosomal aberrations (28), decreased ability to repair damaged DNA (29), and greater ease of transformation by oncogenic viruses (30). It has been suggested that many of the genetic changes that accumulate will do so preferentially in inactive portions of the genome, and thus errors will selectively collect in differentiated cells that divide rarely, if one assumes that repair is most likely to occur during DNA replication. If regulatory genes for cell division are located in the inactive portions of the genome, aging would decrease mitotic efficiency, leading to death for most cells and malignant changes for a few (31).

Epigenetic changes

In Chapter 1 we reviewed the subject of dedifferentiation in cancer at some length. Variable degrees of dedifferentiation coupled with cell proliferation, common to all cancers, tends to make them resemble embryonic tissue. Even so apparently characteristic a feature as metastasis finds analogies in the widespread migrations and invasions by primitive germ cells during embryonic development. Most of the tumor-specific products are also formed by normal cells of undifferentiated embryonic tissues. Thus, there may be said to be little evidence for marked changes in the genome of cancer cells, but considerable evidence from tumor reversibility experiments, studies of cell karyotypes, the many tumor secretion products, and the variable extent of control of tumor growth by endogenous host mechanisms for a pattern of defects in gene expression control (32).

Overall, it is clear that there is no one mechanism of genetic etiology in carcinogenesis. Within the framework of genetic etiology, as in chemical carcinogenesis, there is room for the operation of multiple factors both as initiators and as promotors (25). Inherited traits could clearly be regarded as initiators, and indeed experiments with phorbol esters, which are tumor promoters, show that malignant transformation of fibroblasts from humans with hereditary colorectal adenomatosis requires no further initiation (33). Somatic mutations could function both to promote and to initiate, and it is likely that the resulting genetic variability provides a cell population from which selection of more aggressive cell types may occur. Epigenetic changes also may play a major role in both initiation and promotion. However, many of these somatic mutational and epigenetic changes will represent the terminal results of processes set in motion by other endogenous or exogenous modalities, which we will consider later in this chapter.

PSYCHOLOGICAL ASPECTS OF CANCER ETIOLOGY

When Galen attributed cancer to abnormal unbalanced fluxes of black bile, he was also making an association between the disease and the psychological status of the patient. The term melancholy is derived from the Greek for black bile, and this word was used to describe both the emotional state and the humor responsible for it. Greek medicine had a psychosomatic orientation, one that was retained by Western medicine, steeped as it was in humoral theory, until the eighteenth century. In Greek medical theory, the six non-naturals formed the basis of health and disease, and of these the sixth included emotional disturbance (34). Throughout history, there has been an intuitive belief that emotional disturbances play a role in the etiology of cancer. Thus in the seventeenth century, Johannes Pechlin wrote, "I have seen an affection which was formerly a benign sort of tumor in women's breasts turn into a carcinoma when changed for the worse by fear or sorrow. Indeed, I have never seen a cancer of the breast so thoroughly removed, even after extirpation, that would not, in consequence of fear and sorrow, rather suddenly once again slowly recrudesce and, after long difficulties, at length put an end to life" (35). In the nineteenth century, Sir Astley Cooper wrote that "anxiety of mind, tending to the presence of slow fever and suppressed secretions are the predisposing causes of the complaint. A person, the prey of disappointment from reduced circumstances, and struggling against poverty, when her prospects begin to brighten, finds a malignant tumor in her breast; costive state of bowels, a dry skin, a paucity of other secretions have attended this anxious state of mind, and laid the foundation of that destruction which awaits her" (35). In the 1950's, LeShan and his colleagues reviewed much of the literature and distinguished four traits that might be identified in cancer patients: they suffered the loss of a major relationship prior to onset of their cancer; they were unable to express hostile emotions; they were sexually disturbed; and they had unresolved tensions regarding a parent (36,37). The possible relation between mental state and cancer continues to attract attention (38).

A major problem with the earlier observations, and most of the more recent literature on the psychological factors in cancer development, is that the subjects being studied already had cancer. The knowledge, or even the suspicion, that he or she has cancer could profoundly alter psychological and emotional states. Thus, it is possible to argue that the psychological effect of the disease, not some predisposing mental trait, is disclosed by such studies. Furthermore, in most cases no well-matched control groups were used, so it is not possible to sort out the contribution of such factors as age, race, socioeconomic status, or the fact of being hospitalized from traits that may be strictly related to cancer. It is apparent that definitive answers to the question of a possible psychological etiology of cancer require well-controlled and preferably prospective studies. It is impossible to detail all the more recent work in this area, but we shall summarize some of the better designed studies that illustrate the traits described by LeShan. As will be seen, there is often some conflict and inconsistencies in the data that may reflect the variation in degree of correlation between different forms of cancer and emotional disturbance.

LeShan and Reznikoff (39) compared 250 patients with cancer and 125 patients with other diseases and noted that whereas 64 percent of the cancer patients had suffered a traumatic event, such as loss or death of a parent or sibling during the first 7 years of life, only 10 percent of the controls had experienced a similar loss. The same correlation was seen when 25 patients with breast cancer were compared with 25 matched controls attending a cancer detection clinic (40). Birth of a sibling when the subject is still very young has also been considered a traumatic event for an infant that may be associated with a later cancer (39,40). However, it is hard to see how an event that occurs in the life of so large a fraction of the population could be a specific etiologic factor in this or any other disease. Other workers, such as Muslin (41), have not seen a correlation between early traumatic experiences and cancer, and experiments in rodents subjected to early maternal separation have been contradictory with regard to effects on resistance to transplanted tumors. Major emotional disturbances need not occur in infancy, and indeed, the association between cancer and emotional trauma may be clearer in adults. In those studies compiled by LeShan (37), a consistent finding was loss of a relationship 6 months to 8 years preceding diagnosis of cancer. Widowhood is associated with the highest cancer mortality rate, according to official statistics; divorce appears to be a lesser trauma (37,42). Greene noted that among 61 male patients with leukemia and lymphoma, 57 patients, or 93 percent of the total had suffered personal losses in the 4 years preceding onset of their disease, with a clustering in time of around 1 year (43); no controls were used in this study, presumably because of the convincingly high incidence of losses. Greer (44), like Muslin, was unable to correlate cancer and traumatic events in his controlled study of breast cancer patients. It is possible that some kinds of cancer exhibit such a correlation, whereas others do not. More likely, however, is Bahnson's suggestion (45,46) that it is not the loss itself so much as the patient's reaction to it that is the deciding feature. Hopelessness, in particular, is one reaction to loss that appears especially crucial, to such an extent, indeed, that Schmale and Iker used this as a criterion to predict the presence or absence of cancer with 77 percent accuracy in women predisposed to cancer of the cervix (47).

This brings us naturally to LeShan's second trait, the inability to deal with emotions; once again there is conflict in the data that may stem from differences in the various types of cancer and in the particular emotional behavior being examined. For example, Kissen, in a large study with two groups of matched controls, one for other thoracic disease, found that lung cancer patients had a history of poor emotional outlets, including a lower incidence of childhood behavioral disorders than the controls (48). On the other hand, Hagnell, in a prospective study carried out on 2,550 inhabitants of Essen-Moller, Sweden, performed personality evaluations in 1947, and then in 1957 located 20 men and 22 women from the surveyed population who had developed cancer in the intervening period. Each patient was matched with eight controls, and the only trait that emerged was that a higher proportion of the female cancer patients were substable with a low degree of emotional control (49). Most researchers feel that the major factor is not a general inability to express emotions, but an inability to express hostile feelings. This was apparent in a series of home interviews carried out by Bahnson, who remarked that cancer patients "do not strike back, do not curse and swear, kick and throw things, do not feel tense and restless, do not get excited or keyed up, do not blow up with anger, do not shake or tremble with rage, do not feel like giving up or feel depressed, and especially do not get angry with anyone or with themselves" (50). The controlled, prospective study of Thomas and Greenstreet involved 1,076 students who graduated from John Hopkins Medical School between 1948 and 1962. The students were initially evaluated during their first two years of medical school, and the nine students who later developed cancer had significantly lower anxiety and anger scores than a matched control group of 44 students or the total population of white students (51). It is striking that the inability to express anger was implicated as long ago as 1402 by Maestro Lorenzo Sassoli as a major cause of disease. ". . . let me speak to you regarding the things of which you must most beware. To get angry and shout at times pleases me, for this will keep up your natural heat, but what displeases me is your being grieved and taking all matters to heart. For it is this, as the whole of physic teaches, which destroys our body more than any other cause" (37).

Another characteristic frequently reported in cancer patients is sexual maladjustment (52). Work in this area has mainly involved women who develop cancer of the breast or uterine cervix. An example of this is the work of Stephenson and Grace who compared 100 women with cervical cancer to 100 women with cancer of nonsexual sites, and found indications of sexual maladjustment more frequently in the former group (53). This fits the concept that tumors develop in an organ related to the "frustrated psychophysiological object relationship" (54). In the female this would be the breast or cervix and in the male possibly the prostrate. General application of this concept is impossible, however, in view of such findings as a positive correlation between uterine cervical cancers and sexual activity, with possible involvement of a viral factor. As in all cancer etiology, there is a long sequence of initiating and promoting actions, not all of which are of the same nature.

Many of the findings in this area have implied not only a connection between cancer and sexual maladjustment, but also a connection between sexual maladjustment and relationships with parents. In some cases the association is with a dominant mother (55), in others there was unresolved hostility toward the mother (56). The findings with the Johns Hopkins' students mentioned above disclosed that the cancer patients had the lowest matriarchal dominance and a low closeness to parents scores (57). LeShan's study showed that 38 percent of the 250 patients with cancer had experienced significant tension in their relationships with one or both parents, and this tension reached a new poignancy after the parents' death; only 12 percent of matched controls experienced similar tension (39). There are methodological pitfalls in studies of this type. When Bahnson used a standard Roe-Siegelman Parent Child Relationship Questionnaire, the results suggested that cancer patients viewed their parents as more neglectful and cold than did healthy matched controls or patients with myocardial infarctions (46). Conversely, unstructured interviews tended to show that the cancer patients had very close attachments to a parent early in life, which proved impossible for the patient to transcend (50). Clearly, attention to methodology is needed to establish meaningful correlates.

Thus, we have seen that although the evidence for a psychological etiology of cancer is suggestive, it is not compelling. These results suffer in many cases from inadequate experimental design and lack of matched controls; prospective studies and adequate statistical treatment are needed. In other cases, major differences may reflect the heterogeneity of cancer rather than conflicting data. There is no reason why emotional disturbance or suppression of emotional outlets should be equally involved in the development of all types of cancer.

If we accept what the accumulating body of evidence now suggests, that psychological factors can induce cancer, or much more likely, promote its growth and proliferation, it is appropriate to speculate on the mechanisms that might be involved. The most probable mechanism involves hypothalamic disturbances of the endocrine balance, which, in turn, can affect the body's immune system (58); thus, experimental lesions made in the hypothalamus of guinea pigs have interfered with antibody production (59,60). The hypothalamic-pituitary axis is responsible for elaborating trophic hormones that stimulate the secretion of major hormone classes at peripheral sites. Among these classes of hormones are the adrenocortical steroids, which have a direct cytolytic effect on lymphoid cells, thus depressing the cellular immune system's defense against cancer (61, 62), and prolactin and the estrogens, which are known to influence breast and endometrial cancers (61). There is a positive correlation between levels of anxiety and psychological defensiveness and the secretion of adrenocortical steroids, which increases with intensifying anxiety (63,64). Environmental stimuli, such as stress during infancy and early life, may permanently alter the adrenocortical secretions and immunological defenses, perhaps predisposing to cancer later (64,65). This type of "imprinting" effect is well known in psychology and has been noted in such other areas as drug metabolism, when subjects received hormone therapy at an early age.

Thus, we can see that there is a rational basis for a psychological etiology of cancer, one that involves the mediation of endocrine and immunological mechanisms. However, there is a need for a more adequate evaluation of those psychological factors most closely associated with cancer, and their relationship to physiological functions, before attempting therapeutic or preventive intervention.

IMMUNOLOGICAL ASPECTS OF CANCER DEVELOPMENT

In the preceding section, it was suggested that psychological stress might promote the development of cancer through a circuitous route involving, in turn, the hypothalamic-pituitary axis, the endocrine system, and the immune system. It was pointed out that the necessary steps have been demonstrated experimentally (59–64), but we must now turn to the question of how the immune system might regulate tumor growth in order to complete this pathway. It is first appropriate to review the main types of immune

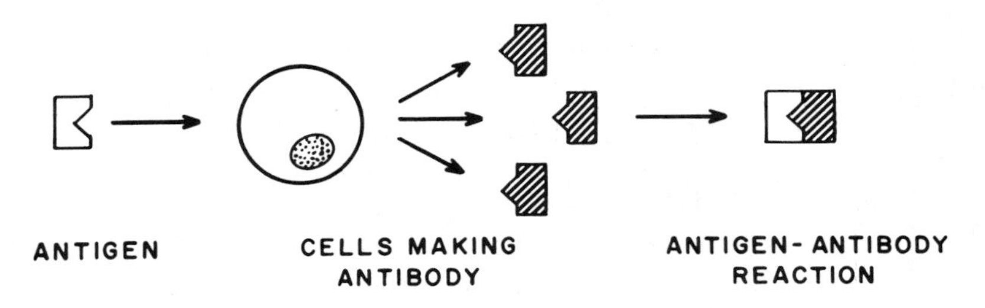

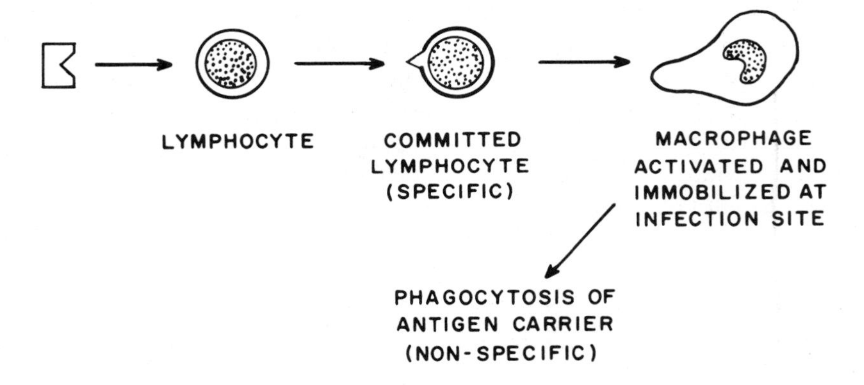

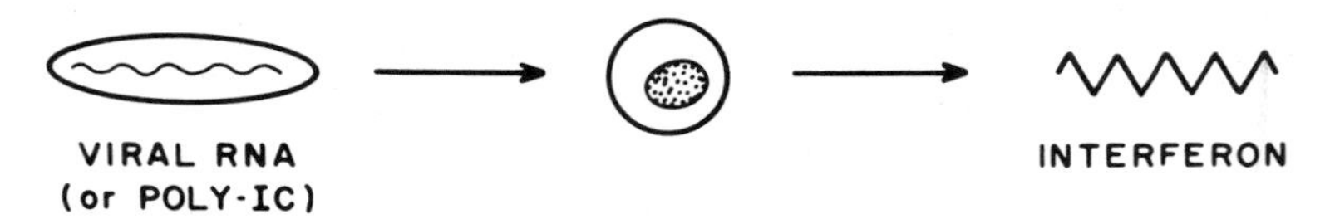

Figure 6-1 Schematic representation of the major types of immune response.

response to foreign material as outlined in Figure 6-1. Here our main concern is with the two major forms of immunity mediated by antibodies and by cells, respectively, although as we shall see these are not completely exclusive mechanisms. The production of interferon, which has recently been shown to inhibit tumor growth, will be considered in Chapter 9 as a research approach to cancer therapy. It is now clear that two different lymphocyte types are primarily responsible for specific immune response, the B-cells, which undergo a bursal equivalent maturation process and secrete antibodies, and the T-cells, which undergo thymus-dependent differentiation and are responsible for specific cell-mediated immunity. In addition, nonspecific lymphoid cells, killer cells or NK-cells, lyse tumor cells with bound antibody, and macrophages may exert cytotoxic effects. The B- and T-cell systems interact by way of helper and suppressor T-cells and monocytes, as illustrated in Figure 6-2. These interactions involve both negative and positive regulation and control the overall functioning of the immune system. Since the primary initiating event for the system is the presence of an antigen, a specific recognizable structure, or a foreign body, for the purposes of this discussion we must first establish that tumors possess distinct antigens that are detected by the immune system, even if the tumor cells originate from normal cells. Next we will deal with the question of how a tumor might be susceptible to immune reactions, and then with the mechanism that might prevent such a reaction from occurring, thus allowing the tumor to grow.

Tumor-specific antigens

Following unsuccessful attempts to vaccinate against cancer early in this century, there was a hiatus in tumor immunology until the early 1940's, when a variety of inbred mouse strains and transplantable neoplasms became available. This overcame the early problem of distinguishing between rejection of tumor grafts due to specific antigens on the tumor and rejection due to a reaction to alloantigens present in both normal and tumor tissue of the donor, but not the recipient animal. These aspects have been reviewed elsewhere in more detail (66). From the early 1950's to the present, many studies have shown that tumors generally possess antigens against which rejection reactions can occur. Tumors induced by a particular virus, such as the polyoma virus, contained the same antigen, so that immunization of mice with polyoma tumor clones that did not release virus could produce immunity to tumor transplantation (67). Similar resistance to transplantation occurs against a methylcholanthrene-induced sarcoma in the primary (*autochthonous*) host after the primary tumor has been removed and irradiated cells from it inoculated repeatedly (68). Such tumor-specific transplantation antigens (*TSTA*) are thus surface antigens, in contrast to others that have been found intracellularly and thus do not nor-

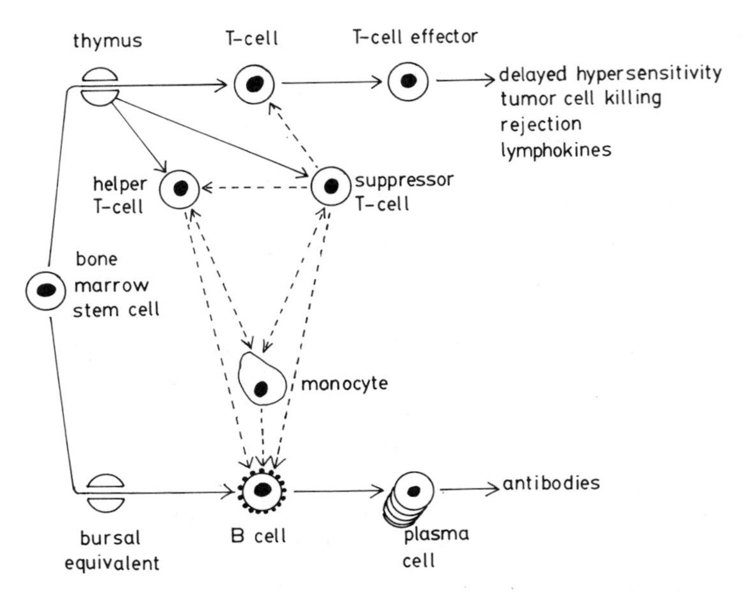

Figure 6-2 Schematic representation of cell regulatory mechanisms in lymphocyte differentiation. Some of the targets of regulatory control are represented by interrupted arrows. Reproduced from Ref. 97.

mally take part in immunological rejection. For some time it appeared that chemically induced tumors had distinct TSTA's for each tumor, in contrast to the virally induced tumors with antigens characteristic of the virus, as concluded from cross-reactivity studies (69–72). Later it became apparent that virally induced tumors might also possess individual antigens in addition to those referable to the virus, but detectability of the former may be affected by expression of the latter. Furthermore, many chemically induced tumors have common antigens (66). It is quite likely that many transplantation antigens, especially those of the unique individual group, may actually be embryonic in nature and reflect varying degrees of gene derepression occurring in different tumors (73). For this reason, such antigens are frequently referred to as *carcinoembryonic antigens* (CEA). Although viral nucleic acid or fragments of it may be detected in tumor cells by hybridization techniques (74), and the same TSTA may appear in several species infected with a virus such as polyoma, this does not mean that the antigen is directly determined by the virus. Trypsinization of normal cells may induce the appearance of TSTA of the same immunological properites as that induced by virus, indicating that the latter does not code directly for the antigen (75). Another phenomenon, *antigenic conversion,* may also lead to common tumor antigen. This is a secondary acquisition due to superinfection by another virus after the cells have already been transformed by the first infective agent (76). Finally, neoplastic transformation may in some way activate genes that are never normally expressed, a process that is known to occur in the case of the TL antigens of mouse leukemias (77). These glycoproteins are similar to the normal H-2 antigens, which may be found in leukemias of both TL-negative and TL-positive mouse strains. In the presence of anti-TL antibody *in vivo,* TL-positive cells may undergo *antigenic modulation,* in which they stop producing antigen and continue to grow even in an immunized host (78).

Immunological surveillance

Whatever the method for their acquisition, essentially all tumors that have been studied immunologically carry some sort of antigens and should be susceptible to immune control. Thus T-cells (79), monocytes (80), and macrophages (81) can recognize and kill malignant cells, which has led to the concept that a system of immune surveillance recognizes and eliminates cancer cells (82). Among the wide variety of evidence for such a system, we might cite the notably increased frequency of cancer in patients undergoing immunosuppressive therapy (83), the higher tumor take in thymectomized mice exposed to polyoma virus, even as adults (84), and the reduction in incidence of tumors and longer latency period before their appearance after specific vaccination with tumor antigens (85) or after nonspecific immunostimulation (86). However, not all the evidence clearly supports such a concept; also, although cell-mediated immune reactions always appear to work for tumor rejection, antibodies might frequently potentiate tumor growth by blocking antigenic sites on the tumor cells (66). Thus, the concept of cells and other immune systems primed to recognize and intercept newly formed tumors no longer fits the evidence best.

Escape from immunological surveillance. It is likely that several mechanisms prevent the immune systems, so effective in killing cancer cells *in vitro,* from eliminating or preventing the formation of tumors *in vivo.* During the early stages of growth, prior to angiogenesis, there may be very little antigen present and none of it reaches the blood circulation, so that there is inadequate stimulation to activate immune defenses. Then, a number of chemical carcinogens are known to function as immunosuppressive agents (87). There is also much evidence of a deficiency in the immune systems of tumor-bearing animals and humans (88,89), which is expressed at the cellular level by decreased mobilization and chemotactic responses of macrophages and monocytes (90,91). In some cases, products of the tumor are apparently responsible for these effects (92), and a recent study suggests that, although systemic activation of monocytes is seen in patients with solid tumors, the tumors themselves produced a heat-stable, low molecular weight material, similar to that in normal serum, which inhibits monocyte activation. Thus, successful tumors are able to protect themselves even if they do elicit a systemic immune reaction (93). The ultimate immune action on the tumor then depends on a balance between stimulation and inhibition. It is interesting to point out that even as ubiquitous a factor as insulin inhibits macrophage function, and insulin-like hormones are secreted by many tumors (94). Another possibility may be loosely categorized under the term *blocking factors.* At one time these were considered to be antibodies (95), but it is now apparent that many other materials, including antibody fragments, soluble antigens, and antigen-antibody complexes, may block the immune response (96). Such materials may block antigenic sites on tumor cells or specifically interfere with lymphocyte reactivity. Suppressor T-cells may act to potentiate tumor growth (97). These suppressor T-cells may regulate either humoral or cellular immune functions, as indicated in Figure 6-2, and generally are quite specific (97). As examples of each of these different types of intervention, we may cite inhibition of so-called "killer" T-cells (98), the production by suppressor cells of factors that inhibit humoral immune responses (99), the apparent blocking of polyclonal lymphocyte maturation in patients with multiple myeloma (100), and the correlation between the presence of suppressor T-cells and the incidence of lung metastases in patients with osteogenic sarcoma (101). There also appears to be a class of non-T suppressor cells which may be B-cells or macrophages; they appear to function in a similar manner to suppressor T-cells (102,103).

The immunology of tumors is clearly complex and far from completely understood. For this reason, attempts at immunotherapy are basically premature, and could be harmful in some cases, since either inhibition or enhancement of tumor growth may be achieved depending on the situation and the methods used. The suppressor cell system could be a fundamental element in the enhancement of cancer growth, since both blocking factors and reduced immunologic reactivity might result from their activity. It is even possible that some of the beneficial therapeutic effects of radiation, chemotherapy, and, in some cases, surgery might result from modulation of the suppressor cell system.

ENDOCRINOLOGICAL ASPECTS OF CANCER DEVELOPMENT

Disturbance in the endocrine balance is another of the endogenous factors that may predispose toward the development of cancer. In the late nineteenth century, Beatson described a link between the ovaries and breast cancer (104), but it was not until the 1940's and 1950's that major advances occurred in this area. Furth was responsible for the elaboration of many major concepts regarding tumor endocrinology. The review of Clifton and Sridharan may be consulted for a more detailed bibliography (105). It is not difficult to see how a normal tissue, such as the endometrial lining of the uterus, whose growth is normally controlled endocrinologically, might undergo a prolonged phase of abnormally rapid growth in the presence of a long-term endocrine imbalance. The steps from hyperplasia, through dysplasia to a tumor that might gradually become malignant have been followed in such conditions as bladder and uterine cervical growth disorders. In endocrine-stimulated disorders, the tumor that arises as a result of a disturbance, such as disruption of a feedback system, will depend on that particular endocrine environment and is thus said to be *hormone dependent.* Furth has discussed this definition as well as endocrinological aspects of tumor progression, whereby the tumor gradually becomes malignant as a result of changes occurring during sustained proliferation, loses its hormone dependence, and eventually becomes *autonomous* (106–108). If the original tissue secreted hormones, the tumor may or may not retain this capability, or it may produce intermediates in the synthetic chain, as for example, the production of an androgen instead of an estrogen. It should also be noted that hormones may be necessary for the growth of a cancer induced by other means, such as a chemical carcinogen, and they might also serve to "prime" or to increase the susceptibility of hormone-sensitive tissues to carcinogens (109). As a background to this discussion it might be helpful to review briefly the structure and mechanism of endocrine control.

Endocrine control

The major element in endocrine control is the hypothalamic-hypophyseal-end organ axis (Figure 6-3). A group of releasing or inhibiting peptides are

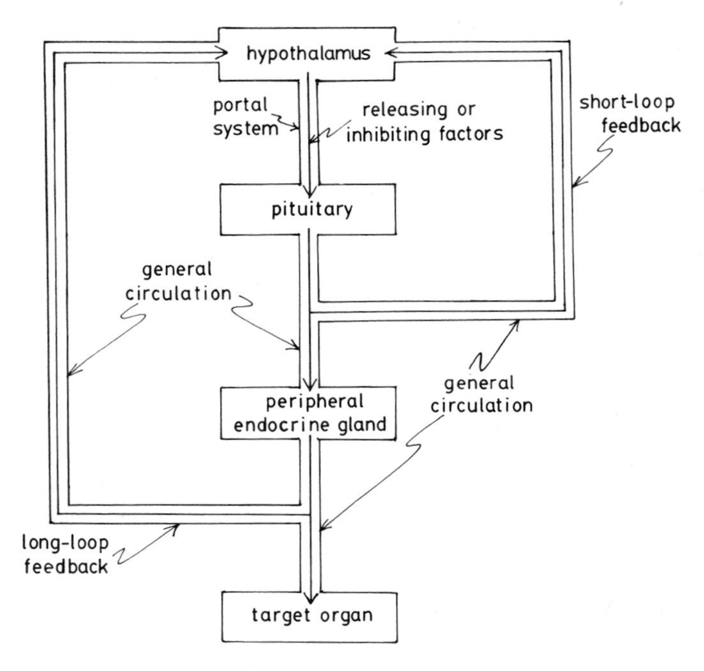

Figure 6-3 Schematic representation of the hypothalamic-hypophyseal-end organ axis for endocrine feedback control.

produced in the neuron cell bodies of the hypothalamus. They are transported along the axons and enter the veins of the hypophyseal portal system, which lead directly to sinusoids in the anterior pituitary. There these factors inhibit or stimulate the formation and release of specific hormones, which enter the blood and are carried to peripheral endocrine organs where they control the release of hormones (110). This control is effected by either short-loop feedback, in which peripheral levels of anterior pituitary factors regulate the activity of the hypothalamus, or long-loop feedback, which involves control of the hypothalamus by the action of hormones from the ultimate target endocrine organs. An example of the short-loop system is the feedback control of hypothalamic thyroid-releasing hormone (TRH) by pituitary thyrotropin (TSH; TtH); of long-loop control, the feedback inhibition of hypothalamic corticotropin regulatory hormone (CRH; ARH) by cortisol.

Hormone receptors

At the level of their action on tissues, hormones specificity depends upon receptors that fall into two distinct classes on the basis of the mechanisms of hormone-receptor interactions. Catecholamines and the peptide hormones, such as insulin, act on cell membrane receptors. Interaction of the hormone with the receptor modulates the formation of cyclic AMP, perhaps through conformational changes in the cell membrane. These changes alter one or more specific enzyme activities, an effect that becomes amplified as changing substrate levels further modulate other enzymes that are not involved directly with the hormone (Figure 6-4). Thus, a hormone, such as insulin, is able to bring about such diverse effects as increased RNA and protein synthesis, glycogen formation, gluconeogenesis, increased glucose utilization, and lipid synthesis, with the predominant action varying from one tissue to another (105).

Steroid and thyroid hormones do not react with surface receptors, but rather enter the cell and combine with a receptor present in the cytosol.

Figure 6-4 Schematic representation of the two principal types of endocrine receptors. Insulin-type receptors, more characteristic of peptide hormones, are mediated by cyclic AMP and are essentially cell-surface receptors. Steroid receptors are generally intracellular and involve interaction of a complex with chromatin and modulation through RNA synthesis.

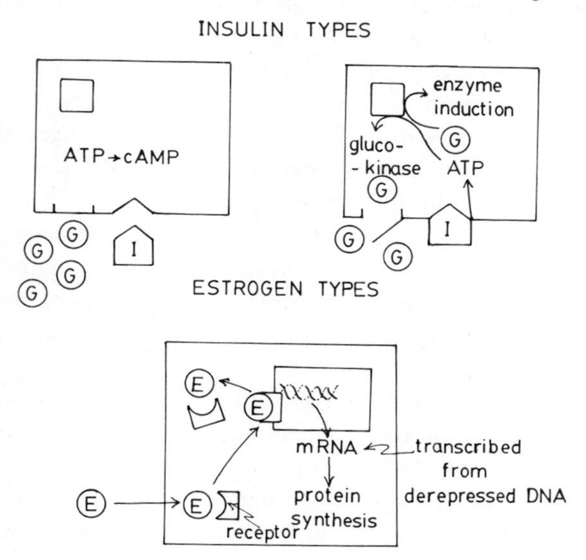

The hormone-receptor complex is then transported into the nucleus where it modulates transcription (111). The best known of this type of receptor is the estrogen receptor, a small cytoplasmic protein with sedimentation properties of 4 or 8S, depending on the medium, which undergoes a rapid non-temperature-dependent binding with estrogen. Transport of the complex into the nucleus does appear to be temperature dependent (112). The multiple actions of estrogens are due to subsequent binding by nuclear protein (5S complex), which associates with the operator loci of specific estrogen operons that contain linked cistrons (functional genes) coding for different derepressor RNA molecules. Thus, estrogen actions generally reflect gene derepression (111). Figure 6-4 presents this in schematic form.

Hormone-dependent tumors—the breast cancer model

In breast cancer, the most common cancer among Occidental women (see Table 2-5, p. 36), endocrine involvement and the value of hormonal therapy have been most definitively established. The primary stimulus for growth and differentiation of normal breast tissue is mammotropin or prolactin (MtH), which is secreted by the anterior pituitary. Secretion of MtH is reduced by a hypothalamic-inhibiting hormone (MIH) and increased by estrogens acting directly on the pituitary or acting indirectly through inhibition of MIH formation. Complete functioning of the breast also requires insulin, cortisol, and perhaps progesterone (105). Since estrogens stimulate MtH release, they could lead to the type of sustained hyperplasia that precedes development of a malignancy. Not surprisingly, therefore, estrogens can induce mammary tumors in rodents (112), and ovariectomy may lead to regression of mammary fibroadenomas (113). In addition, the development of clear cell carcinoma of the vagina in the daughters of women taking the synthetic analog diethylstilbestrol around the time of pregnancy (114), focuses attention on the ability of at least some estrogens to produce growth disorders in other estrogen-sensitive tissue. It is generally agreed that diethylstilbestrol is the most carcinogenic estrogen, with estradiol much less effective, but still more active than estrone; and estriol is inactive.

Recent work on breast cancer has shifted the focus of concern to the anterior pituitary: MtH, and occasionally somatotropin or growth hormone, which is closely related to MtH, can produce hyperplasia, and finally mammary carcinoma, in mice infected with mammary tumor virus, and can also increase the tumor yield in animals treated with methylcholanthrene

(115). Thus, the pituitary factors are in a sense acting as cocarcinogens, presumably by inducing growth. Various drugs that affect the anterior pituitary also are associated with mammary carcinomas. In rodents, the synthetic ergot alkaloid 2-bromo-α-ergocryptine suppresses release of MtH, as well as the biological processes of hyperplasia and carcinogensis (116). In humans, reserpine, which is used primarily for hypertension, increases circulating levels of MtH by inhibiting the release of MIH (117), and it is significant that there is apparently a threefold increase in the incidence of breast cancer in women receiving the drug over long periods (118). This latter finding has, however, been disputed on statistical grounds (119). Thyroid status is also relevant to the effect of MtH on breast cancer. Thyrotropin, the pituitary factor that stimulates thyroid activity, increases the sensitivity of rat mammary epithelium to MtH and also promotes the release of MtH (120). The presence of goiter and other thyroid abnormalities, appears to increase the incidence of breast cancer, which, historically, is higher in the "goiter belts" where iodine intake is low (121). This thyroid effect could, in part, be mediated through thyroid control of steroid hormone formation and metabolism, leading to a lowered urinary 17-hydroxycorticoid/androgen ratio, which appears to be a risk factor for breast cancer (122).

It has been known for a long time that early pregnancy reduces the risk of breast cancer by as much as 70 percent as compared to the risk in nulliparous women. It is the time of the first pregnancy, which should be carried to term, that is critical; further pregnancies offer little or no additional benefit. This suggests that we are dealing with a trigger-like effect that irreversibly changes factors associated with a higher risk. Since a full-term pregnancy is necessary, it appears that the second half, when circulating progestins, MtH, estriol, and placental peptide hormones rise to high levels, is the crucial phase. After age 30, a first pregnancy not only offers no protection, but may lead to a higher incidence of breast cancer than that seen in non-child-bearing women (123).

The relationship of hormones to carcinogenesis is complex. Although hormones themselves may be able to induce cancer, they more often appear to potentiate the carcinogenic action of other agents. In both cases, a sustained high level of cellular proliferation appears to be an important first step (124). Some examples of these carcinogenic actions may be given, in summary. In clear cell carcinoma of the vaginal mucosa, changes induced during fetal life by maternal exposure to diethylstilbestrol apparently remain dormant until activated by endocrine changes at puberty. A similar activation of latent damage may be involved in the development of thyroid adenomas and carcinomas around the time of puberty in subjects who were treated by x-irradiation during early life for thymic enlargement (125). In breast cancer, the proliferative state maintained by prolactin may provide a larger population for selection of malignant cells, especially in response to carcinogenic stimuli. Finally, the endocrine system could link the chain of events that relate psychological status and the development of cancer. In this discussion we have, of necessity, stressed breast cancer, because this is the disease for which the relationship to the endocrine system is clearest. However, many other tumors may have a hormonal component to their etiology. They include ovarian cancer, Leydig cell tumors, renal cortical carcinomas, medullary thyroid carcinomas, and perhaps prostate cancers. Some of these may induce other tumors through their endocrine activity (124).

METABOLIC ASPECTS OF CANCER DEVELOPMENT

There is little direct evidence that metabolic derangements *per se* are carcinogenic. In many cases it is difficult to isolate preexisting metabolic abnormalities from abnormalities related to the metabolism of the tumor. It has been noted, for example, that leukemic subjects frequently have a greater than normal ability to methylate the nucleic acid bases (126), but this could merely reflect the special features of leukemic cells. Of more interest is the possible role of tryptophan metabolites in the genesis of bladder cancer, the etiology of which has been better studied than of most other cancers. Dunning, in 1950, reported that tryptophan stimulated the induction of cancer by 2-acetylaminofluorene in rats (127), and it later became evident that tryptophan, or more probably some metabolite of tryptophan, could induce epithelial hyperplasia and cancer of the bladder (128, 129). Patients with bladder cancer have a number of tryptophan metabolites in larger than normal amounts in their urine (130); these metabolites are indicated in Figure 6-5, and certain of them have been identified as carcinogens in several animal species. It is also evident from Figure 6-5 that pyridoxal phosphate, and hence its dietary precursor pyridoxine, can modify the pattern of tryptophan metabolism through involvement in certain reactions. The principal effect of pyridoxine seems to be a relative increase in the non-carcinogenic metabolites kynurenic and anthranilic acids. It should be pointed out that the bladdder is peculiarly sensitive to many natural and synthetic carcinogens, because, through urinary excretion, the bladder is

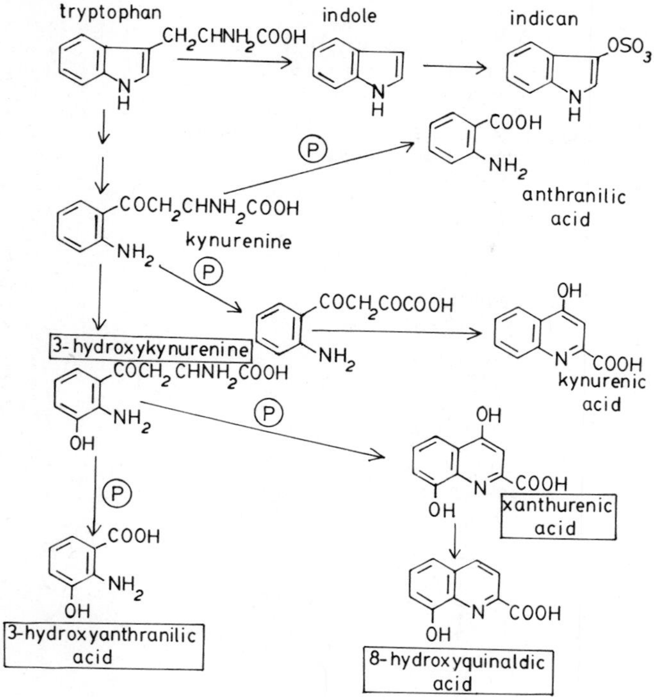

Figure 6-5 Major pathways of tryptophan metabolism: Boxed names, metabolites that are known carcinogens in animal systems; P, reactions dependent on pyridoxal phosphate. Pyridoxal or pyridoxine administration tends to increase primarily the formation of non-carcinogenic kynurenic and anthranilic acids.

exposed to relatively high concentrations of these substances. However, the exogenous carcinogens are chiefly associated with bladder cancer, not the endogenous tryptophan metabolites.

CHEMICAL CARCINOGENESIS

In the late eighteenth century, Percival Pott observed that chimney sweeps were prone to develop cancer of the scrotum as a result of prolonged exposure to soot, a mixture of coal dust, carbon, and coal tar. It was not until 100 years later that Volkman identified coal tar as the carcinogenic component through his studies of workers in the tar industry. Experimental studies of chemical carcinogenesis can only be said to have begun in 1915,

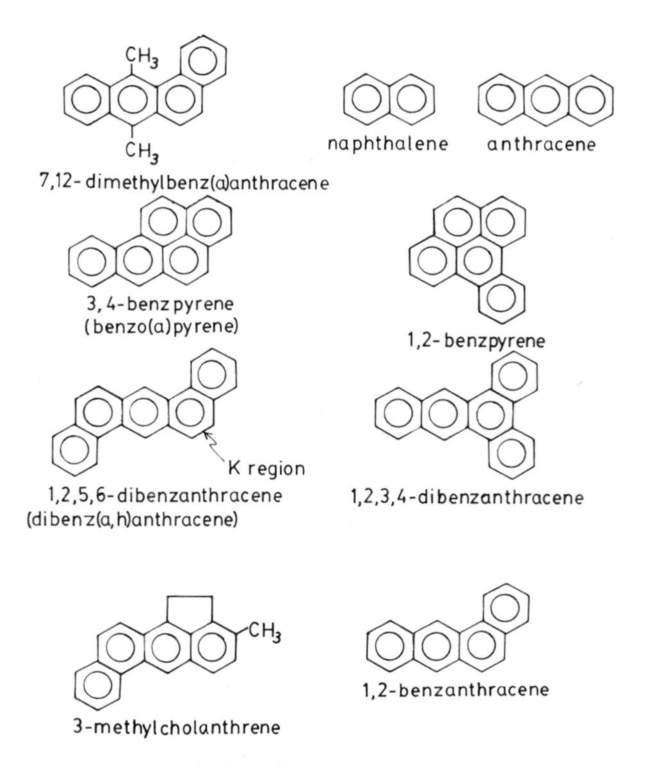

Figure 6-6 Polycyclic aromatic hydrocarbons.

however, when Yamagiwa and Ichikawa induced cancer in rabbits by repeatedly applying coal tar to their ears (131). In 1933, Cook and his associates succeeded in isolating 50 grams of pure carcinogenic 3,4-benzpyrene from 2 tons of tar (132). Thus ended one line of research, extending back over 200 years and leading to the polycyclic aromatic hydrocarbons (Figure 6-6). The distribution of carcinogenic activity among these compounds is interesting. Whereas benzene, naphthalene, authracene, phenanthrene, 1,2-benzpyrene, and 1,2,3,4-dibenzanthracene essentially are not carcinogenic, or only weakly so, 3,4-benzpyrene, 1,2,5,6-dibenzanthracene, 7,12-dimethyl-benzanthracene, 9,10-dimethylanthracene, and β-methylcholanthrene are very active, and 1,2-benzanthracene moderately active. This degree of specificity is very marked and suggests that carcinogenicity depends on the configuration of the molecule and its orientation with respect to the target sites. In experimental carcinogenesis, the ability to induce skin cancer in mice has been a standard method for assaying these agents, but they may induce many other tumors, such as sarcomas, lymphomas, ovarian tumors, and even leukemias; in hamsters, melanomas may be produced. Proof of carcinogenic activity is often a slow, painstaking procedure, and present pressures favoring elimination of carcinogens from the environment requires that some more rapid method for identifying a hazard be available. This is the basic rationale for the *Ames' test,* which determines the ability of a substance to cause mutations in bacteria; in this system, liver homogenate is added to metabolize agents that are inactive without such conversion (133). It would appear that all known carcinogens are potential mutagens, and because of their very short life cycles, bacterial mutants may be evaluated rapidly. Thus, the Ames' test is very useful for initial screening of substances, but its use in no way obviates the need for the usual animal systems to evaluate the carcinogenicity of compounds found to be positive in the Ames test.

While the role of the polycyclic hydrocarbons was being investigated, other types of carcinogens were being discovered. In 1895, Rehn reported an unusual amount of bladder cancer among workers in a dye factory in Frankfurt, and he concluded that the disease was related to aniline (134). It later became evident that it was not aniline itself, but the azo dye structure derived from it that was responsible, together with several other aromatic amines, such as β-naphthylamine. Among the widely used derivatives found to be carcinogenic were the dyes Scarlet Red and Butter Yellow (N,N-dimethyl-4-amino-azobenzene) (135,136). Butter Yellow was once used to color butter and margarine, whereas Scarlet Red was employed to accelerate regeneration of skin tissue in wounds. The aromatic amide 2-acetylaminofluorene, which may be considered along with the amines, also produces a wide variety of tumors, especially bladder tumors and hepatomas. The chemical structures of some of these amines and amides, as well as the two azo dyes discussed above, appear in Figure 6-7.

Much of the present concern over carcinogens stems from the ever increasing production, and the frequently unsatisfactory disposal, of synthetic organic compounds. Figure 6-8 reproduces data, taken from an article by Harris and his coworkers (137), that show the exponential increase in production of organic chemicals and the accompanying rise in cancer death rates. Since a delay of 20 to 30 years is probable for the development of most human cancer after exposure to carcinogens, we probably have not yet seen the full effects of this chemical explosion. The same article reviews the major route whereby carcinogens may reach human populations, that

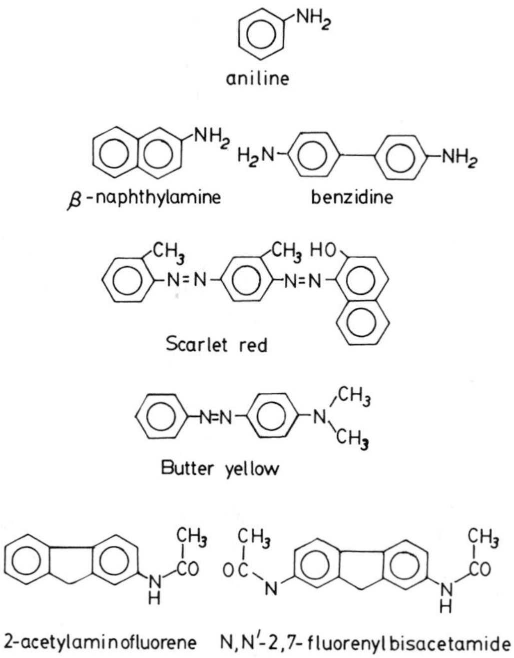

aniline

β-naphthylamine benzidine

Scarlet red

Butter yellow

2-acetylaminofluorene N,N′-2,7-fluorenylbisacetamide

Figure 6-7 Some carcinogenic amines and their derivatives. Aniline itself is not a carcinogen.

Figure 6-8 The rise in cancer death rates and chemical production as a function of time. Reproduced from Ref. 137.

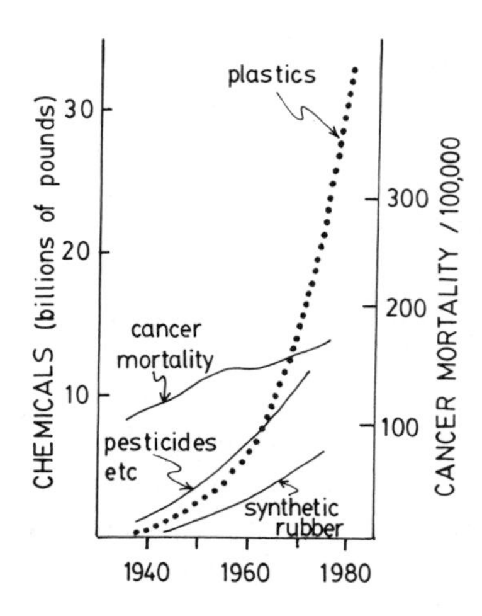

is, in drinking water (137). A major key to this problem is obviously careful control of the disposal of chemical wastes and by-products from the manufacture of such materials as plastics. The natural environment is not a non-saturable sink into which unlimited amounts of chemicals can be poured.

Although synthetic carcinogens are a major concern because their levels in the environment are increasing, it should not be forgotten that there exists a wide variety of natural carcinogens. Among them may be noted shikimic acid, found in the bracken fern, which is eaten in many countries such as Japan with its high incidence of stomach cancer, cycasin derivatives from cycads, betel nut, which is chewed in many tropical areas, plant tannins present in foods and in such beverages as tea, the pyrrolizidine alkaloids, and aflatoxin from peanuts or rice infected with *Aspergillus flavus*, a fungus (Figure 6-9) (138).

Figure 6-9 Naturally occurring carcinogens.

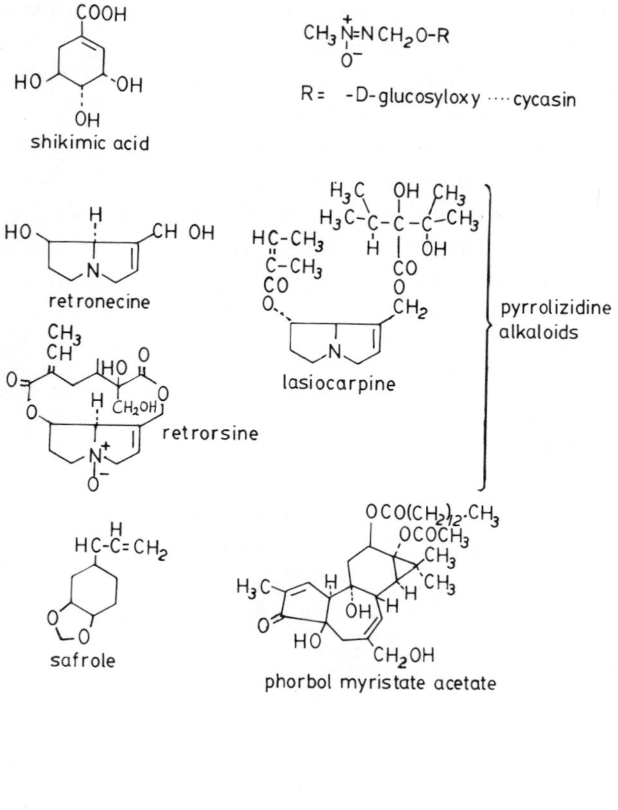

shikimic acid

R= -D-glucosyloxy ···· cycasin

retronecine

lasiocarpine

retrorsine

pyrrolizidine alkaloids

safrole

phorbol myristate acetate

Quantitative aspects of chemical carcinogenesis

As with any pharmacologically active substance, some type of quantitative evaluation of the activity of a carcinogen must be made in order to compare it to other carcinogenic compounds and to evaluate its potential hazard. Plots of tumor yield as percent of animals with tumors against the logarithm of the dose are generally sigmoidal, with approximation to a linear relationship over the middle range (Figure 6-10). These plots enable a comparison to be made between the ED_{50} (dose producing 50% incidence of tumors) for different agents. In the example shown here, 3,4-benzpyrene requires an approximately tenfold higher dose than 20-methylcholanthrene to induce a comparable number of sarcomas. It should be noted that toxicity or lethality not due to tumor growth follow similar dose-response curves, which may be shifted along the dose axis. Yet another indicator of carcinogenic ability is the *Iball index*, a quotient obtained by dividing the tumor yield in percent by the latency period for the appearance of tumors, in days, and multiplying by 100. Of course, to have any meaning, compounds must be administered by the same route to the same species, each at their most effective dose levels. As long ago as 1948, Druckrey and Kuepfmueller obtained data for the induction of liver cancer by N-N-dimethyl-4-aminoazobenzene, in which the total dose required was similar over a range of dose rates, but fell for prolonged treatment with small daily doses (139). In studies in which dimethylnitrosamine was used as the carcinogen, it was evident that the dose required is a function of the daily dose and a power of the time such that $dt^n =$ constant. This type of relation implies that time is also an element in carcinogenesis, which may be viewed as an accelerated process analogous to acceleration in classical physics (140). A

Figure 6-10 Dose-response curves for tumor induction in mice by subcutaneous injection of 20-methylcholanthrene or 3,4-benzpyrene. Reproduced from Suss, Kinzel, and Scribner: *Cancer—Experimental Concepts,* Berlin: Springer-Verlag, 1973.

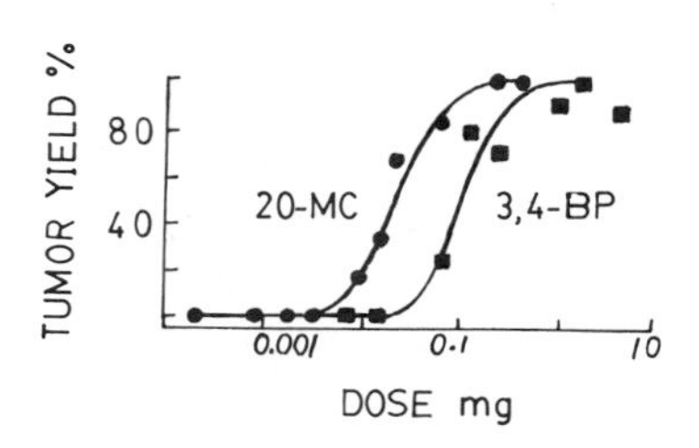

double logarithmic plot of dose versus latent period for such a relationship would be linear, with a slope of n. Furthermore, there would be no threshold value below which no tumors are produced, but rather an extension of the latent period exceeding the life-span of the animals. This, of course, presents a major problem in deriving safe threshold values for environmental carcinogens.

Metabolism of carcinogens

Before dealing with the mechanisms of chemical carcinogenesis, we need to consider the form of the carcinogen. Many carcinogens are biologically active in themselves and require no metabolic conversion for expression of their carcinogenic potential. Carcinogens of this class are typically reactive compounds, the best known examples being the nitrogen mustard type of alkylating agent used in cancer chemotherapy (141). These will be discussed later when we consider therapeutic approaches to cancer. There is a larger group of carcinogens that in themselves cannot induce cancer, but can induce it only after conversion to active derivatives. For example, in the experiments of Bonser, direct implantation of β-naphthylamine pellets into the bladder only rarely produced tumors, whereas inclusion of the amine in the diet produced a high incidence of bladder cancers (142). Pathways for the metabolism of carcinogens typically involve many of the reactions associated with the metabolism of drugs, and the hepatic microsomal enzyme system figures prominently among the systems carrying out this metabolism (143). Typical known reactions are shown in Figure 6-11. For the polycyclic aromatic hydrocarbons and aflatoxin, the primary mechanism for activation appears to be epoxide formation. In the intact animal, epoxides are detoxified by the action of such enzymes as epoxide hydrase and glutathione transferase, leading to a phenol, a dihydrodiol, and an amino acid conjugate, all non-carcinogenic, though toxic. The activities of the components of this series of reactions vary considerably, not only between species, but also among individuals of one species because of genetic variation (144), so sensitivity to these hydrocarbons will also vary widely. For amines and amides, of which 2-acetyl-aminofluorene may be taken as an example, N-hydroxylation is the common first step, to be followed by conversion to an ester form (sulfate, acetate, or hydroxylamine ester). Other compounds are believed to give rise to carbonium ions, which represent the active structure. Typical of this are the pyrrolizidine alkaloids, which are widely distributed in nature and hazardous to livestock, and the nitro-

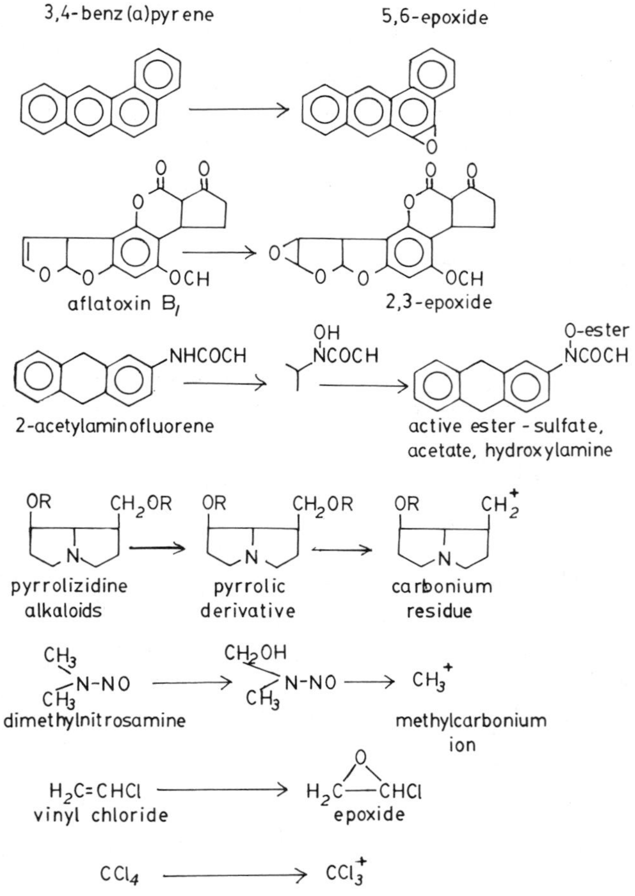

3,4-benz(a)pyrene → 5,6-epoxide

aflatoxin B_1 → 2,3-epoxide

2-acetylaminofluorene → active ester - sulfate, acetate, hydroxylamine

pyrrolizidine alkaloids → pyrrolic derivative → carbonium residue

dimethylnitrosamine → methylcarbonium ion

$H_2C{=}CHCl$ vinyl chloride → H_2C—$CHCl$ epoxide

CCl_4 → CCl_3^+

Figure 6-11 Typical reactions that activate carcinogens.

samines, which have earned some notoriety because of their possible formation from nitrites in processed foods. Interestingly, many carcinogenic alkylating agents also give rise to carbonium ions during activation. Vinyl chloride and carbon tetrachloride are common environmental carcinogens, both of them having been found widely distributed in drinking water; they are metabolized by epoxide formation and dechlorination to an active ion, respectively. The naturally occurring carcinogen safrole (Figure 6-9) follows the same metabolic pathway as the amines, being hydroxylated at the 1′-

position of the side chain and then esterified. Nitro compounds, such as 2-nitronaphthalene, are first reduced to the hydroxylamino derivatives and then esterified. Methylnitrosourea (closely related to the nitrosoureas used in therapy) and ethyl carbamate are activated to carbonium ions (143). Finally, it should be noted that, like the barbiturates, some carcinogens, particularly of the polycyclic hydrocarbon class, are able to induce the microsomal enzymes that metabolize them. This is true for 3,4-benzpyrene, and apparently for cyclamate, which is metabolized to release cyclohexylamine, thought to be the active carcinogen, although this is far from certain (145).

Sites of action of carcinogens

Despite the fact that binding to proteins is widespread among the carcinogens, and was once thought to be relevant to their mechanism of action, it is now generally agreed that their primary action is interaction with nucleic acids (146). Although the N-7 position of the guanine base appears to be the favored site for such interactions, other positions, and all four bases, are subject to attack by carcinogens, but the quantities of these various products are small when it is considered that 60 to 90 percent of the reaction products involve the 7-position of guanine. Both the position of guanine in the wide groove of DNA (147) and wave mechanical reasoning (148) have been used to explain this reactivity. Certain alkylating agents of the SN_1 type (see Chapter 7) also react significantly with the phosphate backbone of DNA. In the case of the polycyclic hydrocarbons, the portion of the carcinogen that reacts with DNA is believed to be a more reactive region—the K region—of the molecule (149), and it is here that epoxide formation occurs.

Binding to RNA has also been studied and occurs with a variety of agents; it usually occurs at sites similar to those involved in binding to DNA. Such binding (and intercalation) would be expected to exhibit the sort of stereo-specificity that carcinogens exhibit.

In addition to the covalent type of interaction that produce alkylated bases, there are also noncovalent interactions. These include internal binding, or *intercalation*, in which the carcinogen is inserted between the base pairs, and external binding, or *adlineation*, in which the agent interacts at sites not involved in base pairing and in which it is usually bound perpendicular to the plane of the bases (150). Some polycyclic hydrocarbons are believed to intercalate, but although actinomycin D, a potent intercalator, is somewhat carcinogenic, the relationship between intercalation, and for that matter the weaker adlineation, and carcinogenesis is not entirely clear at present.

Little or nothing is known of how these interactions effect carcinogenesis. Some of the damage will be reversed during the course of repair processes that involve recognition and incision by an endonuclease, removal of the lesion by an exonuclease, repair replication by a polymerase, and rejoining by a polynucleotide ligase. Miscoding due to incorporated covalently bound carcinogen and abnormal replication and chromosome breaks due to intercalation and errors in repair could all increase the pool of mutants and the possibility of selections that favor unrestrained growth. Aneuploidy and breaks are far more common in cancer cells than in normal cells, and carcinogens would produce just such abnormalities.

Initiation and promotion

The concept that some carcinogens act as initiators of malignant transformation, whereas other compounds promote the manifestation of this change, is a long-standing one in carcinogenesis (25). Even though a multistep process is now the favored model, many agents can be broadly classed as promoters, the phorbol esters (Figure 6-9) being among the best known examples; they occur in croton oil. As we have seen, other agents may play the role of initiator, genetic features among them, whereas promoters include not only chemicals, but also time itself, immune defects or psychological and other forms of stress. Viral and other infections may also play similar roles and it is to them that we will now turn.

VIRAL ETIOLOGY OF CANCER

In Chapter 2 we discussed the growth of certain bird tumors that are associated with viruses and that exhibit a proliferative pattern involving conversion of normal host cells into tumor cells. Beginning in 1908, with the discovery of chicken myeloblastosis virus by Ellerman and Bang and the subsequent isolation of chicken sarcoma virus by Rous, a steadily increasing number of viruses able to induce tumors in a range of animals have been identified, until by 1970, a total of 110 such viruses were known (Table 6-2) (151). The pace of discovery has slowed somewhat since then, but the sheer number of these viruses, and the ability of many of them to transform cultured human cells into lines behaving like malignant cells, provides strong suggestive evidence that viruses play a role in the development of

Table 6-2 Viruses that induce neoplasms in animals.

Common name of virus	*Number of major isolates*	*Host of origin*	*Produces tumors in*	*Tumor type*
Mouse leukemia (NKV)*	16	Mouse	Mouse, rat, hamster	Leukemia, lymphoma
Mouse sarcoma (MSV)	6	Mouse	Mouse, rat, hamster, cat, tissue culture	Sarcomas
Polyoma (Py)	2	Mouse	Mouse, hamster, tissue culture	All types except leukemia
Mammary tumor (MTV)	2	Mouse	Mouse	Carcinoma
Chicken leukemia (ALV)	4	Chicken	Chicken, tissue culture	Leukemia
Twiehaus	1	Chicken	Chicken, quail, hamster	Reticuloendotheliosis
Chicken sarcoma (Rous et al.)(RSV)	9	Chicken	Chicken, quail, turkey, duck, hamster, monkey snake, tissue culture	Sarcoma
Marek's (MHV)	1	Chicken	Chicken	Lymphoma
CELO	1	Chicken	Hamster	Sarcoma
Cat leukemia (FLV)	4	Cat	Cat	Leukemia, lymphoma
Cat sarcoma (FSV)	3	Cat	Cat, rat, dog, monkey, tissue culture	Sarcoma
Guinea pig leukemia	1	Guinea pig	Guinea pig	Leukemia
Guinea pig herpes	1	Guinea pig	Guinea pig	Sarcoma
Deer fibroma	1	Deer	Deer	Fibroma
Squirrel fibroma	1	Squirrel	Squirrel	Fibroma
Shope fibroma	1	Rabbit	Rabbit	Fibroma
Dog sarcoma	1	Dog	Dog, tissue culture	Sarcoma
Dog mast cell	1	Dog	Dog	Carcinoma
Lucké	1	Frog	Frog	Carcinoma
Human adenovirus †	31	Man	Hamster, mouse, tissue culture	Sarcoma-lymphoma
Wart	1	Man	Man	Papilloma
Hybrids ‡	7	Monkey Man Cat Mouse	Hamster, cat, tissue culture	Sarcoma-lymphoma
Yaba	1	Monkey	Monkey, man	Histiocytoma
H. saimiri	1	Monkey	Monkey	Lymphoma
Simian adenovirus	6	Monkey	Hamster, tissue culture	Sarcoma-lymphoma
SV40¶	1	Monkey	Hamster, mouse, tissue culture	Lymphosarcoma
Graffi hamster	2	Hamster	Hamster	Lymphoma, papilloma
Bovine papilloma	1	Cow	Cow, horse, mouse, hamster	Papilloma, fibroma, sarcoma
Bullhead papilloma		Fish	Fish (bullhead catfish)	Papilloma
	110			

Reproduced from J. F. Holland and E. Frei, III, *Cancer Medicine*, p. 16, 1973, with permission of the publisher Lea & Febiger.

*Strains of mouse leukemia virus (MLV) are usually designated by the names of the original investigator: GLV, Gross leukemis virus; FLV, Friend leukemia virus; RLV, Rauscher leukemia virus.

† As of May 1970 approximately 12 of 31 human adenoviruses induce malignancies in hamsters. These 12 and the remaining 19 induce discrete foci of transformed (apparently cancerous) cells in tissue cultures.

‡ Hybrid, Genotypic recombinates of two different viruses, e.g., SV40 + adeno; cat leukemia + mouse sarcoma.

¶ Simian virus 40.

human cancer. However, there is no means of assessing by current methodology just what the risk of viral cancer actually is. The difficulty in making such an assessment does not mean that the association between viruses and cancer is negligible, but rather that the relationship is complex and that factors in addition to an infecting virus are generally required. For example, cells from patients with several of the genetic conditions that predispose toward cancer, such as Down's syndrome, may show as much as a 100-fold increased susceptibility to viral transformation (152). A hamster cell line infected with an RNA viral strain is similarly much more susceptible to transformation by chemical carcinogens (153). These examples suggest a co-carcinogenic role in which the viral genome contributes some key element needed for carcinogenesis to occur.

Biology of oncogenic viruses

Before considering the nature of the key contribution by viruses to carcinogenesis, we should briefly survey their biology. Both RNA and DNA viruses may be oncogenic; the most common types are listed in Table 6-3. In some respects, the specificity of these tumor viruses is low, in that different viruses may induce similar tumors, whereas one virus may give rise to a range of tumor types. On the other hand, the host cell-virus interaction is specific in that cells may be *permissive* for a certain virus, allowing viral replication and a high frequency of neoplastic transformation, or they be *non-permissive,* in which case infection occurs, but with no viral replication and a very low incidence of transformation. Most of the naturally occurring viral neoplastic diseases are associated with the medium-sized, membrane-enclosed RNA type. Examination of infected cells reveals virions, about 100 mμ in diameter, consisting of a core surrounded by a double lipo-protein membrane. Such virions have been classified as *C-particles* by Bernhard (154). Type *B-particles* are essentially similar, except that the external spikes on the membrane are more pronounced and the central core is frequently eccentric (155). For both types of virus, the core has a shell with subunits that surrounds the nucleoid, a nucleoprotein complex. Apart from the components of the RNA-directed DNA polymerase (*reverse transcriptase*), virions from mammalian cells contain four polypeptides and two glycoproteins; avian viruses have an additional polypeptide. Other minor components may be present in variable amounts, and it would appear that these proteins are of both viral and host cell origin (156). The RNA viruses operate through the formation of a DNA copy of the viral

Table 6-3 Types of oncogenic viruses.

Classification of virion	Popular group designation	Site of maturation	Prototype virus	Type of lesion	Proliferative lesion transmitted under natural conditions
DNA					
Large					
Membrane-bound	Pox	Cytoplasmic inclusion	Shope rabbit fibroma	Near-neoplasia	Yes
Medium					
Membrane-bound	"Herpes-type"	Nucleus	Lucké frog kidney carcinoma*	Solid malignant neoplasia	Yes
			EBV	Lymphoma and solid malignant neoplasia	Yes
Naked	Adeno	Nucleus	Adenovirus 12	Solid malignant neoplasia	No
Small					
Naked	Papova	Nucleus	Human wart	Near-neoplasia	Yes
			Shope rabbit papilloma	Solid benign neoplasia	Yes
			S-E polyoma	Solid malignant neoplasia	No
RNA					
Medium					
Membrane-bound	"Myxo-like"†	Cytoplasm	Rous sarcoma	Solid malignant neoplasia	—‡
			Bittner mouse mammary cancer	Solid malignant neoplasia	Yes
			Avian leukosis	Leukemia and solid lymphoma	Yes
			Gross mouse leukemia	Aleukemic leukemia	Yes

Reproduced from J. F. Holland and E. Frei, III, *Cancer Medicine*, p. 19, 1973, with permission of the publisher Lea & Febiger.

* Frog kidney carcinoma virus of Lucke'. Tentative classification on a basis of (a) reproduction and maturation in the nucleus; and (b) morphological similarity to "herpes-like" viruses, known to be of DNA type.

† So called because of budding from cell membranes, as is characteristic of the myxoviruses. Hemagglutination, which is characteristic of the myxoviruses, does not occur with the RNA tumor viruses.

‡ Laboratory strain isolated from a particular spontaneous tumor. Other similar tumors occur spontaneously in chickens with low frequency, but the relationship among etiological agents is known.

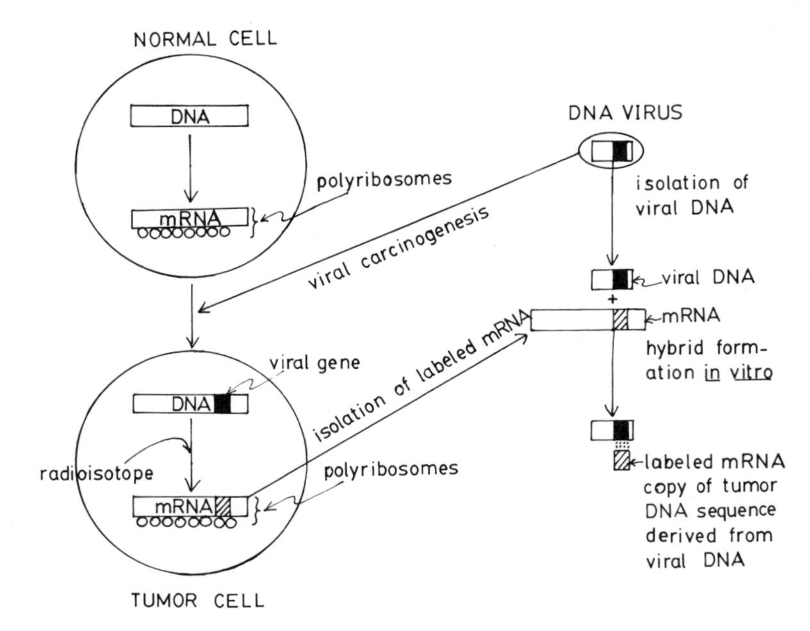

Figure 6-12 Principles behind the testing for viral genes in cancer cells. The incorporated viral sequence gives rise to a messenger RNA (*m*RNA) sequence, which because of its affinity for corresponding viral DNA, may be annealed to it during hybridization. Radioisotopic incorporation into the tumor cell enables the sequence to be identified. Reproduced from Ref. 74.

genome, made within the first 12 hours of infection, which is integrated into the host DNA to form a provirus (157). These integrated sequences are detectable by such techniques as *molecular hybridization* (Figure 6-12). Proviral sequences serve as templates for the synthesis of viral RNA during replication. This step operates through the normal host cellular mechanisms for RNA synthesis. Core formation occurs in the cytoplasm, and the envelope is acquired from the host during budding of viral particles through the cell membrane (156) (see Figure 6-13). How the incorporated viral sequences transform cells is not understood, but there is the possibility that errors in transcription, the formation of unusual products, and also new genetic information that overrides normal control of cell maturation could all contribute. In non-permissive cells the proviral sequences are present, but their expression is blocked.

Three general types of DNA viruses may be distinguished, the papovaviruses, the adenoviruses, and the herpesviruses. The DNA is double-stranded in all these, but it is circular and superhelical in the papovaviruses, and linear in the other types. Structurally there is a DNA-containing core (the DNA is doughnut shaped in herpes, with a central protein) surrounded by a coat. In herpesvirus, the coat consists of three layers, the capsid, tegument, and envelope (158). Infection of cells by these DNA viruses involves "uncoating," possibly within the cell nucleus, and the association of the viral DNA with the cell genome. Except for small papovaviruses, which may be incorporated entire, only certain segments of the viral DNA actually become integrated into host DNA (159). Since purified viral DNA is infectious, it appears that the virus carries with it no enzymes needed for its replication, but makes use of the host cell enzymes for its synthetic purposes. Replication of papovavirus DNA is bidirectional, beginning and ending at a unique point of this circular molecule. For adenovirus, and particularly for herpesvirus, there is evidence that gaps form in single-strand regions of the DNA, permitting replication from multiple initiation sites (159). The more complex nature of these viruses is reflected in the fact that there is a definite sequence for the synthesis of different species of RNA and protein. Viral RNA synthesized in the nucleus using host polymerase is of very high molecular weight; it is processed into a cyto-

Figure 6-13 Model for the control of oncogenes and virogenes. These are normally repressed, but further viral infection or other trauma may derepress these innate sequences. Reproduced from Ref. 162.

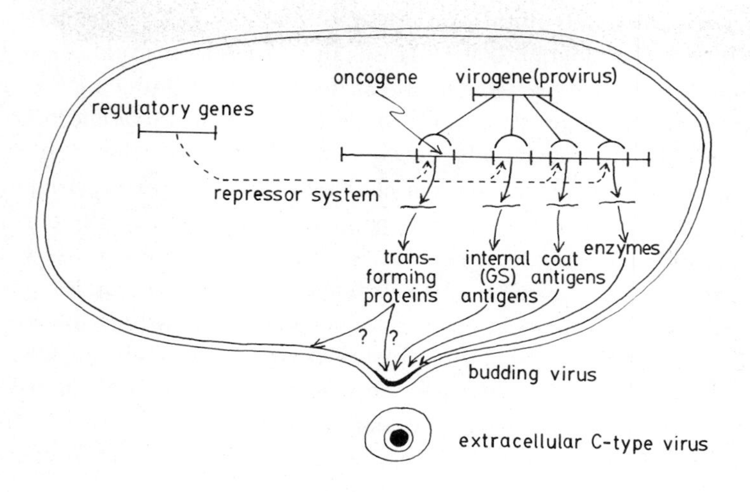

plasmic messenger RNA. Proteins are formed on polyribosomes in the cytoplasm and then transported into the nucleus where the virions are assembled. As with the RNA viruses, it is not yet possible to explain how transformation occurs, but it is manifested by the appearance of proteins and antigenic markers not present on normal cells, which may arise *de novo* or by gene derepression.

Viruses and human cancer

It would take too long to discuss all the reports of viral particles associated with human tumors. In some cases it is probable that the reported viruses are "passengers" infecting tumors with whose etiology they have no connection, but in many other cases a causal relationship is likely. Among early definitive examples of viral inclusions are the finding of EBV viral etiology for Burkitt's lymphoma (160) and nasopharyngeal carcinoma, the association of herpes simplex type 2 with uterine cervical cancer (161), and the presence of B and C type particles in milk and breast tissue from women of families with a high incidence of breast cancer (19, 151).

Viral oncogenes. The concept of a *viral oncogene* has been proposed as part of a theory of carcinogenesis (162). Regions of close resemblance or complete identity between viral nucleic acids and host cell DNA provide evidence for either an incorporation of viral genome or for the acquisition by the virus of host cell sequences. Such sequences are the oncogenes associated with neoplastic transformation, and although they are not normally expressed, infection with the appropriate virus having the same genes, thus permitting recombination that increases the oncogene content, or an actual mutation by physical or chemical means to give tumor-inducing sequences, may promote the expression of these carcinogenic factors. The oncogenes may be transmitted vertically through the reproductive cells. It is clear that apparently uninfected normal cells may not only reveal virus-like sequences in their genomes, but may also produce C-particles under appropriate conditions. An oncogene, which represents cistrons of the viral genome that carry information to bring about transformation, may be distinguished from a *virogene*, which encodes for the whole infectious virus. Since cancer does not develop universally, although oncogenes are considered to be ubiquitous, it is apparent that if the concept has some basis in fact, oncogene activity is normally repressed (Figure 6-13), and viral infection or other stresses may represent mechanisms for derepression. In a recent report, high molecular weight DNA from normal or spontaneously transformed 3T3 cells did not transform recipient cells. Sonicated DNA from both cell lines could transform normal cells, however, and high molecular weight DNA from these transformed cells was a highly effective transforming agent. During sonic fragmentation, transforming genes may become separated from neighboring repressor or regulator sites, and oncogene activity manifested (163). Whether cancer is the only manifestation of their action, or whether oncogenes play a role in the interchange of informational RNA molecules between cells, particularly during embryonic development, as suggested by Temin (164), remains to be seen, but clearly more work needs to be done to evaluate the role and control of oncogenes.

RADIATION CARCINOGENESIS

Radiation has been a known carcinogen for more than 70 years, mainly because of the development of cancer among early radiologists (165). Although these early cases were principally epidermoid carcinomas of exposed regions, such as the hands, most tissues can yield neoplasms as a result of intensive radiation, with leukemia (except chronic lymphocytic leukemia), osteosarcoma, thyroid and lung tumors, and lymphomas the most frequently encountered forms (166). Although radiologists are no longer uniquely at risk due to improvements in radiological equipment and practices, data from these earlier experiences, together with more recent information on uranium miners, survivors of the atomic bombs in Japan, Marshall islanders accidentally exposed to nuclear fallout, watch dial painters who had ingested luminous paint containing radium, and patients who developed cancer as a result of diagnostic or therapeutic irradiation, give some idea of the susceptibility of humans to radiation-induced tumors. First, it is evident that there is a long latent period between exposure and clinical evidence of solid tumors. Typical examples are the thyroid tumors, which require an average of 10 to 20 years, with an incidence of one case per 10^6 person-years per rad, or about three per 1,000 during a 15-year period after 200 rads (125). On the other hand, leukemias show a much earlier peak. In the Japanese survivors, incidence peaked 4 to 8 years after exposure, although the frequency remained above normal for more than 20 years (167); in the case of children exposed to x-rays prenatally, leukemia incidence peaked between ages 3 and 5, and was average by age 7 (168). Dose-response curves are particularly difficult to establish for humans, in large part because the delivered dose has frequently been very uncertain, but also because of the low incidence of significant radiation exposure, the long latent period, the complications of the underlying disease for which the patient received radiation, and numerous genetic and demographic variables. When taken in conjunction with better-defined animal studies, certain features may be identified. Dose-response curves are curvilinear with increasing slope progressing from low to intermediate doses and a plateau, or even a decline, in cancer incidence at very high doses. Interpretations suggest the operation of repair processes at low doses, of enhancement or promotion at intermediate doses, and excessive injury and cell death reducing neoplastic transformation at high doses (166). It is the low dose range that has attracted most attention, because environmental hazards fall in this region. Although most experimental data suggest a declining slope of the dose versus incidence curve as the dose declines, some experiments have suggested a linear relationship (169), and for the sake of prudence as well as convenience in estimating risks, this has much merit and has been adopted officially (170). Whatever the actual nature of the curve at low doses, it is clearly advisable to limit all radiation exposures, whether environmental or medical. The use of x-rays for treating such benign conditions as inflamed tonsils and adenoids, or for fitting shoes, practices of some years ago, clearly cannot be condoned. Caution with regard to exposure to sunlight is also warranted; in animals there is a clear relationship between skin cancer and ultraviolet radiation (171), and the geographical incidence of such cancers in humans correlates well with sunlight intensity (172).

Molecular basis of radiation carcinogenesis

In a multistep theory of carcinogenesis, radiation may contribute to one or more steps, and the likelihood of neoplastic transformation and the dose required are related to other factors. The effects of radiation may be exerted either directly on macromolecules, which are damaged by the ionized and free radical species produced by radiation, and indirectly through interactions at a site distant from that at which the tumor arises. Since DNA is a prime target for radiation, it is here that other factors may potentiate the carcinogenic action. This is seen in xeroderma pigmentosum, in which a genetic defect is a major contributor to the action of ultraviolet light in inducing skin cancer (10). In other cases, radiation may interact with an oncogenic virus, whether to potentiate its ability to transform cells (173) or to derepress an oncogene (174). Somatic mutations may arise directly through the ability of radiation to break strands, which may or may not be repaired correctly, or indirectly through injury to endocrine glands or the lymphoid system to create hormonal or immunological disturbances favoring tumor growth.

MISCELLANEOUS MECHANISMS OF CARCINOGENESIS

A number of other agents have been implicated in the development of cancer. Among them are various forms of trauma and inflammation, certain parasitic infections, and dietary defects, notably lack of fiber.

Trauma. This is probably the most frequently cited mechanism, but certainly the most difficult to establish (175). Perhaps the most definitive example is the relationship between burns and skin cancer; in a study of 2,465 cases of epidermal cancer, 2 percent of the epidermoid carcinomas and 0.3 percent of the basal cell carcinomas arose on skin that had suffered thermal trauma (176). Other examples of thermal etiology include the wearing of the hot kairo box, a tin box containing hot coals for warmth, in Japan, which may lead to epidermoid cancer of the abdomen, and the association between esophageal cancer and hot drinks, although in the latter case the combined use of alcohol and tobacco is also implicated (175).

Parasites. Although a number of parasitic infestations have been considered to be etiological factors in cancer (177), the best documented case is the association between schistosomiasis and bladder cancer (177,178). In parts of Egypt and such other countries as Tanzania and Uganda, the incidence of bladder infection by *Schistosoma hematobium* is so high that red urine is regarded as normal for young males. This hematuria arises from an inflammatory cystitis provoked by the mass of eggs, large numbers of which may become calcified in the bladder wall. In the same populations, the incidence of bladder cancer is high, with age of occurrence and intracystic distributions rather different from those seen in the usual form of the disease. The predisposing factors are believed to be chronic inflammation, urinary retention, especially in conjunction with increased levels of such carcinogens as the tryptophan metabolites mentioned earlier in the chapter, *Salmonella* bacteriuria, and immunosuppression (178). Infection with another schistosome, *S. mansoni,* which invades the liver and intestine, may be associated with hepatomas and colonic polyposis, but the relationship is less clear than for bladder cancer (178); an association with lymphoma and leukemia has also been reported (179). Suppression of schistosome infection, and control of the snail that is the intermediate host, are clearly needed to control this carcinogenic hazard.

Diet. Only two dietary aspects will be discussed here, the increased risk of colon and breast cancer that accompanies diets deficient in fiber or high in animal fat, respectively. In Chapter 8, a number of other dietary factors will be considered against the background of their largely unproven use in nutritional therapy advocated as part of a natural control program for cancer. Fiber has a major role in maintaining large bowel function. It increases stool output, dilutes the contents of the colon, affects the absorption and metabolism of the intestinal contents, ensures a faster rate of passage through the gut, and helps retain water in the stools. There appear to be two classes of fibers, those that are digestible, such as cabbage, carrot, or apple fiber and pectin, which do not survive transit through the gut, but greatly stimulate the growth of bacteria, the main component of stool, and indigestible fiber from wheat or other cereals, which survive digestion and retain water. In both cases the bulk of the intestinal contents is increased (180). Colonic disease, including cancer, may be more common in those with small stool output, who are likely to suffer constipation and to have long gut transit times (181). Related to this is the evidence of an association between breast cancer and diets high in total fat, animal protein, and animal calories (closely correlated together), as well as refined sugar (182). In this latter case it is probable that such a diet would also be low in fiber, which is mainly of vegetable origin. Thus, these two examples could be part of the same phenomenon. It has been suggested that retention in the gut allows greater metabolism of the contents, especially the bile pigments, to occur, and enhances the possibility that carcinogens are produced and concentrated in the reduced stool bulk (183). Absorption of these products with systemic as well as local colonic action might then occur.

CONCLUSION

We have seen that a wide variety of factors may operate to induce cancer. Genetic factors and viral oncogenes may be inheritable and thus beyond the possibility of control, unless genetic engineering reaches unexpected levels. On the other hand, we have seen that the expression of these factors that are present in the cell genome depends, in most cases, on further steps in an often complex chain of events. Thus, even an inherited trait may not be manifested if these other factors, including chemical carcinogens, radiation, the endocrine and immune systems, psychological status, and parasitic infestations, can be controlled. Even in so well established a relation as that between cigarette smoking and lung cancer, variations in sensitivity strongly suggest a genetic basis (184). Measures aimed at reducing exposure to environmental carcinogens or manipulating the endocrine and immune systems would serve to reduce the risk of expression of genetic or viral cancer, while decreasing the risk from cancer not related to these endogenous types of disease. A large number of hazardous substances are encountered in daily life and in the workplace, and of these, 1,900 show evidence of carcinogenicity. The Occupational Safety and Health Administration (OSHA) has issued threshold limits for only 17 of the known chemical carcinogens, including asbestos, coke oven emissions, naphthylamine, vinyl chloride, and N-nitrodimethylamine (185). With radiation, medical procedures remain the chief hazards, with a probably small, but uncertain risk of nuclear accidents following behind. Control of parasites is attainable, and certainly more likely to be successful than attempts to cure the tumors associated with the organisms; in this connection, though, some of the antiparasitic drugs, such as metronidazole, are known to carry some risk of inducing cancer. Finally, personal attention to health and habits, stopping smoking, cutting down on alcohol use, eating appropriate diets, and reduction of stress may contribute most to reducing the cancer death toll.

REFERENCES

1. C. O. Nordling: A new theory on the cancer inducing mechanism. Br. J. cancer *7:*68–72, 1953.
2. P. Armitage and R. Doll: The age distribution of cancer and multistage theory of carcinogenesis. Br. J. Cancer *8:*1–12, 1954.
3. S. H. Moolgavkar: The multistage theory of carcinogenesis and the age distribution of cancer in man. J. Natl. Cancer Inst. *61:*49–52, 1978.
4. A. G. Knudson: Mutation and human cancer. Adv. Cancer Res. *17:*317–352, 1973.
5. R. D. Jensen and R. W. Miller: Retinoblastoma: epidemiologic characteristics. New Eng. J. Med. *285:*307–311, 1971.
6. R. J. Gorlin, R. A. Vickers, E. Kelln, and J. J. Williamson: The multiple basal-cell nevi syndrome. Cancer *18:*89–104, 1965.
7. B. C. Morson and H. J. R. Bussey: Predisposing causes of intestinal cancer. *In Current Problems in Surgery.* Chicago: Year Book Medical Publishers, Feb., 1970, pp. 50.
8. E. J. Gardner and R. C. Richards: Multiple cutaneous and subcutaneous lesions occurring simultaneously with hereditary polyposis and osteomatosis. Am. J, Human Genet. *5:*139–147, 1953.
9. J. F. Fraumeni, Jr.: Genetic factors. *In Cancer Medicine,* J. F. Holland and E. Frei, III, eds., Philadelphia: Lea & Febiger, 1973, pp. 7–15.

10. W. B. Reed, B. Landing, G. Sugarman, J. E. Cleaver, and J. Melnyk: Xeroderma pigmentosum. Clinical and laboratory investigation of its basic defect. J. Am. Med. Assoc. *207:*2073–2079, 1969.
11. R. W. Miller: Persons with exceptionally high risk of leukemia. Cancer Res. *27:*2420–2423, 1967.
12. J. German: Oncogenic implication of chromosomal instability. *In Medical Genetics*, V. A. McKusick and R. Claiborne, eds., New York: HP Publishing Co., 1973, pp. 39–50.
13. R. B. Setlow: Repair deficient human disorders and cancer. Nature *271:*713–717, 1978.
14. R. A. Gatti and R. A. Good: Occurrence of malignancy in immunodeficiency diseases. Cancer *28:*89–98, 1971.
15. R. W. Miller: Deaths from childhood leukemia and solid tumors among twins and sibs in the United States, 1960–67. J. Natl. Cancer Inst. *46:*203–209, 1971.
16. S. Kurita: Familial leukemia. Acta Haematol. Jap. *31:*748–755, 1968.
17. H. T. Lynch: *Recent Results in Cancer Research*, Vol. 12, New York: Springer-Verlag, 1967, pp. 186.
18. D. E. Anderson: A genetic study of human breast cancer. J. Natl. Cancer Inst. *48:*1029–1034, 1972.
19. D. H. Moore, J. Charney, B. Kramarsky, E. Y. Lasfargues, N. H. Sarkar, M. J. Brennan, J. H. Burrows, S. M. Sirsat, J. C. Paymaster, and A. B. Vaidya: Search for a human breast cancer virus. Nature *229:*611–615, 1971.
20. W. G. Smith: The cancer-family syndrome and heritable colonic polyps. Dis. Colon Rectum *13:*362–367, 1970.
21. F. P. Li and F. J. Fraumeni, Jr.: Rhabdomyosarcoma in children: epidemiologic study and identification of a familial cancer syndrome. J. Natl. Cancer Inst. *43:*1365–1373, 1969.
22. W. Haenszel and M. Kurihara: Studies of Japanese migrants. I. Mortality from cancer and other diseases among Japanese in the United States. J. Natl. Cancer Inst. *40:*43–68, 1963.
23. I. Aird and H. H. Bentall: A relationship between cancer of the stomach and the ABO blood groups. Br. Med. J. *1:*799–801, 1953.
24. T. Boveri: *Zur Frage der Enstehung maligner Tumoren*, Jena: Fisher, 1914 (English translation—M. Boveri: *The Origin of Malignant Tumors*, Baltimore: Williams & Wilkins, 1929).
25. I. Berenblum: A speculative review: The probable nature of promoting action and its significance in the understanding of the mechanism of carcinogenesis. Cancer Res. *14:*471–477, 1954.
26. S. R. Wolman and A. A. Horland: Genetics of tumor cells. *In Cancer: A Comprehensive Treatise*, Vol. 3, F. F. Becker, ed., New York: Plenum Press, 1975, pp. 155–198.
27. P. A. Jacobs, M. Brunton, W. M. Court Brown, R. Doll, and H. Goldstein: Change of human chromosome count distributions with age: Evidence for a sex difference. Nature *197:*1080–1081, 1963.
28. E. Saksela and P. S. Moorhead: Aneuploidy in the degenerative phase of serial cultivation of human cell strains. Proc. Natl. Acad. Sci. U.S.A. *50:*390–395, 1963.
29. R. W. Hart and R. B. Setlow: Correlation between deoxyribonucleic acid excision-repair and life-span in a number of mammalian species. Proc. Natl. Acad. Sci. U.S.A. *71:*2169–2173, 1974.
30. G. J. Todaro, S. R. Wolman, and H. Green: Rapid transformation of human fibroblasts with low growth potential into established cell lines by SV-40. J. Cell Comp. Physiol. *62:*257–265, 1963.
31. K. Lemone Yielding: A model for aging based on differential repair of somatic mutational damage. Perspect. Biol. Med. *17:*201–207, 1974.

32. A. C. Braun: Differentiation and dedifferentiation. *In Cancer: A Comprehensive Treatise*, Vol. 3, F. F. Becker, ed., New York: Plenum Press, 1975, pp. 3–20.
33. L. Kopelovich, N. E. Bias, and L. Helson: Tumour promoter alone induces neoplastic transformation of fibroblasts from humans genetically predisposed to cancer. Nature *282:*619–621, 1979.
34. L. J. Rather: The six things non-natural, Clio Medica *3:*337–347, 1968.
35. L. J. Rather: *The Genesis of Cancer*, Johns Hopkins University Press, Baltimore, 1978, p. 182.
36. L. I. LeShan and R. E. Worthington: Personality as a factor in the pathogenesis of cancer: A review of the literature, Br. J. Med. Psych. *29:*49–56, 1956.
37. L. I. LeShan: Psychological states as factors in the development of malignant disease, a critical review. J. Natl. Cancer Inst. *22:*1–17, 1959.
38. C. Holden: Cancer and mind. Science *200:*1363–1369, 1978.
39. L. I. LeShan and M. Reznikoff: A psychological factor apparently associated with neoplastic disease. J. Abnormal Psychol. *60:*439–440, 1960.
40. M. Reznikoff: Psychological factors in breast cancer. Psychosomatic Med. *17:*96–108, 1955.
41. H. L. Muslin, K. Gyarfas, and W. J. Pieper: Separation experience and cancer of the breast. Ann. N.Y. Acad. Sci. *125:*802–806, 1966.
42. L. I. LeShan: An emotional life-history pattern associated with neoplastic disease, Ann. N.Y. Acad. Sci. *125:*780–793, 1966.
43. W. A. Greene: The psychosocial setting of the development of leukemia and lymphoma, Ann. N.Y. Acad. Sci. *125:*794–802, 1966.
44. S. Greer and T. Morris: Psychologic attributes of women who develop breast cancer. J. Psychosomatic Res. *19:*147–153, 1975.
45. C. B. Bahnson: Epistemological perspectives of physical disease from the psychodynamic point of view. Am. J. Public Health *64:*1034–1040, 1974.
46. C. B. Bahnson: Psychophysiological complemetarity in malignancies—past work and future vistas. Ann. N.Y. Acad. Sci. *164:*319–333, 1969.
47. A. H. Schmale and H. P. Iker: Hopelessness as a predictor of cervical cancer. Social Sci. Med. *5:*95–100, 1971.
48. D. Kissen: The significance of personality in lung cancer in men. Ann. N.Y. Acad. Sci. *125:*820–825, 1966.
49. O. Hagnell: The premorbid personality of persons who develop cancer in a total population investigated in 1947 and 1957. Ann. N.Y. Acad. Sci. *125:*846–855, 1966.
50. C. B. Bahnson and M. B. Bahnson: Role of ego defense: Denial and repression in the etiology of malignant neoplasms. Ann. N.Y. Acad. Sci. *125:*827–945, 1966.
51. C. B. Thomas and R. L. Greenstreet: Psychological characteristics in youth as predictors of 5 disease states: suicide, mental illness, hypertension, coronary heart disease and tumor. Johns Hopkins Med. J. *132:*16–43, 1973.
52. D. W. Abse, M. M. Wilkins, R. L. Van de Castle, W. D. Buxton, J. P. Demars, R. S. Brown, and L. G. Kirschner: Personality and behavioral characteristics of lung cancer patients. J. Psychosomatic Res. *18:*101–113, 1974.
53. J. H. Stephenson and W. J. Grace: Life stress and cancer of the cervix. Psychosomatic Med. *16:*287–294, 1954.
54. G. Booth: General and organic specific object relationships in cancer. Ann. N.Y. Acad. Sci. *164:*568–577, 1969.
55. M. Tarlau and I. Smalheiser: Personality patterns in patents with malignant tumors of the breast and cervix. Psychosom. Med. *13:*117–121, 1951.
56. R. E. Renneker, R. Cutler, J. Hora, C. Bacon, G. Bradley, J. Kearny, and M. Cutler: Psychoanalytical explorations of emotional correlates of cancer of the breast. Psychosom. Med. *25:*106–123, 1963.

57. C. B. Thomas and K. R. Puszynski: Closeness to parents and the family constellation in a prospective study of 5 disease states: suicide, mental illness, malignant tumor, hypertension and coronary heart disease. Johns Hopkins Med. J. *134:*251–270, 1974.
58. R. E. Kavetsy, N. M. Turkevich, R. N. Akimova, I. K. Khayetsky, and Y. D. Matveichuck: Induced carcinogenesis under various influences on the hypothalamus. Ann, N.Y. Acad. Sci. *164:*517–518, 1969.
59. M. Stein, R. C. Schiavi, and T. J. Luparello: The hypothalamus and immune process. Ann. N.Y. Acad. Sci. *164:*464–471, 1969.
60. M. Stein, R. C. Schiavi, and M. Camerino: Influence of brain and behavior on the immune system. Science *191:*435–440, 1976.
61. S. Margolin, moderator: Panel discussion I: The neuroendocrinologic aproach. Ann. N.Y. Acad. Sci. *164:*611–619, 1969.
62. C. Southam: Emotions, immunology and cancer: How might the psyche influence neoplasia? Ann. N.Y. Acad. Sci. *164:*373–375, 1969.
63. D. Kissen and L. G. S. Rao: Steroid excretion patterns and personality in lung cancer. Ann. N.Y. Acad. Sci. *164:*476–481, 1969.
64. G. F. Solomon and R. H. Moos: Emotions, immunity and disease. Arch. Gen. Psychiatry *11:*657–674, 1974.
65. S. W. Tromp: The possible effect of metereological stress on cancer and its importance for psychosomatic cancer research. Experimentia *30:*1474–1478, 1974.
66. H. F. Oettgen and K. E. Hellström: Tumor immunology. *In Cancer Medicine*, J. F. Holland and E. Frei, III, eds., Philadelphia: Lea & Febiger, 1973, pp. 951–990.
67. H. O. Sjogren: Studies on the specific transplantation resistance against polyoma virus-induced tumors. III. Transplantation resistance against genetically compatible polyoma tumors induced by polyoma tumor homografts. J. Natl. Cancer Inst. *32:*645–659, 1964.
68. G. Klein, H. O. Sjogren, K. Klein, and K. E. Hellström: Demonstration of resistance against methylcholanthrene-induced sarcomas in the primary autochthonous host. Cancer Res. *20:*1561–1572, 1960.
69. G. Klein: Tumor antigens. Ann. Rev. Microbiol. *20:*223–252, 1966.
70. L. J. Old and E. A. Boyse: Immunology of experimental tumors. Ann. Rev. Med. *15:*167–186, 1964.
71. R. T. Smith: Tumor specific immune mechanisms. New Eng. J. Med. *278:*1207–1326, 1968.
72. K. E. Hellström and I. Hellström: Cellular immunity against tumor antigens. Adv. Cancer Res. *12:*167–233, 1969.
73. R. J. Brown: Possible association of embryonal antigen with several primary 3-methylcholanthrene-induced murine sarcomas. Int. J. Cancer *6:*245–249, 1970.
74. M. Green, K. Fujinaga, M. Piña, and D. C. Thomas: Molecular basis of viral oncogenesis. *In Exploitable Molecular Mechanisms and Neoplasia.* 22nd Ann. Symp. Fundamental Cancer Res. Baltimore: Williams & Wilkins, 1969, pp. 479–506.
75. P. Häyry and V. Defendi: Surface antigen(s) of SV-40 transformed tumor cells. Virology *41:*22–29, 1970.
76. H. O. Sjogren and I. Hellström: Induction of the polyoma specific transplantation antigen in Moloney leukemia cells. Exp. Cell Res. *40:*208–212, 1965.
77. E. A. Boyse, L. J. Old, and E. Stockert: The TL (thymus leukemia) antigen. A review. *In Immunopathology.* IV Intern. Symposium, P. Grabar and P. A. Miescher, eds. Basel: Schwabe and Co., 1965, pp. 23–40.
78. L. J. Old, E. Stockert, E. A. Boyse, and J. H. Kim: Antigenic modulation. Loss of TL antigen from cells exposed to TL antibody. Study of the phenomenon *in vitro.* J. Exp. Md. *127:*523–539, 1968.
79. A. C. Allison: Immunological surveillance against tumor cells. *In Cancer: A Comprehensive Treatise*, Vol. 4, F. F. Becker, ed., New York: Plenum Press, 1975, pp. 237–258.

80. J. B. Hibbs, L. H. Lambert, and J. S. Remington: Possible role of macrophage mediated nonspecific cytotoxicity in tumour resistance. Nature New Biol. *235:*48–50, 1972.
81. M. H. Levy and E. F. Wheelock: The role of macrophages in defense against neoplastic disease. Adv. Cancer Res. *20:*131–163, 1974.
82. R. T. Smith and M. Landy, eds.: *Immune Surveillance.* New York and London: Academic Press, 1970, pp. 536.
83. I. Penn, C. G. Halgrimson, and T. E. Starzl: *De novo* malignant tumor in organ transplant recipients. Transplant. Proc. *3:*773–778, 1971.
84. R. C. Ting and L. W. Law: Thymic junction and carcinogenesis. Prog. Exp. Tumor Res. *9:*165–191, 1967.
85. A. J. Girardi: Prevention of SV-40 virus oncogenesis in hamsters. I. Tumor resistance induced by human cells transformed by SV-40. Proc. Natl. Acad. Sci. U.S. *54:*445–451, 1965.
86. H. O. Sjogren and J. Ankerst: Effect of BCG and allogeneic tumour cells on adenovirus 12 tumor-genesis in mice. Nature *221:*863–864, 1969.
87. R. T. Prehn: Function of depressed immunologic reactivity during carcinogenesis. J. Natl. Cancer Inst. *31:*797–805, 1963.
88. F. R. Eilbert and D. L. Morton: Impaired immunologic reactivity and recurrence following cancer therapy. Cancer *25:*362–367, 1970.
89. L. Helson, C. Ramos, H. F. Oettgen, and M. L. Murphy: DNCB-reactivity in children with neroblastoma. Proc. Am. Assoc. Cancer Res. *12:*86, 1971.
90. S. J. Norman and E. Sorkin: Cell-specific defect in monocyte function during tumor growth. J. Natl. Cancer Inst. *57:*135–140, 1976.
91. D. A. Boetcher and E. J. Leonard: Abnormal monocyte chemotactic response in cancer patients. J. Natl. Cancer Inst. *52:*1091–1099, 1974.
92. R. Snyderman, L. Meadows, W. Holder, and S. Well, Jr.: Abnormal monocyte chemotaxis in patients with breast cancer: Evidence for a tumor-mediated effect. J. Natl. Cancer Inst. *60:*737–740, 1978.
93. J. Rhodes, M. Bishop, and J. Benfield: Tumor surveillance: How tumors may resist macrophage-mediated host defense. Science *203:*179–182, 1979.
94. T. Hyodo, K. Megyesi, C. R. Kahn, J. P. McLean, and H. G. Friesen: Adrenocortical carcinoma and hypoglycemia: Evidence for production of nonsuppressible insulin-like activity by the tumor. J. Clin. Endocrinol. Metab. *44:*1175–1184, 1977.
95. I. Hellström: Cellular immunity against tumor antigens. Adv. Cancer Res. *12:*167–223, 1969.
96. R. W. Baldwin, M. R. Price, and R. A. Robbins: Blocking of lymphocyte mediated cytotoxicity for rat hepatoma cells by tumour specific antigen-antibody complexes. Nature New Biol. *238:*185–187, 1972.
97. S. Broder, L. Muul, and T. A. Waldmann: Suppressor cells in neoplastic disease. J. Natl. Cancer Inst. *61:*5–11, 1978.
98. C. A. Savary and E. Lotzova: Suppression of natural killer cell cytotoxicity by splenocytes from *Corynebacterium parvum* injected, bone marrow tolerant, and infant mice. J. Immunol. *120:*239–243, 1978.
99. T. Tada, M. Taniguchi, and T. Takemori: Properties of primed suppressor T cells and their products. Transplant. Rev. *26:*106–129, 1975.
100. S. Broder, R. Humphrey, M. E. Durm, M. Blackman, B. Meade, C. Goldman, W. S. Frober, and T. Waldmann: Impaired synthesis of polyclonal (non-paraprotein) immunoglobulins by circulating lymphocytes from patients with multiple myeloma: Role of suppressor cells. New Eng. J. Med. *293:*887-–892, 1975.
101. A. Yu, H. Watts, N. Jaffee, and R. Parkman: Concomitant presence of tumor-specific cytotoxic and inhibitor lymphocytes in patients with osteogenic sarcoma. New Eng. J. Med. *297:*121–127, 1977.

102. R. M. Gorczynski: Immunity to murine sarcoma virus-induced tumors. II. Suppression of T-cell mediated immunity by cells from progressor animals. J. Immunol. *112:*1826–1838, 1974.
103. H. Kirchner, T. M. Chused, R. B. Herberman, H. T. Holden, and D. H. Lavrin: Evidence of suppressor cell activity in spleens of mice bearing primary tumors induced by Moloney sarcoma virus. J. Exp. Med. *139:*1473–1487, 1974.
104. G. T. Beatson: On treatment of inoperable cases of carcinoma of the mamma: Suggestions for a new method of treatment, with illustrative cases. Lancet *2:*104, 1896.
105. K. H. Clifton and B. N. Sridharan: Endocrine factors and tumor growth. *In Cancer: A Comprehensive Treatise,* Vol. 3, F. F. Becker, ed., New York: Plenum Press, 1975, pp. 249–285.
106. J. Furth: Conditioned and autonomous neoplasms: A review. Cancer Res. *13:*477–492, 1953.
107. J. Furth: A meeting of ways in cancer research: Thoughts on the evolution and nature of neoplasms. Cancer Res. *19:*241–258, 1959.
108. J. Furth, U. Ki, and K. H. Clifton: On evolution of the neoplastic state: Progression from dependence to autonomy. Natl. Cancer. Inst. Monogr. *2:*148–177, 1960.
109. K. H. Clifton: Hormones and experimental oncogenesis: Mammary and mammotropic tumors. *In Proc. Fourth Natl. Cancer Conf. 1961,* Philadelphia: Lippincott, pp. 41–50.
110. C. D. Turner and J. T. Bagnara: *General Endocrinology,* Philadelphia: Saunders, 1971.
111. B. W. O'Malley and A. Means: Molecular biology and estrogen regulation of target tissue growth and differentiation. *In Estrogen Target Tissues and Neoplasia,* T. L. Dao, ed., Chicago, University of Chicago Press, 1972, pp. 3–22.
112. K. H. Clifton: Problems in experimental tumorigenesis of the pituitary gland, gonads, adrenal cortices and mammary glands: A review. Cancer Res. *19:*2–22, 1959.
113. C. Huggins, G. Briziarelli, and H. Sutton: Rapid induction of mammary carcinoma in the rat and the influence of hormones on the tumors. J. Exp. Med. *109:*25–42, 1959.
114. A. I. Herbst, U. Ulfelder, and D. C. Poskanzer: Adenocarcinoma of the vagina. New Eng. J. Med. *284:*878–881, 1971.
115. J. Furth, G. Ueda, and K. H. Clifton: The pathophysiology of pituitaries and their tumors. Methodological advances. *In Methods in Cancer Research,* Vol. 10, H. Busch, ed., New York: Academic Press, 1973, pp. 201–277.
116. C. W. Welsch and C. Gribler: Prophylaxis of spontaneously developing mammary carcinoma in C3H/HeJ female mice by suppression of prolactin. Cancer Res. *33:*2939–2946, 1973.
117. J. Meites, K. H. Lu, W. Wuttke, C. W. Welsch, H. Nagasawa, and S. K. Quadri: Recent studies on functions and control of prolactin secretion in rats. Recent Progr. Hormone Res. *28:*471–526, 1972.
118. Boston, British and Finnish cooperative reports on reserpine and breast cancer. Lancet *2:*669–677, 1974.
119. D. Kodlin and N. McCarthy: Reserpine and breast cancer. Cancer *41:*761–768, 1978.
120. I. Mitra: Mammotropic effect of prolactin enhanced by thyroidectomy. Nature *248:*525–526, 1974.
121. G. M. Bogardus and J. W. Finley: Breast cancer and thyroid disease. Surgery *49:*461–468, 1961.
122. R. D. Bulbrook, J. L. Hayward, and C. C. Spicer: Relation between urinary androgen and corticoid excretion and subsequent breast cancer. Lancet *2:*395–398, 1971.
123. B. MacMahon, P. Cole, and J. Brown: Etiology of human breast cancer: A review. J. Natl. Cancer Inst. *50:*21–42, 1973.
124. J. Furth: Hormones as etiological agents in neoplasia. *In Cancer: A Comprehensive Treatise,* Vol. 1, F. F. Becker, ed., New York: Plenum Press, 1975, pp. 75–120.

125. L. H. Hempelmann: Risk of thyroid neoplasms after irradiation in childhood. Science *160:*159–163, 1969.

126. R. W. Park, J. F. Holland, and A. Jenkins: Urinary purines in leukemia. Cancer Res. *22:*469–477, 1962.

127. W. F. Dunning, M. R. Curtis, and M. E. Maun: The effect of added dietary tryptophane on the occurrence of 2-acetylaminofluorene-induced liver and bladder cancer in rats. Cancer Res. *9:*454–459, 1950.

128. J. L. Radomski, E. M. Glass, and W. B. Deichmann: Transitional cell hyperplasia in the bladders of dogs fed DL-tryptophan. Cancer Res. *31:*1690–1694, 1971.

129. G. T. Bryan, R. R. Brown, and J. M. Price: Incidence of mouse bladder tumors following implantation of paraffin pellets containing certain tryptophan metabolites. Cancer Res. *24:*582–585, 1964.

130. S. Gailani, G. Murphy, G. Kenny, A. Nussbaum, and P. Silvernail: Studies on tryptophan metabolism in patients with bladder cancer. Cancer Res. *33:*1071–1077, 1973.

131. K. Yamagiwa and K. Ichikawa: Experimental study of the pathogenesis of carcinoma. J. Cancer Res. *3:*1–21, 1918.

132. J. W. Cook, C. L. Hewett, and I. Hieger: Isolation of a cancer-producing hydrocarbon from coal tar. I. Concentration of the active substance. J. Chem. Soc. p. 395, 1933.

133. B. N. Ames, W. E. Durston, E. Yamasaki and F. D. Lee: Carcinogens are mutagens: A simple test system combining liver homogenates for activation and bacteria for detection. Proc. Natl. Acad. Sci. *70:*2281–2285, 1973.

134. L. Rehn: Blasengeschwülste bei Fuchsin—Arbeitern. Arch. Klin. Chir. *50:*588–600, 1895.

135. B. Fischer: Die experimentelle Erzeugung atypischer Epithelwucherungen und die Entstehung bösartiger Geschwiilste. Munch. med. Wschr. *53:*2041–2047, 1906.

136. R. Kinoshita: The cancerogenic chemical substances. Trans. Soc. Pathol. Japan. *27:*665–725, 1937.

137. R. H. Harris, T. Page and N. A. Reiches: Carcinogenic hazards of organic chemicals in drinking water. *In Origins of Human Cancer*, Book A, H. H. Hiatt, J. D. Watson, and J. A. Winsten, eds., Cold Spring Harbor Laboratory, 1977, pp. 309–330.

138. N. R. Farnsworth, A. S. Binel, H. H. S. Fong, A. A. Saleh, G. M. Christenson, and S. M. Saufferer: Oncogenic and tumor-promoting spermatophytes and pteridophytes and their active principles. Cancer Treatment Rep. *60:*1171–1214, 1976.

139. H. Druckrey and K. Küpfmüller: Dose and effect. Contribution to theoretical pharmacology. Pharmazie Ergänzungsband *1:*515–645, 1949.

140. R. Süss, V. Kinzel, and J. D. Scribner: *Cancer: Experiments and Concepts*. New York-Heidelberg-Berlin: Springer-Verlag, 1973, p. 47.

141. R. H. Adamson and S. M. Sieber: Antineoplastic agents as potential carcinogens. *In Origins of Human Cancer*, Book A, H. H. Hiatt, J. D. Watson, and J. A. Winsten, eds., Cold Spring Harbor Laboratory, 1977, pp. 429–443.

142. G. M. Bonser, L. Bradshaw, D. B. Clayson, and J. W. Jull: A further study of the carcinogenic properties of orthohydroxyamines and related compounds by bladder implantation in the mouse. Br. J. Cancer *10:*539–546, 1956.

143. J. H. Weisburger and G. M. Williams: Metabolism of chemical carcinogens. *In Cancer: A Comprehensive Treatise*, Vol. 1, F. F. Becker, ed., New York: Plenum Press, 1975, pp. 185–234.

144. A. H. Conney: Carcinogen metabolism and human cancer. New Eng. J. Med. *289:*971–973, 1973.

145. I. I. Kessler and J. P. Clark: Saccharin, cyclamate and human cancer: No evidence of an association. J. Am. Med. Assoc. *240:*349–355, 1978.

146. D. S. R. Sarma, S. Rajalakshmi, and E. Farber: Chemical carcinogenesis: Interactions

of carcinogens with nucleic acids. *In Cancer: A Comprehensive Treatise,* Vol. 1, F. F. Becker, eds., New York: Plenum Press, 1975, pp. 235–287.
147. B. Reiner and S. Zamenhof: Studies on the chemically reactive groups of deoxyribonucleic acids. J. Biol. Chem. *228:*475–486, 1957.
148. B. Pullman and A. Pullman: The electronic structure of the purine pyrimidine pairs of DNA. Biochim. Biophys. Acta *36:*343–350, 1959.
149. E. D. Bergmann and B. Pullman, eds.: *Physiochemical Mechanism of Carcinogenesis,* Jerusalem: Israel Academy of Sciences and Humanities, 1969.
150. J. C. Arcos and M. F. Argos: Molecular geometry and carcinogenic activity of aromatic compounds: New perspectives. Adv. Cancer Res. *11:*305–471, 1968.
151. F. J. Rauscher and T. E. O'Connor: Virology. *In Cancer Medicine,* J. F. Holland and E. Frei, eds., Philadelphia: Lea & Febiger, 1973, pp. 15–44.
152. G. Todaro, H. Green, and M. R. Swift: Susceptibility of human cells to transformation by SV40. Science *153:*1252–1254, 1966.
153. A. E. Freeman, P. J. Price, R. J. Bryan, R. J. Gordon, R. V. Gilden, G. J. Kelloff, and R. J. Huebner: Transformation of rat and hamster embryo cells by extracts of city smog. Proc. Natl. Acad. Sci. U.S. *68:*445–449, 1971.
154. W. Bernhard: The detection and study of tumor viruses with the electron microscope. Cancer Res. *20:*712–727, 1960.
155. R. C. Nowinski, L J. Old, N. H. Sarkar, and D. H. Moore: Common properties of the oncogenic RNA viruses (oncornaviruses). Virology *42:*1152–1157, 1970.
156. J. M. Bishop and H. E. Varmus: The molecular biology of RNA tumor viruses. *In Cancer: A Comprehensive Treatise,* Vol. 2, F. F. Becker, ed., New York: Plenum Press, 1975, pp. 3–48.
157. H. M. Temin: The RNA tumor viruses—background and foreground. Proc. Natl. Acad. Sci. U.S.A. *69:*1016–1020, 1972.
158. B. Roizman and D. Furlong: The replication of herpes viruses. *In Comprehensive Virology,* Vol. 3, H. Fraenkel Conrat and R. R. Wagner, eds., New York: Plenum Press, 1974, pp. 229–403.
159. F. Rapp and M. A. Jerkofsky: DNA viruses: Molecular biology. *In Cancer: A Comprehensive Treatise,* Vol. 2, F. F. Becker, ed., New York: Plenum Press, 1975, pp. 209–239.
160. H. zur Hausen and H. Schulte-Holthausen: Presence of nucleic acid homology in a "virus-free" line of Burkitt tumor cells. Nature *227:*245–248, 1970.
161. G. R. Dreesman, J. Burek, E. Adam, R. H. Kaufman, J. L. Melnick, K. L. Powell, and D. J. M. Purifoy: Expression of herpes virus-induced antigens in human cervical cancer. Nature *283:*591–593, 1980.
162. G. J. Todaro and R. J. Huebner: The viral oncogene hypothesis: New evidence. Proc. Natl. Acad. Sci. U.S.A. *69:*1009–1015, 1972.
163. G. M. Cooper, S. Okenquist, and L. Silverman: Transforming activity of DNA of chemically transformed and normal cells. Nature *284:*418–421, 1980.
164. H. M. Temin: The protovirus hypothesis: Speculations on the significance of RNA-directed DNA synthesis for normal development and for carcinogenesis. J. Natl. Cancer Inst. *46:*111–VII, 1971.
165. A. Frieben: Demonstration eines Cancroids des rechten Handnickens das sich nach langdauernder Einwirkung von Roentgenstrahlen entwickelt hatte. Fortschr. Gebiete Roentgenstrahlen Nuklearmed. *6:*106, 1902.
166. A. C. Upton: Physical carcinogenesis: Radiation—History and Sources. *In Cancer: A Comprehensive Treatise,* Vol. 1, F. F. Becker, ed., New York. Plenum Press, 1975, pp. 387–403.

167. O. J. Bizzozero, K. G. Johnson, and A. Çicocco: Radiation-related leukemia in Hiroshima and Nagasaki, 1946–1964. New Eng J. Med. *274:*1095–1101, 1966.
168. B. MacMahon: Prenatal X-ray exposure and childhood cancer. J. Natl. Cancer Inst. *28:*1173–1191, 1962.
169. J. B. Storer: Radiation carcinogenesis. *In Cancer: A Comprehensive Treatise,* Vol. 1, F. F. Becker, ed., New York: Plenum Press, 1975, pp. 453–483.
170. International Commission on Radiological Protection. Radiosensitivity and spatial distribution of dose. ICRP Publication 14, Oxford: Pergamon Press, 1969.
171. N. Waterman: Observations on the carcinogenic effect of ultra-violet rays of different wavelengths on the skin of mice with some remarks on carcinogenesis. Geneesk. BI *50:*297–347, 1963.
172. D. Gordon, H. Silverstone, and B. S. Smithhurst: The epidemiology of skin cancer in Australia. *In Melanoma and Skin Cancer,* W. H. McCarthy, ed., Sydney: NSW Government Printer, 1972.
173. E. J. Pollack and G. J. Todaro: Radiation enhancement of SV40 transformation in 3T3 and human cells. Nature *219:*520–521, 1968.
174. L. J. Cole and P. C. Nowell: Radiation carcinogenesis: The sequence of events. Science *150:*1782–1786, 1965.
175. J. F. Gaeta: Trauma and inflammation. *In Cancer Medicine,* J. F. Holland and E. Frei, eds., Philadelphia: Lea & Febiger, 1973, pp. 102–106.
176. N. Treves and G. T. Pack: The development of cancer in burn scars. Surg. Gnec. Obstet. *51:*749–782, 1930.
177. P. Mustacchi: Parasites. *In Cancer Medicine,* J. F. Holland and E. Frei, eds., Philadelphia: Lea & Febiger, 1973, pp. 106–112.
178. A. W. Cheever: Schistosomiasis and neoplasia. J. Natl. Cancer Inst. *61:*13–18, 1978.
179. G. M. Edington, F. Von Lichtenberg, I. Nwabuebo, J. R. Taylor, and J. H. Smith: Pathologic effects of schistosomiasis in Ibadan, Western State of Nigeria. I. Incidence and intensity of infection: Distribution and severity of lesions. Am. J. Trop. Med. Hyg. *19:*982–985, 1970.
180. A. M. Stephen and J. H. Cummings: Mechanism of action of dietary fibre in the human colon. Nature *284:*283–284, 1980.
181. D. P. Burkitt, A. R. P. Walker, and N. S. Painter: Effect of dietary fibre on stools and transit-times, and its role in the causation of disease. Lancet *11:*1408–1412, 1972.
182. G. Hems: The contribution of diet and childbearing to breast-cancer rates. Brit. J. Cancer *37:*974–982, 1978.
183. M. J. Hill, J. S. Crowther, B. S. Drasar, G. Hawksworth, V. Aries, and R. E. O. Williams: Bacteria and aetiology of cancer of the large bowel. Lancet *1:*95–100, 1971.
184. J. M. Hopkin an H. J. Evans: Cigarette smoke-induced DNA damage and lung cancer risks. Nature *283:*388–390, 1980.
185. D. Schottenfeld and J. F. Haas: Carcinogens in the workplace. CA-A Cancer J. for Clinicians *29:*144–168, 1979.

7. Treatment

The advice given in the Hippocratic writings that patients with occult cancers would live longer if left untreated, coupled with Galen's belief that cancer arose from an excess of black bile, doubtless discouraged attempts to treat the disease. Only medicinal treatment, based for the most part on herbals and folk remedies, was used for tumors that were not superficial until the eighteenth century. Between 1704 and 1769, the concept was developed successively by Valsalva (1), LeDran (2), and then Morgagni (3) that initially cancer was a local disease that could be cured by surgery if detected before it became disseminated. From that time, surgery has remained the chief form of treatment for malignant as well as benign tumors. Radiotherapy, beginning almost immediately after Roentgen's discovery of x-rays, has come to be the second most effective form of therapy. Its major limitations are the radiosensitivity of the tumor and the need to keep dosages at a level that does not damage normal tissues excessively. A modern, more rational heir to the medicinal approach, chemotherapy has achieved limited success, although it is now applied widely. Immunotherapy is currently an experimental method; its future role is unclear. What is now emerging is an interdisciplinary approach, coordinating the three major treatment modalities for maximum benefit to the patient, while the attempt is made to minimize disability, disfigurement, and side effects. We shall review the major modalities of treatment, pointing out their successes and limitations and how newer concepts of tumor biology are altering them.

SURGERY

It was only after the concept of an initial phase of local cancer growth was developed that the possibility of a surgical cure seemed realistic. As surgical techniques improved during the nineteenth and twentieth centuries, more complex operations became feasible. Surgery thus came to occupy center stage with respect to cancer, not only as a means of cure, but also for biopsies, palliative treatment, laparotomy, and removal of endocrine glands to modify the hormonal status and suppression of pain by neurosurgical procedures. It is unfortunate that major developments in the surgical approach to cancer predated knowledge of tumor biology, for in the absence of such knowledge, there is always the possibility of a faulty basis for therapy. Many surgeons deeply involved in cancer treatment now believe that this did occur in the form of a trend toward ever more radical operations (4). It is interesting to see how this occurred.

Radical surgery

The late nineteenth century saw the development of Halsted's concepts regarding the type of surgery appropriate for breast cancer (5), concepts that were to dominate the surgical treatment of all forms of cancer for about 70 years. Halsted, an American surgeon, adopted the views of Handley on how metastasis occurs (6). According to this view, cancer extends by infiltration and lymphatic spread, as well as along the planes of fascia, uninterruptedly, so as to produce a region of essentially continuous disease. Dissemination of tumor cells by the vascular system was not considered significant, despite the demonstration, as early as 1869 (7), of cancer cells in the blood. Acceptance of such a view, when wedded to the perceived need to eradicate all cancer cells, led to the definition of a "satisfactory cancer operation" as one in which the primary tumor, along with regional lymphatics, lymph nodes, and adjacent normal structures, were removed *en bloc*. This meant that large amounts of skin, muscle, and bone, together with lymphatics, would be dissected out, frequently creating severe psychological, functional, and cosmetic problems for the patient, but not necessarily improving the chance of cure. The data reproduced in Table 7-1 clearly show that even in a group of patients with breast cancer that is considered potentially surgically curable, radical mastectomy failed to provide cures for most of the patients with positive nodes, despite extensive dissection. Thus, we may conclude that in these patients metastasis had

Table 7-1 Treatment failures in patients 5 and 10 years after radical mastectomy.

Status of nodes *	*Treatment failures (percent)* (*5 years*)	(*10 years*)
Negative nodes	18	24
One to three positive nodes	50	65
Four or more positive nodes	79	86

These data reproduced in part from Ref. 4, with permission of the publisher, Plenum Press.
*The number of nodes with cancer in the resected area.

already occurred well beyond the local region, and the positive nodes reflected this, rather than merely marking the extent to which the disease had spread. As we saw in Chapter 3, a tumor can shed blood-borne metastatic cells as soon as angiogenesis occurs, when the size of the tumor is far below that at which clinical detection is possible. In a sense, then, radical surgery has a questionable theoretical basis, since it is unlikely ever to deal with metastases, although it may effectively extirpate local and extensively infiltrative disease. What then are the newer definitions of the role of surgery in curative management? We can begin by enumerating the factors from tumor biology that need to be considered and then give examples of what is emerging as cancer surgery with a biological rather than a purely anatomical basis (4).

Biological factors in cancer surgery

Data such as those shown in Table 7-1 reflect the fact that although cancer may start as a local disease, it very soon becomes systemic. This does not mean, however, that the galenical attitude that prevailed prior to the eighteenth century was correct. A local approach may still be curative, but other factors involved, which may be operative during and after surgery, may deal with systemic disease. Obviously no surgical operation can remove micrometastases to distant regions, so what then is actually controlling them? As we have seen, the growth of cancer is not an entirely uncontrolled process, and most disseminated cells do not establish metastases. When the primary tumor is removed, in many cases the balance appears to be tipped in favor of the host; neuroblastoma and renal carcinoma are diseases in which removal of the primary tumor has led to the regression of metastases (7A).

Chief among the effects of surgery are modulations of the immune system (4). In both experimental animals and human patients, reduction of the tumor burden has led to a precipitous fall in "blocking antibody" activity (8–10), to recovery of cell-mediated immune functions (9,11–14), and to the appearance of specific immunizing antitumor antibodies (15). With respect to these immunological findings, however, it should be pointed out that reports at variance with the cited references have appeared. These reports involved animal model systems in which tumor resection led to loss of immunity and growth of metastases (16) and to loss of *in vitro* cytotoxicity by macrophages in bone marrow cultures from animals after tumor removal (17). Such variation is to be expected in view of much experimental evidence for the heterogeneity of metastases and the variable influence of immune factors on their growth (18). Surgery itself, with its own trauma leading to hormone changes, together with the effects of anesthesia and other drugs, may act on tumor immune responses both positively and negatively (4).

Another area in which removal of the primary tumor affects metastases is that of cell kinetics. There is evidence that the primary tumor and its metastatic foci behave in some respects as a unity, and may show synchronous slowing of growth rates as the total mass evolves further along the Gompertzian growth curve (19). Reduction of the tumor mass by surgery or other methods may increase the growth fraction in the remaining tumor foci, thus elevating growth rates and making the residual metastatic tumor more sensitive to chemotherapeutic agents (20,21); this constitutes an argument for the use of so-called *adjuvant chemotherapy*.

In Chapter 3 we discussed the role of the lymph node as a partial barrier to tumor spread, certainly not the effective barrier once believed, but one that is capable of interfering with the growth of tumor cells (22), provided it is not overwhelmed with too many circulating cells. In a given region, the difference between positive and negative nodes (in terms of the presence of tumor cells) may reflect differential ability to kill cells entering various nodes; the extent of the challenge, which might exceed the nodal cytotoxic ability; a bypassing of the node by tumor cells; or even cell traversal through the node. Thus nodal distribution may give little definitive information about the extent of disease, although it may demonstrate the existence of metastases and indicate the prognosis (4).

Multicentric tumors present a special surgical problem (23). Here, many tumors may develop at different loci within an organ. Common sites for this are the oral cavity in pipe and cigar smokers, the colon in cases of familial polyposis or ulcerative colitis, the bladder, and the lungs. Related to this are bilateral tumors of paired organs. There is said to be a 10 to 20 times greater risk of finding cancer of the contralateral breast in subjects who have had one breast removed because of a neoplasm (24), and bilateral ovarian carcinoma occurs in 40 to 50 percent of all cases (23). A complication in such figures is that occult lesions found by autopsy or by random biopsies may occur far more frequently than overt clinical breast cancer, for example (25,26). It is of course much more likely that such occult nodules will be found in a woman who has had a mastectomy, because she most likely will be under more intensive scrutiny than other females, but what happens to most of these lesions? A likely explanation is that most do not progress further, or may even regress, rather as do childhood neuroblastoma, thyroid carcinomas, and carcinoma of the prostate, none of which show as high an incidence of overt tumors as random pathological material or other tests would suggest (27).

Trends in curative cancer surgery

While there has been a general trend toward less radical surgery, this has been most marked in the case of breast cancer. Lack of evidence of significantly greater survival following extended radical mastectomy, as contrasted with more conservative procedures (28), consideration of biological findings, and the wish to avoid needless disfigurement have altered the approach to this disease. Total mastectomy has come into favor as appropriate surgery for most breast cancer, whereas segmental mastectomies or "lumpectomies," in which only a portion of the breast is removed, are being performed increasingly for what appears to be limited disease (29). The aim of such surgery is not to attempt to extirpate all cancer cells, but to reduce the tumor burden to a level that can be handled by various control mechanisms of the host, or alternatively, to render the remaining tumor cells more sensitive to other modalities, notably chemotherapy, because of alterations in cellular kinetics (4). Curative surgery is increasingly associated with more imaginative use of breast prostheses and cosmetic surgery to improve the patient's appearance and morale (30). In some cases, a primary surgical approach has been abandoned in favor of radiotherapy of breast lesions, using both radioactive implants and external beam irradiation (31). This has been done most frequently in very young women with limited disease. However, extreme caution is needed in using such treatment extensively, in preference to well-tried surgical procedures. A final aspect of breast cancer surgery concerns bilateral disease. Many surgeons have routinely performed simple mastectomy of the contralateral breast whenever they performed a radical mastectomy (32). Unless there is clear evidence of disease in the contralateral breast, however, it is probably not necessary to go to such lengths, but certainly frequent followup is essential (23). At present not enough is known to be able to determine which lesions may progress and which regress, and thus to make a rational decision for or against contralateral mastectomy.

Osteosarcoma, primarily a bone disease of the young, most frequently affects the lower extremities. Since the tumor is not notably radiosensitive, and since it invades bone and bone marrow, preferred treatment has been amputation (33). Recently, there has been much experimentation aimed at preserving the limb. These approaches use such measures as artificial bone implants (34), cadaver bone, after sterilizing it with heat or high dose irradiation and reimplanting it (35). Such implants do not have the same strength as native, unprocessed bone, but enable the patient to avoid the trauma of amputation. This has been a consideration behind Marcove's studies using bone autografts.

Wilms' tumor (36), an embryonal kidney tumor that originates in the fetal metanephrogenic blastoma, is the second most common abdominal malignant childhood tumor in the United States. At the time of discovery the tumor is frequently very large, weighing up to 5 kilograms and usually demarcated from renal parenchyma by a thin pseudocapsule of connective tissue. However, invasion of neighboring structures and blood vessels is very common. The treatment of this tumor is the best example of a coordinated, multi-modal therapeutic approach that involves surgery, radiation, and chemotherapy. Total removal of the tumor is the essential first step, but when this is not possible, the use of chemotherapeutic drugs to shrink the tumor may then be followed by successful surgery. The tumor bed is irradiated immediately with 200 to 500 rads per day over about a 3-week period. Finally, chemotherapy with actinomycin D is started at the same time as the other modalities. Vincristine also is effective in this disease. This multi-modal approach has led to a 5-year survival rate of around 90 percent.

Palliative surgery

Surgeons are frequently called upon to perform operations that are not curative, but rather serve to lesson the pain or the complications of the disease. Such palliative surgery, even if it is non-curative, fulfills a major role in helping to ease the life of a patient with incurable disease. Thus, primary tumors may be removed even if it is clearly established that there is metastatic disease. Examples might be ulcerating sarcomas of the limb or primary breast cancers, where amputation or simple mastectomy may reduce pain, bleeding, and the chance of infection, but would probably not alter the eventual outcome. In some cases the debulking of total tumor burden that results may improve the response of metastases to chemotherapy, probably because of cell kinetic factors discussed previously. There are even a few cases in which the palliative removal of primary tumor has led to regression of metastatic disease (7A,37). Presumably the tumors no longer overwhelmed the immune capacity of the host.

For tumors of the gastrointestinal and genitourinary tracts, obstruction is a major problem, for which palliative surgery, in the form of bypasses, gastroenteric anastomoses, colostomies, and decompression with the help of tubes, may relieve the acute situation. Hemorrhages of the alimentary tract, especially the stomach, may result from lymphomas, and surgical intervention may be necessary to stop blood loss. Compression of the spinal cord due to epidural disease, that is, tumor arising in the membranes, may also be relieved surgically, although radiotherapy is frequently used despite the fact that it tends to produce edema that sometimes worsens the situation.

Surgery is frequently used to modify hormone status in patients with disease that is responsive to hormones. At the present time it is essential to determine the endocrine responsiveness of the tumor by surveying excreted steroids and measuring hormone-binding activity, which reflects the number of receptors, in samples of the tumors. Thus, ovariectomy is commonly used in the treatment of premenopausal women with breast cancer (38); hypophysectomy (removal of the pituitary) with a number of cancers, including thyroid carcinoma; and orchiectomy with prostatic cancer (39).

The disfiguring nature of many cancer operations, especially those for tumors of the breast, head, and neck, makes reconstructive surgery a useful adjunct that can contribute greatly to the patient's well-being.

Finally, such procedures as cordotomy, the interruption of spinothalamic tracts within the spinal cord, local nerve blocks, sensory rhizotomy, chemical rhizotomy by intrathecal administration of phenol in glycerol, irrigation of the subarachnoid space with saline, and intracerebral surgery have been used to control intractable pain (40). Problems that arise from such procedures include inadvertent more widespread neurological damage and, more frequently, injuries due to burns and lacerations that result from decreased sensory perception by the patient.

It is beyond the scope of this book to discuss the actual techniques used in cancer surgery. For this the reader is referred to several excellent texts (41–44).

RADIOTHERAPY

Overview

Radiation therapy began within months of Roentgen's discovery of x-rays so that, by 1899, the first report of the cure of a basal cell epithelioma appeared. This was followed by a succession of impressive responses of superficial cancers that generated great enthusiasm. However, it soon became apparent that there were major problems with this new modality. Delivered as a single massive dose, the damage to normal tissues was so severe that significant numbers of patients died, and in most cases when the treatment itself was not fatal, the tumor recurred (45,46). Equipment was primitive, unreliable, and of low voltage, and in the absence of any method of dosimetry, radiotherapists were forced to test the working of their apparatus by such hazardous procedures as observing the degree of redness (erythema) of their own and their patient's skin. No advance was possible until Claude Regaud and his colleagues showed that fractionated doses could permanently eradicate testicular spermatogenesis, whereas single massive doses created intolerable damage to the skin for the same biological effect on the testis (47). These findings were then applied to cancer radiation therapy, in which Regaud perceived the same problem of selectively killing rapidly dividing cells without causing excessive damage to normal tissues (48).

The next phase of development began with Coolige's hot cathode vacuum x-ray tube with its reliable kilovolt energies (up to 250 kVp). Further progress followed the adoption of the roentgen as the unit of radiation dose, a standard based on the extent of ionization of air by the radiation, since all clinically used radiation is able to excite and eject electrons from the target. Initially, ionization chambers were used to measure radiation dose, but thermoluminescent detectors are now most common. Other methods include oxidation of salts of metals that exist in more than one valency state and calorimetry, in which heat production by the irradiation is measured. These improvements led to more consistent cures of skin, oral, laryngeal, and uterine cervical cancers.

Despite such progress, however, damage to superficial tissues and skin remained a severe limitation to the dose that could be delivered. Sloughing of skin to give a virtually permanent non-healing sore, which was a major

Table 7-2 Improved survival of patients treated with megavoltage therapy.

Type of cancer	*Five-year survivals (percent)* (*kilovoltage x-rays*)	(*megavoltage x-rays*)
Bladder	0–5	25–35
Cervix	35–45	55–65
Hodgkin's disease	30–35	70–75
Nasopharynx	20–25	45–50
Ovary	15–20	50–60
Prostate	5–15	55–60
Retinoblastoma	30–40	80–85
Testis (embryonal)	20–25	55–70
Testis (seminoma)	65–70	90–90
Tonsil	25–30	40–50

Data derived from the Report of the Panel of Consultants on the Conquest of Cancer, U.S. Government Printing Office, Washington, D.C., 1970.

site of infection, resulted from too high a dose. The post-World War II era brought new developments. One of these was the production of radiocobalt (^{60}Co), which could be used both for internal implants (giving a new alternative to radium) and for external beam therapy by virtue of the high energy γ-rays of 1.1 and 1.3 MeV, nearly an order of magnitude more energetic than hitherto possible. Other developments in physics led to the construction of betatrons, which accelerate electrons in a circular path up to energies of 5 to 40 MeV, and linear accelerations, which transfer energy from microwaves to electrons moving in a linear path with energies of 5 to 35 MeV. In both cases, the electrons may be used either as they are, or they are allowed to strike a target and generate high energy x-rays (up to 25 MeV), which have much greater penetrative ability than electrons. Linear accelerators generate more of these energetic x-rays than do betatrons. The results obtained with linear accelerators far surpass kilovoltage x-rays (Table 7-2). Attempts are now being made to use even higher energy particles, as well as to modify the action of radiation by enhancing or protective agents, and to combine radiation therapy with surgery and chemotherapy.

Physics of radiation (49)

The types of radiation used or studied experimentally in radiation therapy include short wavelength electromagnetic radiation (x-rays, γ-rays), electrons, neutrons, α-particles (helium nuclei), and some other heavy particles (protons, π-mesons, heavy ions). All have in common the ability to generate certain ions in the target tissue, that is, they are all ionizing radiation. Neutrons are a special case in that they cause ionization only indirectly through their ability to generate protons and α-particles when interacting with hydrogen, carbon, and oxygen atoms in the target tissue. The rates at which the different forms of radiation transfer their energy to targets by ionization vary widely, depending on the type, energy level, and nature of the ions they produce. Heavy, highly charged particles, such as α-rays, interact very readily with atoms because of their comparable size and transfer their energy within a short distance; their penetration is thus very limited, but local ionization is very intense. On the other hand, γ-rays, with high energy, negligible mass, and no charge, interact less readily and give a lower density of ionization. These radiations of lower ionization density act to a large extent by displacing electrons. Neutrons are also very penetrating because they have no charge, but they generate density-ionizing particles. X-rays with lower energy levels are poorly penetrating, despite low mass and no charge. The initial energy of other high-energy particles carries them some distance before they reach the most intensively ionizing portions of their track, the *Bragg peak region.* These properties are illustrated in Figure 7-1, where it can be seen that increase in energy delivers a larger fraction of the dose at a greater depth. Thus, the superficial tissues may be spared, while most of the cytotoxic damage occurs in the underlying tumor. This is most pronounced with pion therapy, in which very localized intense dosages may be delivered.

Figure 7-1 Percent of maximum dose delivered at various depths for radiations of different energies. Derived from Ref. 49.

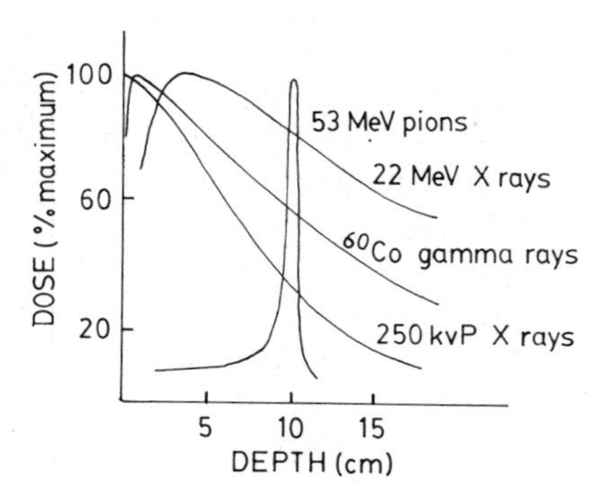

In describing the density of ionization produced by radiation, the term *linear energy transfer* (LET) is used. This is the average energy imparted per unit of distance traveled, expressed in kiloelectron volts per micrometer (KeV/μm). However, ionization may occur very non-uniformly along the track, and since the average ionization may be calculated either by dividing the track into equal lengths (track average) or by dividing the track into sections of identical energy transfer (energy average), figures that are quoted may show marked discrepancies. Thus for ^{60}Co γ-rays, the LET values for track and energy averages are 0.27 and 0.32 KeV/μm, whereas for 14 McV neutrons, these values are 12 and 75 KeV/μm, respectively. α-Particles, which are very densely ionizing, have LET values of 120 KeV/μm for 2.5 MeV particles (50).

In the case of local irradiation, sometimes termed brachytherapy, as opposed to external beam therapy, radioisotopes are placed in such body cavities as the peritoneal cavity, the vagina, or the cervical channel, or implanted directly in the target tissue in the form of needles. Radium-226, radon-222, cesium-137, iridium-192, iodine-125 or iodine-131, and gold-198 are the most commonly used isotopes, and some work has been done with californium-252. Gold, used as a colloidal preparation for abdominal and other ascites, is not removed after use, but allowed to decay. The properties of these isotopes are shown in Table 7-3. With brachytherapy, the absorbed dose falls rapidly with distance, being reduced to around 10 percent at 1.5 cm and 1 percent at 4 cm from the source. These values do not vary too widely for the different isotopes, since geometry is the important factor.

From the point of view of advantages and disadvantages of different forms of radiation, the higher energy particles have very favorable dose-depth relations for deep-seated tumors. However, the size of the machines needed to generate protons and π-mesons (pions), problems with focusing and generating high energy neutrons (large cyclotrons are needed), and the sharpness of the ionizing field, which entails precise knowledge of the tumor location, present difficulties. Despite these problems, much effort is being directed into developing higher energy particles not only because of the dose-depth relations, but also because of evidence that the oxygen effect is diminished.

We mentioned above that the roentgen (R) was the unit of radiation dose. This has been defined as the dose that produces, by ionization, one electrostatic unit of electricity per cm^3 of air, or that deposits 100 ergs per cm^3. The unit more commonly employed in practice is the rad, which is

Table 7-3 Properties of radioisotopes used in radiotherapy.

Isotope	Half-life	Energy of radiation (MeV) α	β	γ
Californium-252	2.65 years	6.119*		0.043*
		6.076		0.100
		5.975		0.160
Cesium-137	30.23 years	0.511*		0.662
		1.176		
Iodine-125	60 days (electron capture)			0.035
Iodine-131	8.07 days		0.257	0.080
			– 0.806	– 0.723
			0.606*	0.364*
Iridium-192	74 days		0.24	0.136
			0.536	– 1.062
			0.672*	0.317*
			+ 0.24†	
Gold-198	2.693 days		0.280	0.412*
			0.961*	0.676
			1.374	1.088
Radium-226	1,600 years	4.160		0.186
		– 4.781		– 0.61
		4.781*		0.186*
Radon-222	3.823 days	4.824		0.51
		4.984		
		5.486*		

Data derived from CRC Handbook of Chemistry and Physics 1972–73. Where more than three discrete particle energies exist a range is given.

* Most intense.

† Positron.

defined as the dose that deposits 100 ergs per gram of tissue; it is between 0.92 and 0.96 times the exposure measured in roentgens.

Radiochemical interactions

The initial products of radiation in its interaction with matter are ionized species, but these then interact with other molecules to generate free radicals (Figure 7-2). Since the predominant molecular species in tissues is water, radicals derived from water are the most important. A feature of free radicals is that they can undergo chain reactions with other molecules, in which free radicals are continuously regenerated. Thus, the initial ioni-

Water reactions:

$$H_2O \xrightarrow[\text{excitation}]{\text{radiation}} H_2O^* \longrightarrow H^\bullet + OH^\bullet$$

$$H_2O \xrightarrow[\text{ionization}]{\text{radiation}} H_2O^+ + e^-$$

$$H_2O^+ + H_2O \longrightarrow H_3O^+ + OH^\bullet$$

$$e^- + H_2O \longrightarrow e^-_{aq} \longrightarrow OH^- + H^\bullet$$

$$e^- + H_3O^+ \longrightarrow H_2O + H^\bullet$$

$$2OH^\bullet \longrightarrow H_2O_2$$

$$2H^\bullet \longrightarrow H_2 \xrightarrow{OH^\bullet} H_2O + H^\bullet$$

$$H_2O_2 \xrightarrow{H^\bullet} H_2O + OH^\bullet$$

In presence of O_2:

$$H^\bullet + O_2 \longrightarrow HO_2^\bullet \longrightarrow H_2O_2 + O_2$$

$$HO_2 + e^- \longrightarrow HO_2^- \xrightarrow{H^+} H_2O$$

With organic molecules:

$$R + OH^\bullet \longrightarrow ROH^\bullet$$

$$R + OH^\bullet \longrightarrow R^\bullet + H_2O$$

$$R^\bullet + O_2 \longrightarrow RO_2^\bullet \longrightarrow R + O_2^\bullet$$

$$RO_2^\bullet \xrightarrow{R'H} RO_2H + R'^\bullet$$

Figure 7-2 Excited species and radicals derived from the interaction of radiation with water and with organic molecules. In the presence of oxygen, additional species are formed.

zation may give rise to a prolonged formation and diffusion of reactive species. Such radicals are responsible for most of the biological damage resulting from ionizing radiation (51). Direct damage due to radiation acting on macromolecules, such as DNA, without other intermediate radicals, doubtless occurs, but is much less likely because most of the molecules in the path of the radiation will be water. It is of major biological import that, in the presence of oxygen, a wider variety of radical species is formed, and in addition, peroxides, which are themselves reactive; other toxic substances are also produced. This additional formation of reactive species forms the basis of the oxygen effect.

Radiobiological damage

The amount of biological damage that radiation produces directly reflects the number of active radical species generated. The simplest measure of damage, the fraction of cells killed by radiation, will vary depending on the type of radiation for any given dosage. The biological effectiveness of a particular form of radiation is frequently compared to the effectiveness of 250 kVp x-rays, and this ratio of the dose of x-rays to the dose of the other radiation needed to give the same effect is termed the *relative biological effectiveness* (RBE). Additionally, since extra reactive species are formed in the presence of oxygen, more damage will occur. The ratio of the dose under hypoxic to that under aerobic conditions required to produce a given amount of damage is known as the *oxygen enhancement ratio* (OER). Like the RBE, the OER varies with the LET value of the radiation. Although the actual shape of the curves depends upon the type of high energy particles used, it is clear that the oxygen effect diminishes and disappears at high LET values, whereas the RBE increases to a maximum around 100 KeV/μm (Figure 7-3). This means that the oxygen effect should be lower for high energy particles and neutrons than for lower energy radiations. Since, as we saw earlier, the interior of a tumor may be hypoxic and thus less sensitive to conventional radiation, there is a theoretical advantage in using high LET radiation. The advantage may, in fact, be less than theory suggests, because of the phenomenon of "*reoxygenation*," by which the original fraction of hypoxic cells tends to be reestablished by better oxygen supply to previously hypoxic cells as a result of reduction in tumor mass and hence distance from capillaries (52). Since radiation is always given in fractionated doses, this phenomenon may enhance the effectivenes of subsequent doses.

Figure 7-3 The variation of the oxygen enhancement ratio (OER) and the relative biological efficacy (RBE) as functions of the value of the linear energy transfer (LET) of α particles. Biological data represent killing of T_1 kidney cells in culture. From Barendsen, G.W., *In Proceedings of the Conference on Particle Accelerators in Radiation Therapy*. U.S. Atomic Energy Commission, Technical Information Center, LA-5180-C, pp. 120–125, 1972.

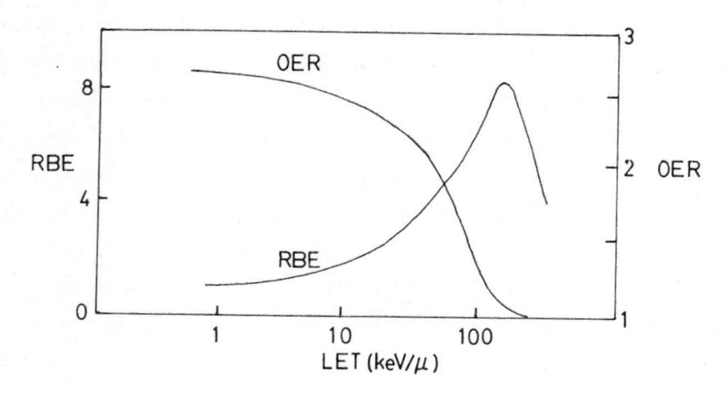

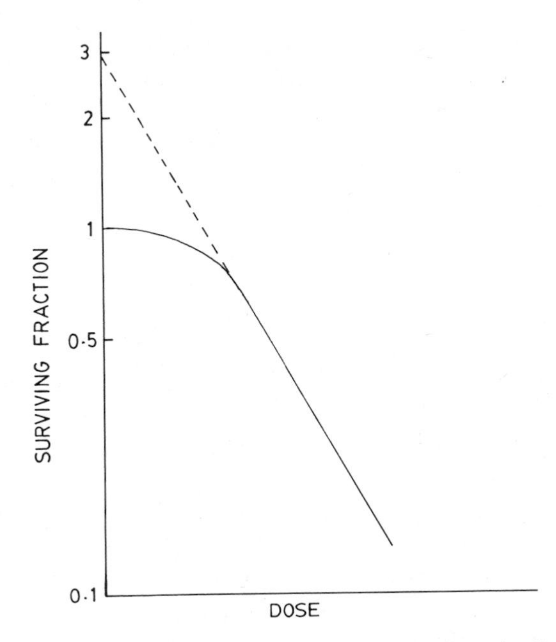

Figure 7-4 Typical dose-response curve for the survival of irradiated cells.

Cytotoxicity. Cytotoxicity is a very definitive and easily measured end point, yet one which is the result of a complex series of events. Survival curves for irradiated cells generally have the features shown in Figure 7-4. The major portion represents exponential or logarithmic kinetics of cell kill, in other words, during this phase a given dose of radiation will kill a fixed fraction of the population, no matter what the initial number of cells; many chemotherapeutic agents show similar kinetics of lethality. Extrapolation of this linear portion of the curve back to the ordinate gives a value known as the *extrapolation number n.* This number, in large measure, reflects the size of the initial portion of the curve, the *shoulder.* It is generally considered that the shoulder represents the dosage region in which damage created by radiation may still be repaired completely. At higher doses, repair processes cannot keep up with the increased amount of damage. The reciprocal of the slope of the linear portion of the curve is D_0. Although radiation may kill cells no matter what their proliferative state, there is no question that cells committed to division are more sensitive than those not in the cell cycle (53). The initial effect on dividing cells is mitotic delay, with cells blocked in the G_2 phase and thus unable to enter mitosis. There appears to be a delay of about one-tenth of a cell cycle per 100 rads, that is, of the order of 1 hour per 100 rads for rapidly dividing epithelial cells and 7 hours for skin. Cell death commonly occurs at a mitosis subsequent to the mitotic arrest, except for lymphocytes, which are extraordinarily sensitive and die in interphase (54). As for the sensitivity of the phases of the cell cycle, there is preferential kill of those in mitosis and G_2 (Figure 7-5), with G_1 and early S phase cells of intermediate sensitivity, and those in late S most resistant to radiation (55).

Damage to DNA. This is considered to play a central role in the overall effect of radiation on cells. The correlation between chromosome volume or DNA content and radiosensitivity, the effect of base composition on sensitivity to radiation, which decreases with increasing adenine-thymine content, the greater sensitivity of bacterial mutants deficient in DNA repair, and the sensitizing action of such analogs as 5-bromo-2′-deoxyuridine when they are incorporated into DNA all argue for a major role for this macromolecule (56). Studies of the effects of ultraviolet light, which is a non-ionizing radiation, also implicate a DNA with an ultraviolet absorption

Figure 7-5 Cell survival curves for Chinese hamster cells irradiated at different stages of the cell cycle. Taken from W. R. Sinclair: Cyclic x-ray responses in mammalian cells *in vitro*, Radiation Res. *33*:620, 1968.

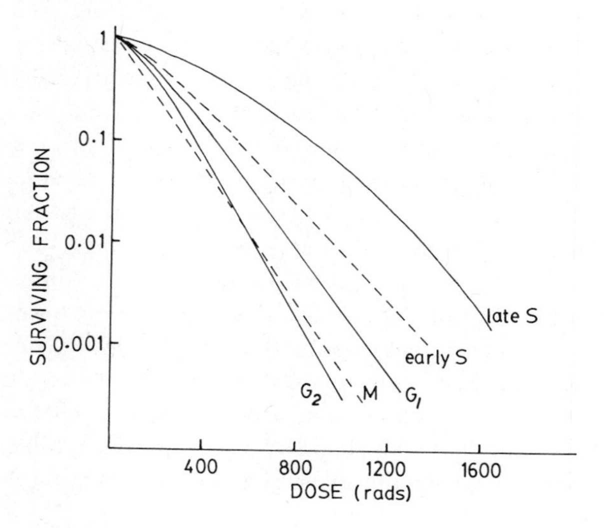

spectrum that corresponds with the action spectrum for biological damage. However, it seems unlikely that DNA represents a single simple target on the basis of several findings. First, the OER for isolated DNA does not exceed 1.5, whereas typical values for cells are around 3.0. Second, acriflavin, which intercalates between the base pairs of DNA and inhibits repair of DNA damage, is a better sensitizer of hypoxically irradiated bacterial cells than of those irradiated in the presence of oxygen. Third, there is a correlation between sensitivity to ultraviolet light, sensitivity to x-rays under hypoxia, the magnitude of the OER, and the size of the RBE such that repair-deficient bacteria are highly sensitive to both ultraviolet and x-rays and have low OER values; and the opposite is true of ultraviolet-resistant strains. Alper has suggested that such data are consistent with a two-target model, DNA itself (type N) and a DNA-membrane complex, which is mostly responsible for the oxygen effect (type O) (57,58). Such a concept agrees with the data, such as that the site of attachment of DNA to membranes is the location for strand separation and initiation of replication, that radiation damage to membranes, measured by enzyme release, shows OER values of 5 or more, and that lipid-containing membranes are very subject to peroxide formation by irradiation under aerobic conditions (56). Type N effects would thus be dominant under hypoxic conditions and in repair-deficient cells with ultraviolet and radiation sensitivity.

The actual molecular damage created by radiation seems to be primarily in the form of DNA *strand breaks*, principally single-strand breaks, but with additional double-strand breaks at a relative frequency of 1:25 (56). Such breaks occur because the energy transferred during each absorption is about 60 eV, enough to break any molecular bond. Single-strand breaks include both overt strand cleavage and lesions that are manifested only after exposure to alkaline conditions. At lower doses (< 800 rads) that allow a high degree of cell survival, a limited number of breaks occur in DNA and in the DNA-membrane complex, permitting the release of fairly high molecular weight single-stranded DNA and leading also to conformational changes in the form of a relaxed degree of supercoiling. With increasing dosage of radiation, the sedimentation profile by sucrose density gradient analysis, indicates the appearance of DNA of clearly lower molecular weight reflecting more extensive strand breakage (59). When irradiated cells are incubated at 37°C prior to density gradient analysis, these changes are partly or wholly reversed, as shown in Figure 7-6. This temperature-dependent reversal reflects the action of repair enzymes, which underlies the phenomenon of the shoulder on dose-response curves for cell survival.

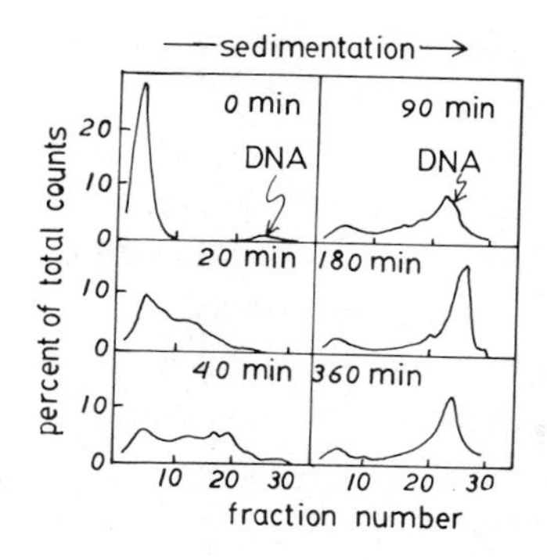

Figure 7-6 Sedimentation profile of DNA from V79 Chinese hamster cells at various times after the end of the irradiation with 2,890 rads, to show the course of repair, which is essentially complete at 360 minutes. Reproduced from M. M. Elkind and C. M. Chang-Liu: Repair of a DNA complex from x-irradiated Chinese hamster cells. Int. J. Radiation Biol. *22*:75, 1972.

It is likely that double-strand as well as single-strand breaks are repaired, though perhaps less readily and with more possibility of errors. With respect to the DNA strand, excision of damaged sections, resynthesis of those sections, and rejoining are the three major steps, followed by reassociation of the DNA with its lipid-membrane complex. This repair process is very efficient in that thousands of breaks may have to be repaired in each surviving cell. For example, x-rays may create about 1,000 single-strand and 40 double-strand breaks per D_0 per cell, and in fluorescent light exposure of cells containing bromodeoxyuridine, up to 50,000 breaks per D_0 may be formed (56). In addition to DNA strand repair, repair of damage to DNA-associated protein and lipid structures may probably also be necessary. It is possible that this ubiquitous repair system (60) arose as an evolutionary adaptation to the background of naturally occurring radiation and chemicals to which living things have always been exposed.

However, if DNA repair is so efficient, there must be a reason for cell death, and this is most likely to be found in errors in repair. This includes not only failure to close the breaks, but also insertion of faulty sequences or reassembly, to a different confrontation. The DNA is then non- or poorly functional or miscodes to a degree incompatible with survival. It is important to stress here that certain chemotherapeutic agents, notably such antibiotics as actinomycin D, might become intercalated into the region undergoing repair and prevent the restoration of DNA superstructure. This could be the mechanism for the additive cell killing that occurs with such chemotherapy (61).

Other biochemical damage. Among other damage known to occur is inhibition of sulfhydryl enzymes and reduction of sulfhydryl content after high doses (62), interference with mitochondrial (63) and nuclear (64) oxidative phosphorylation after low to moderate doses, changes in membrane permeability (65), and peroxidation of biomolecules, especially lipids (66). The relation of such effects to cytotoxicity is much less clear than in the case of damage to DNA, but certain effects, such as the inhibition of phosphorylation, would be expected to have repercussions on metabolic processes, such as DNA synthesis.

Principles of radiation therapy

Damage to normal tissue is still a major problem in radiotherapy, despite the improved depth-dose relations of the newer types of radiation. Although in theory, any localized tumor mass is curable, in practice, its dose-response curve may be so situated with respect to that of a neighboring normal tissue as to make the needed dosage for cure prohibitively damaging to the tissue. Optimal therapy necessitates the choice of a dose that provides the closest to maximum tumor response while minimizing tissue toxicity (Figure 7-7). The issue is complicated by the fact that there are three distinct types of damage to normal tissues: transient changes during therapy; early injury; and late injury, which often is manifested years later. The choice of appropriate dosage rests to a large extent on empirical findings and the experience and judgment of the radiotherapist, but a certain amount of quantitative information is available as a guide. Table 7-4 lists some of these data. Transient early changes occur during or very soon after therapy. In addition to those listed, radiation sickness in the form of nausea, vomiting, and anorexia occurs in most patients, but its severity usually declines over the course of the therapy. Depression of the white blood cells and platelets also may occur, and dose adjustments should be made to ensure that the granulocyte count does not fall below 600 per mm^3. These early changes are easily seen and usually readily controlled, and the dose can be adjusted if necessary. It is in this area of the early injury occurring up to one year that the greatest contribution from the radiotherapist's experience may be made. Late injury is less predictable and less can be done to avoid it therefore. Fibrosis is one of the commonest forms

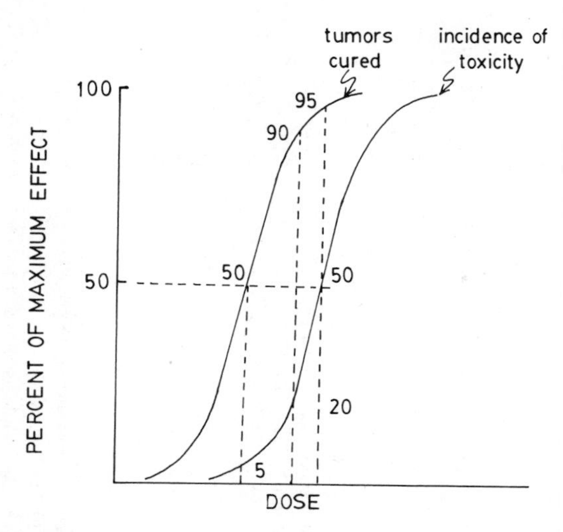

Figure 7-7 Schematic dose-response curves for effects of radiation on tumor and on normal tissue. In raising the tumor cure rate from 50 to 90 percent, the incidence of normal tissue damage rises from 5 to 20 percent. Further increase in antitumor effect will be minimal as the dose is increased, but there will be a dramatic increase in toxicity.

of late injury. A possible explanation for it is that an early effect, increased permeability of the capillaries, may lead to edema, which tends to give rise to fibrosis when it is of long duration. The increase in cures and long-term remissions that has resulted from improved radiotherapeutic technique has greatly accentuated the problems of delayed effects on normal tissue (68). These may be manifested in more generalized form as altered growth and learning impairments. Another long-term effect of radiation not listed in Table 7-4 is the induction of second cancers. This topic, mentioned in Chapter 6, may be expected to become more prominent as long-term survivorship increases.

Fractionated dosage has been the standard radiotherapeutic practice since the 1920's. This has permitted a relative increase in the therapeutic index by favoring recovery of normal tissues. The principle appears to be that similar damage may be inflicted on the tumor and on normal dividing cells, but the latter have a somewhat greater ability to repair damage and thus recover sooner (69). As a result, when a series of doses are given at the intervals used in the clinic (24 to 48 hours), the tumor undergoes a greater net loss of cells, reflecting higher cell kill and slower recovery (Figure 7-8). It is important to stress that fractionation of doses does not mean

Table 7-4 Radiation damage to normal tissues.

Organ	*Transient damage*	*Early injury*	*Delayed injury**	*Tolerated dose (k rads)*
Bladder	Cystitis	Contracture (7 to 8 months)	Atrophic ulcers (year +)	6–8
Bone marrow	Leukopenia	Pancytopenia	Fibrosis	0.25–0.45
Brain	Edema		Necrosis (1 to 2 years)	6–8
Colon and rectum	Diarrhea, colic	Diarrhea, necrosis (6 to 12 months)	Stenosis, fibrosis (2 to 3 years)	4.5–7
Endocrine glands		Loss of function	Fibrosis	4.5–30
Esophagus	Pain	Ulceration	Stenosis (1 to 5 years)	6–7.5
Eyes			Cataracts (>2 years)	0.5–1.2 (lens) 5–7 (cornea)
Fetus		Death		0.2–0.4
Heart			Pericarditis (1 to 2 years)	4.5–5.5
Intestine	Diarrhea, colic	Obstruction (6 to 12 months)	Obstruction (1 to 11 years)	4.5–6.5
Kidney		Sclerosis (6 to 12 months)	Nephritis (1.5 to 3 years)	1.5–2.5
Liver	Abnormal function (7 to 12 months)			2.5–4
Lung	Pneumonitis (3 months)		Fibrosis (8 months to 2 years)	3–3.5
Oral mucosa	Mucositis	Atrophy (2 to 3 months)	Fibrosis (0.5 to 1 year) Necrotic (1 to 5 years) Ulcers	6–7.5
Ovary		Sterilization		0.2–0.6
Skin	Erythema, desquamation	Desquamation, pigmentation (2 months)	Deep fibrosis, ulceration (0.5 to 5 years)	5.5–7
Spinal cord	Edema	Compression, pain	Myelitis, paraplegia (1 to 2 years)	4.5–5.5
Testes		Sterilization		0.5–2
Ureters			Fibrosis, obstruction (1 to 2 years)	7.5–10

Reproduced from Table 2, Ref. 67, with permission of the publisher Plenum Press.

* Secondary cancer is also a risk of irradiation.

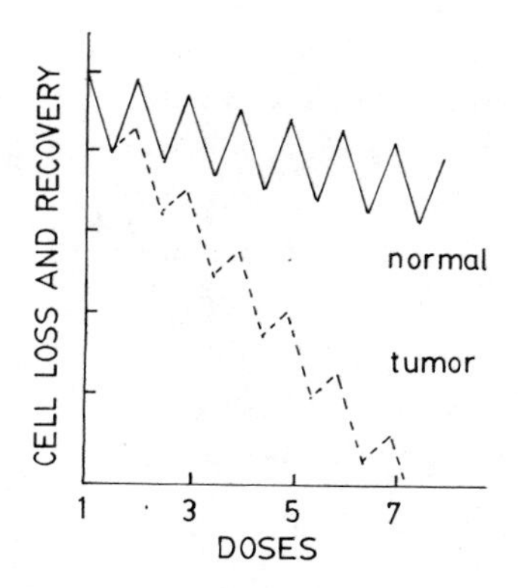

Figure 7-8 Cell loss (kill) and recovery. The percentage of cell kill may be similar for normal tissues and tumor, but in the latter, recovery is slower.

that one dose is merely divided into equal smaller doses. The total dose administered must increase as the number of fractions and the time of duration increase; the number of fractions is the more critical parameter. This is expressed by the formula for nominal standard dose (NSD) devised by Ellis (69):

$$\text{Total dose} = \text{constant} \times (\text{time})\ 0.11 \times (\text{fraction number})\ 0.24$$

This has been modified by Kirk (70) to allow for the exponential decay of radiation injury with time, thus changing the (time) term in what is known as the cumulative radiation effect (CRE) formula; many other schemes have been proposed or used. As a result, maximum tolerable dosages follow relations of the type shown in Table 7-5 with respect to different fractionation

Table 7-5 Typical radiotherapeutic regimes for treatment of laryngeal and pharyngeal carcinomas.

Fractionation	*Total dose** *(rads)*
10 in 3 weeks	4,500
15 in 3 weeks	5,000
20 in 4 weeks	5,500
18 in 6 weeks	5,750
30 in 6 weeks	6,500

*Doses are generally considered those maximally tolerable and may be reduced according to size and situation. In North America, the customary treatment schedule involves five doses per week given on weekdays. Reproduced from Table 5, Ref. 67, with permission of the publisher Plenum Press.

schemes. This effect of repair processes on the total required dose extends not only to dose fractionation, but also to the rate of delivery of radiation. Repair can proceed even during the course of irradiation at low dose rates in the range of 0.1 to 1 rad per minute obtained with implants of such radioisotopes as radium, but has little chance to make significant differences at the 50 to 300 rads per minute used with external beams. Finally, if radiation is fractionated over long time periods, not just repair, but cellular repopulation can occur; this, of course, is definitely not a therapeutically desirable result if it occurs in the tumor.

Palliative radiotherapy. This is given for inoperable primary tumors and metastatic disease. Here the crucial indication is not the size of the tumor, but the problems it creates in the form of pain, obstruction, compression of normal structures, or ulceration. Dosages used may be in the therapeutic dose range, as if curative treatment were being undertaken, or they may be at a reduced level, especially if significant amounts of nervous tissue or bone are included in the field. Steroids may be administered to prevent swelling of the tumor mass during treatment, if it impinges on such vital structures as nerves or major blood vessels.

Modification of radiation effects. In an attempt to improve the therapeutic index of radiation, efforts have been made to modify the underlying biological interaction between radiation and tissue (71). Since tumors are typically hypoxic relative to normal tissues (except cartilage), which are generally well oxygenated due to better perfusion with blood, most attempts at modifying radiation effects have addressed this phenomenon. Generating hypoxic or anoxic conditions may reduce the magnitude of the oxygen effect, bringing tissue sensitivity into line with that of the tumor. In practice this has been limited to limbs where a tourniquet can be applied, but there is little evidence of efficacy. Exposure to hyperbaric oxygen at 3 atmospheres, or even oxygen at normal pressure, before and during irradiation increases the oxygen tension in the blood and potentially in the tumor. However, a reflex vasoconstriction that occurs during the breathing of oxygen may reduce the blood flow and thus limit the amount of additional oxygen that can reach the tumor.

In most respects, the effect of oxygen can be described as the result of its affinity for the electrons produced during ionization, leading to the formation of reactive radicals. Thus the ejected electrons are trapped and unable to reassociate with the biological cation. Attempts to provide oxygen substitutes (electron affinic sensitizers) that can diffuse into hypoxic tumor cells and sensitize them in the same way as oxygen does, have recently acquired great impetus. Most interesting have been the family of agents known as 4-nitroimidazoles, of which the most familiar is the well-known antiparasitic agent metronidazole (Figure 7-9). More promising is misonidazole (RO-07-0582), which is able to inhibit sublethal repair processes. These drugs have entered clinical trial as radiosensitizers on the basis of their promise *in vitro* (72).

Among other attempts to sensitize cells are the incorporation of analogs, such as the halogenated pyrimidine IUDR, into their DNA and the exposure of cells to such compounds as N-ethylmaleimide and diamide (Figure 7-9), which react with sulfhydryl-containing compounds that normally protect cells from radiation damage through scavenging for radicals (71).

In the opposite direction, radioprotective agents have been developed to decrease radical formation in normal tissues. Most attention was initially

Figure 7-9 Radiosensitizers and protectors.

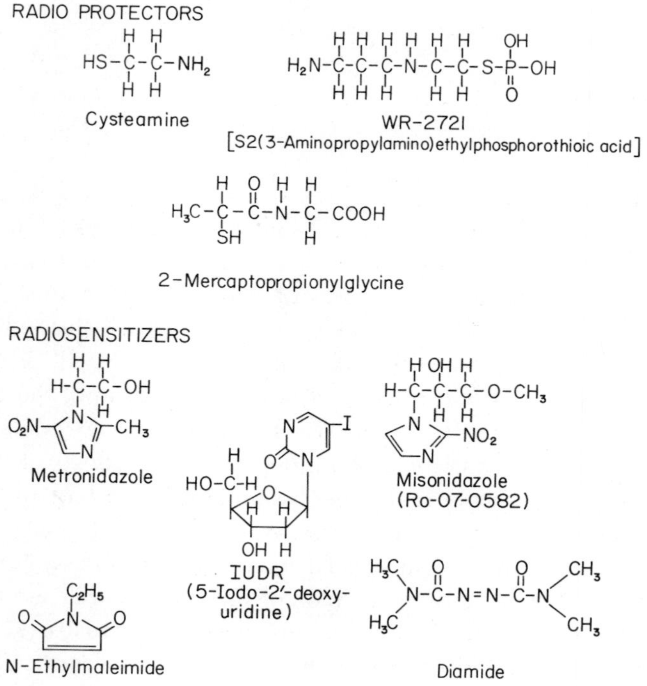

RADIO PROTECTORS

Cysteamine

WR-2721
[S2(3-Aminopropylamino)ethylphosphorothioic acid]

2-Mercaptopropionylglycine

RADIOSENSITIZERS

Metronidazole

IUDR
(5-Iodo-2′-deoxyuridine)

Misonidazole
(Ro-07-0582)

N-Ethylmaleimide

Diamide

given to such simple sulfhydryl compounds as cysteamine (Figure 7-9), but *in vivo* results were much less promising than studies with cell suspensions (73). Recently, other thiol compounds have been developed, notably such phosphorothioate derivatives as WR-2721 and other possibly less toxic material, such as 2-mercaptopropionylglycine (74).

Hyperthermia

Application of temperatures of 40 to 45°C, with or without concomitant ionizing radiation, is an approach to cancer that is now under intensive scrutiny (67). Based on early observations of tumor regression in patients with fevers, as well as on laboratory studies, it is evident that this approach can greatly enhance radiation damage both to tumors and to normal tissue, but by an appropriate choice of radiation, this enhancing action may be made more selective. It is likely that the higher temperatures lead to an acceleration of chemical reactions, and this increases the amount of radiation damage. Since normal as well as tumor tissues would experience greater damage as a result, the approach with the best chance of success would be local irradiation through implants, rather than external beams that must necessarily traverse normal tissues.

CHEMOTHERAPY

History

Although the use of plant preparations to treat cancer goes back more than three thousand years, and inorganic substances containing such heavy metals as mercury and silver were used several hundred years ago, the first detailed example of cancer therapy was Lissauer's report in 1865 of a favorable response in a patient with leukemia treated with potassium arsenite (75). If we exclude substances such as bloodroot, which will be discussed in the next chapter, there was a gap of nearly 80 years until the beginning of modern chemotherapy. In World War I, mustard gas, or sulfur mustard, was used for chemical warfare. Among the many side effects of this corrosive material were leukopenia and the dissolution of lymphoid tissue. Little attention was paid to this finding, even though in 1931 Adair and Bagg used sulfur mustard to treat superficial squamous carcinomas (76). The development of nitrogen mustard as part of further research into chemical warfare, and its use against lymphosarcoma in the early 1940's (77), marked the beginning of modern cancer chemotherapy, and, specifically, of the class of alkylating agents.

Beatson's observation, in 1896, that removal of the ovaries benefited some women with breast cancer (78) represented the earliest step toward endocrine therapy of cancer, but it was the work of Huggins and his colleagues on prostate cancer in the early 1940's (79) that constituted the first systematic use of this approach. Endocrine therapy has proven valuable in a number of different cancers in which individual hormone dependence can be demonstrated. Soon after, there followed the development of the first antimetabolites, the antifolates, of which one of the earliest, amethopterin, or methotrexate (80), has been a mainstay of chemotherapy for over 30 years. Other antimetabolites include the fluorinated pyrimidine 5-fluorouracil (81) and the purine derivative 6-mercaptopurine (82). It is likely that the success of the sulfonamides in antibacterial chemotherapy stimulated the early development of the antimetabolites. Antibiotics used in antimicrobial chemotherapy are usually identified during random screening of soil and other samples for fungi. Among the agents discovered in this way, some proved rather toxic to mammalian cells, and thus less desirable for use against bacteria, but it is from this group that the antitumor antibiotics have been recruited. The prototype of this class is actinomycin D, used by Farber in 1954 to treat Wilms' tumor (83), and it is still the primary drug for this disease. Higher plants have been the source of a number of drugs, principally alkaloids, that have made their way into the clinic. Of these, the vinca alkaloids, first isolated in the late 1950's (84,85), have been the most effective.

The rate of discovery and application of new anticancer drugs escalated during the late 1960's, but has since slowed considerably. Apart from the development of new drugs, the main emphasis in chemotherapy today is on drug combinations with a rational basis and on integration of chemotherapy with surgery and radiation therapy into a comprehensive regimen with enhanced chance of radical cures.

Features of chemotherapy

In the absence of demonstrable features unique to cancer cells that could be exploited selectively, in the same way as the penicillins act specifically on the bacterial cell wall, cancer chemotherapy has primarily been directed at the process of cell division. There is a fundamental distinction, however, between the way hormones affect cell division and the action of other classes of antitumor drugs. Whereas hormones interact with receptors to form complexes that normally modulate cell division and maturation, and thus endocrine manipulation is essentially the application of natural mechanisms, other forms of chemotherapy are primarily cytotoxic and depend upon inhibition of normal pathways and destruction or malfunction of biomolecules. We shall consider the principles of endocrine therapy under that specific heading and devote the rest of this discussion to cytotoxic drugs.

Cell kill. This generally follows the same type of logarithmic relationship to dose as occurs with radiation (Figure 7-4). However, three broad types of variation on this pattern may be distinguished (Figure 7-10). The first, typified by cyclophosphamide, nitrogen mustard, and other alkylating agents, shows a single slope for both normal and tumor cell kill, with a low, but consistent selectivity for tumor cells. Analysis of such curves suggests that the drugs kill both proliferating resting cells, but are somewhat more toxic for the former. In the second example, of which 5-fluorouracil and Adriamycin (or other antibiotics) are prime examples, the survival curves have a similar shape to those seen with alkylating agents, but there is a marked difference in the slope between curves for bone marrow and tumor. This reflects a greater degree of selectivity for proliferating tumor cells. Finally, a large number of drugs, including methotrexate (and most other antimetabolites) and vinblastine, show biphasic curves for cell survival, which indicates a high degree of selectivity for a subset of the population.

Figure 7-10 Fraction of normal marrow (N) and transplanted lymphoma (L) colony-forming units (CFU) surviving 24 hours after drug administration, 1 week after tumor inoculation. Suspensions of the femoral marrow from treated mice were injected into lethally irradiated mice, which were killed 10 days later, and the number of colonies in the spleen counted. Taken from Ref. 86.

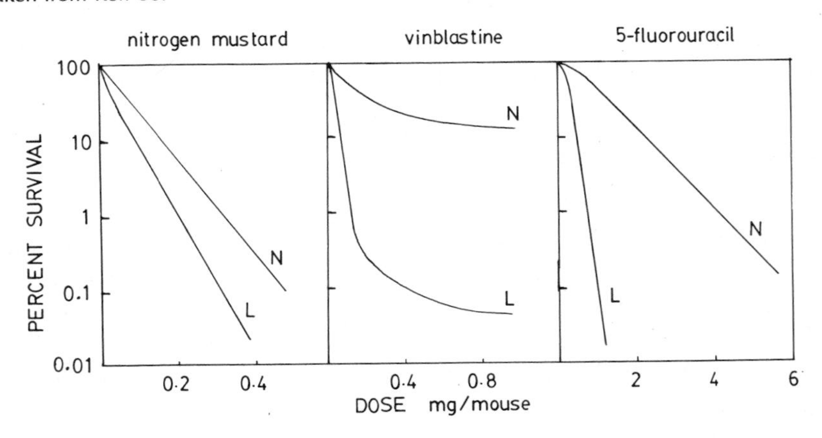

The explanation for these findings lies in the *cell-cycle kinetic selectivity* of the drugs. Alkylating agents are able to kill both resting and proliferating cells, but since proliferating cells must undergo complete repair very quickly in order to resume division, whereas non-dividing cells do not have the pressure to complete repair rapidly, the fraction of cells in cycle will be killed somewhat selectively. Agents of the second class are still very cytotoxic for proliferating cells, since they interfere with processes needed for cell division, but they have much less effect on the non-proliferating compartment. The third class of drugs act during specific phases of the cell cycle only, and thus their targets represent small fractions of the total cell population. Basically, drugs have two types of action on cells in cycle: either they block cell progress through the cycle or they kill the cells. These two effects may occur during one or more phases of the cycle. The more phases affected, the more the dose-response curves for survival resemble the second, cycle-active pattern discussed above. Table 7-6 lists the sites of the blocking and lethal actions of some of the more common drugs.

As in the case of radiation, *dose fractionation* of anticancer drugs has

Table 7-6 Sites of action of anticancer drugs in the cell cycle.

Drug	*Block*	*Lethality*
Actinomycin D	$G_1/S, S/G_2, G_2$	$M, G_1/S$
Adriamycin		S
Azacytidine	S/G_2	S
BCNU	Delay	$M, G_1/S$
Bleomycin	G_2	G_2/M
CCNU		M, G_1
Chlorambucil		M, G_1
Cytarabine		S
Ellipticine		M, G_1
Fluorouracil	G_1/S	S, G_1, G_2
Hydroxyurea	G_1/S	S
Matulane		G_1/S
Melphalan		M, G_1
Methotrexate	G_1/S	G_1/S-S, early G_1
Mitomycin C	S/G_2	M, G_1, or G_2
Nitrogen mustard	G_2	$M, G_1/S$
Thio TEPA		M, G_1
Vinblastine	M	S, late G_1, M
Vincristine	M	S

Derived from Madoc-Jones, H. and Mauro, F., *In Antineoplastic and Immunosuppressive Agents*, Vol. 1. A. C. Sartorelli and D. G. Jones, eds., Heidelberg: Springer-Verlag, 1974, pp. 205–219.

generally proved to be the more effective means of delivery. Two factors are important. Scheduling is obviously of great importance if we are to take advantage of the cell cycle kinetic features of tumors. For example, with agents that act only during S phase, optimal response would be achieved by ensuring that all the proliferating cells are eventually exposed to drug during this phase. This demands continuous exposure or very frequent administration, as the data of Skipper for L1210 mouse leukemia treated with cytosine arabinoside would suggest (Table 7-7). However, interruption in the schedule is also necessary to allow for recovery of normal tissues, which brings us to the second factor. Normal tissues appear to recover more quickly from the damage caused by cytotoxic drugs (and radiation) than do malignant tissues. Even incomplete recovery is sufficient to enable a normal tissue to come through with acceptable damage, whereas the more slowly recovering tumor will become less viable with each successive dose. This is similar to the pattern for radiation in Figure 7-8.

Resistance to drugs. Resistance is a common phenomenon among tumors, and one that is closely analogous to resistance in antimicrobial chemotherapy. This resistance is probably never absolute, but reflects a relationship between the dose-response curves for tumor and critical normal tissues that does not allow any usable selectivity for the tumor. Two forms of resistance may be distinguished, innate and acquired. Innate resistance is immediately apparent in a failure to respond to initial treatment at appropriate, tolerable dosage levels. Acquired resistance, on the other hand,

Table 7-7 Schedule-dependence of the response of mouse L1210 leukemia to cytosine arabinoside.

Number of cells inoculated	*Drug dose (mg/kg body weight)*	*Schedule, begun on day 2 after inoculation*	*Cures (percent)*
10^5	3,000	Single dose	0
	30	Every day (× 15)	0
	500	Every 2 days (× 8)	0
	1,500	Every 4 days (× 4)	0
10^5	15	Every 3 hours (× 8) day 2	0
	15	Every 3 hours (× 8) days 2,6	32
	15	Every 3 hours (× 8) days 2,6,10	93
	15	Every 3 hours (× 8) days 2,6,10,14	86

Data derived from Skipper (87). Cytosine arabinoside, as an S-phase-specific drug, will only kill cells in cycle at the phase during the time that the drug and its intracellular nucleotides are at adequate levels. Intense 24-hour courses spaced 4 days apart to allow for normal tissue recovery are most effective.

Table 7-8 Biochemical mechanisms of resistance to some cancer chemotherapeutic agents.

Drug	*Mechanism*
Actinomycin D	↓ Transport ↓ Retention by cells ↓ Interaction with DNA
Adriamycin	↓ Transport or interaction with DNA ↑ Inactivation
Alkylating agents	↑ Repair of alkylated DNA ↓ Transport
Asparaginase	↑ Asparagine synthetase ↑ Immune clearance
Cytosine arabinoside	↓ Activation by kinase ↑ Inactivation by deaminase
5-Fluorouracil	↓ Uridine phosphorylase ↓ Uridine kinase ↓ Pyrimidine phosphoribosyl transferase ↑ Degradation of active metabolites Altered thymidylate synthetase
6-Mercaptopurine	↓ Hypoxanthine-guanine phosphoribosyl transferase ↑ Alkaline phosphatase
Methotrexate	Altered dihydrofolate reductase ↓ Transport
6-Thioguanine	↓ Hypoxanthine-guanine phosphoribosyl transferase ↑ Guanine deaminase ↑ Alkaline phosphatase ↓ Ribonucleotide reductase

appears in an initially responsive patient during treatment as the reduction and eventual loss of tumor response in the face of unchanged toxicity of the drug. Both forms of resistance arise from the same basic mechanisms. These include inadequate uptake and activation of drug, metabolic degradation, alteration of inhibitory kinetics due to selection of alternate forms of an enzyme or increased levels of normal metabolites, elevated levels of target enzyme, and increased repair of damage. Table 7-8 lists some of these mechanisms for a number of drugs. In general, host tolerance to a drug, which may be analogous to tumor resistance, is a much less frequently encountered phenomenon, since the cancer cell is usually more "plastic" biochemically than normal cells and is, in a sense, evolving genetically. When it is encountered, host tolerance usually results from hepatic enzyme induction leading to increased drug metabolism.

We have spoken of *drug toxicity*, and it is important to stress that because the anticancer drugs depend for their specificity only on quantitative differences in cell proliferation, their therapeutic indices, the ratios between their median toxic doses and their median effective doses (e.g., TD_{50}/ED_{50}), will be low. As a result, most patients receiving chemotherapy will experience relatively severe side effects, such as leukopenia, anemia, ulceration of the mucosa, nausea, vomiting, diarrhea or constipation, hair loss, interference with nerve function, and kidney malfunction. The effects on the bone marrow, manifested as leukopenia, thrombocytopenia, or anemia, are especially critical because they lead to life-threatening hemorrhages and infections. In addition to these rather generalized effects on normal tissues, especially those that are proliferating, particular agents will have very specific toxic side effects. As we deal with the major classes of drugs, we will indicate the types of toxicity encountered. In addition, toxicity is perhaps the most critical factor in the design of regimens of combination chemotherapy, which we will discuss after considering the classes of drugs.

The status of the patient. This needs to be taken into account, not only before placing him or her on chemotherapy, but also in terms of evaluating progress during therapy. It is the intent of all therapy not merely to shrink tumors or to improve laboratory tests, but to cure the cancer, or at the very least improve the subject's well-being and quality of life. Therapy that produces minor effects on the tumor and does not improve the patient's overall status, while subjecting the individual to repeated severe side effects is worthless or even unethical and likely to be rejected by the patient. This might very well be the primary reason many patients seek unorthodox or "quack" remedies.

A commonly used criterion for the performance status of patients is that drawn up by the late David Karnofsky (Table 7-9), in which he attempted to put patient performance on a numerical basis. Such an evaluation must be combined with physical, cytological, and radiological examination to assess response to therapy adequately. On the Karnofsky scale, patients of status below 40 percent are unlikely to receive significant benefit from chemotherapy. One must also consider the discomfort brought about by drugs, the side effects of which are likely to be greater in debilitated individuals in whom physiological functions may be marginal, or whose liver,

Table 7-9 The Karnofsky scale of patient performance status.

Definition	*Percent*	*Criteria*
Able to carry on work and normal activity; no special care needed.	100	Normal, no complaints, no evidence of disease
	90	Only minor signs of disease
	80	Normal activity with effort, some symptoms of disease
Unable to work, but can live at home and care for most needs; some assistance needed.	70	Cares for self, but cannot carry on normal activity and work
	60	Requires some assistance, but can take care of most needs
	50	Requires frequent assistance and medical care
Unable to care for self, requiring institutional or hospital care; disease progressing rapidly.	40	Disabled, requires special care
	30	Severely disabled, requires hospitalization
	20	Very sick, hospital care and active supportive treatment needed
	10	Near death, vital functions deteriorating

Derived from Ref. 88.

for example, may be compromised by tumor involvement that reduces its ability to metabolize drugs. Immunological function is also an important aspect of patient status. It has been found, for example, that patients who are immunocompetent at the start of therapy, in terms of cell-mediated immunity, or who achieve this status during therapy, enter remission, whereas those whose immune function is depressed are unlikely to enter remission (89). This is another example of the general concept mentioned earlier that treatment removes the bulk of a tumor, but host control mechanisms must intervene if the remaining cells are to be destroyed.

Chemotherapy agents

Table 7-10 lists the major anticancer drugs, which we shall now briefly review from the point of view of their mechanisms of action and biological properties. For a more complete discussion, the reader is referred to the text by Pratt and Ruddon (90); pharmacokinetic data may be found there and in the text by Creasey (91).

Alkylating agents. The alkylating agents are highly reactive chemicals that form covalent links with biomolecules containing groups that readily donate

Table 7-10 Alternate names for anticancer drugs in common use.

Generic name	*Common name*	*American brand name*
Alkylating agents		
Busulfan		Myleran
Carmustine	BCNU	
Chlorambucil		Leukeran
Cyclophosphamide		Cytoxan
Dacarbazine	DTIC, DIC	
Lomustine	CCNU	CeeNU
Mechlorethamine	Nitrogen mustard, HN_2	Mustargen
Melphalan	L-PAM	Alkeran
Triethylenethiophosphoramide	Thio-TEPA	Thiotepa
Antimetabolites		
Cytarabine	Cytosine arabinoside, ara-C	Cytosar
Fluorouracil	5-FU	
Mercaptopurine	6-MP	Purinethol
Methotrexate	Amethopterin, MTX	
Thioguanine	6-TG	
Antibiotics		
Bleomycin		Blenoxane
Dactinomycin	Actinomycin D	Cosmegen
Daunorubicin	Daunomycin, rubidomycin	
Doxorubicin		Adriamycin
Mithramycin		Mithracin
Mitomycin	Mitomycin C	Mutamycin
Alkaloids		
Vinblastine	VLB	Velban
Vincristine	VCR	Oncovin
Miscellaneous		
Hydroxyurea		Hydrea
Procarbazine		Matulane
Mitotane	*o,p'*-DDD	Lysodren

protons (92). These include the widely distributed -SH, $-NH_2$, and -OH groups, and thus the alkylating agents will attack most biopolymers as well as low molecular weight compounds. As a result, an alkyl or substituted alkyl group is linked to the biomolecule, hence the term alkylating agent. Although alkylation may occur extensively, the alkylation of DNA, with its major implication for the cell's genetic information, is the most critical (93). About 90 percent of the alkyl substituents are located at the 7-position of the guanine bases. In addition, the sugar phosphate backbone and the cytosine bases are alkylated, and the lesser amount of damage at these positions may nevertheless cause biological damage equal to that resulting from substitution on guanine, this because such damage gives rise to chain breaks and faulty transcription of the information in DNA (93). The types of damage caused to DNA include single alkylations of a base, alkylation of two bases so as to cross-link them, either within the same or different strands, single- or double-strand breaks, and depurination. Single substitutions may lead to errors in DNA function, or they, as well as cross-linked regions, may undergo repair. This repair process involves an initial phase of "nicking" by an endonuclease and excision of the section by an exonuclease, a second phase in which repair polymerase synthesizes a new segment, and a final phase in which a ligase links up the newly formed segment to give the original double-stranded DNA. These reactions are outlined in Figure 7-11. Incomplete repair may lead to strand breaks, and the repair process may not be efficient in highly alkylated and cross-linked

Figure 7-11 Schematic outline of the repair processes occurring in DNA exposed to radiation or to alkylating agents.

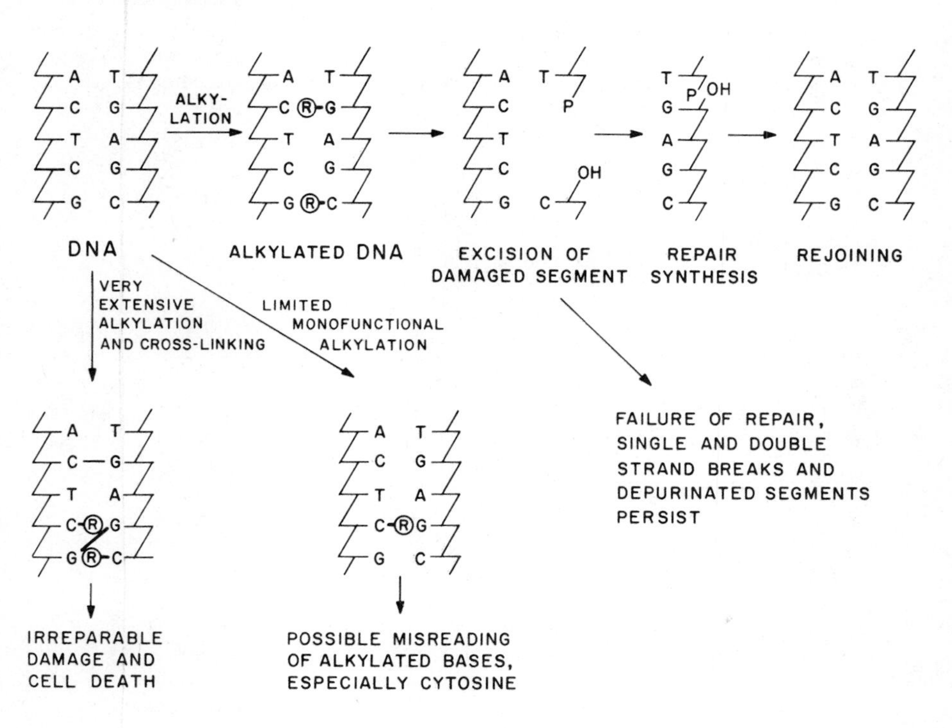

regions. Single base alkylations that are not repaired may relate to mutations, since 7-substituted guanine residues may undergo anomalous base pairing with thymine rather than cytosine (95). Cross-links can only be formed by the action of bifunctional or "two-armed" alkylating agents, which includes most of the clinically used agents. These links can be inter- or intra-strand or they may join DNA to protein molecules. Cytotoxicity is closely related to cross-linkage, as is suggested by the much greater cell kill that occurs following treatment with bifunctional rather than monofunctional alkylators (96). Damage to DNA is manifested by diminished ability to act as a template for DNA and RNA synthesis, which occurs at 100 times lower concentrations of drug than those required to affect ribosomes or the polymerase enzyme systems (90).

The actual reaction of alkylation usually involves an initial conversion to an active intermediate, which frequently is a carbonium ion (Figure 7-12). In the case of the mustards, this step is a first-order (S_N1) intramolecular cyclization that is followed by a second-order (S_N2) nucleophilic substitution

Figure 7-12 A, Formation of imonium and then carbonium ions from nitrogen mustard, and the reaction with guanine; B, metabolic activation of cyclophosphamide to yield phosphoramide mustard and acrolein; C, generation of active species from the nitrosourea BCNU.

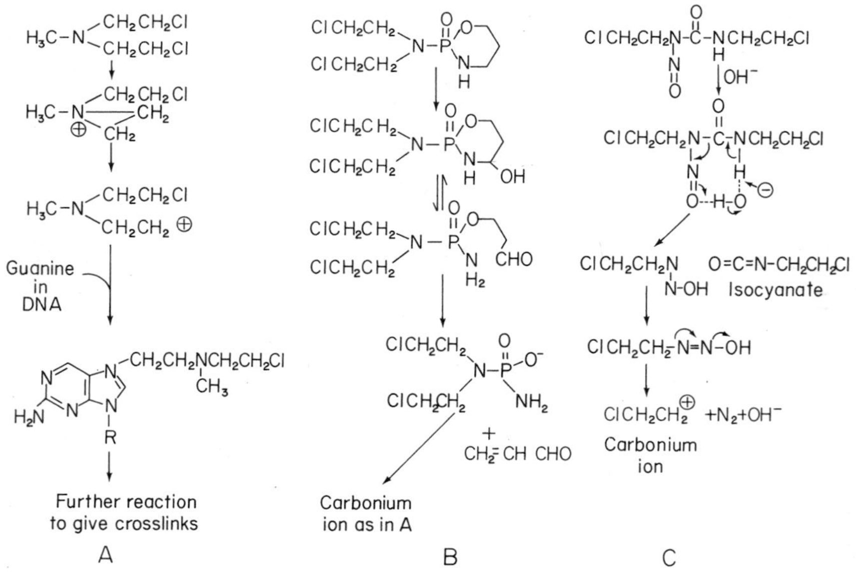

reaction. Unlike most mustards, cyclophosphamide must undergo an initial metabolic hydroxylation by microsomal mixed function oxidases in the liver; subsequent nonenzymatic reactions lead to the cytotoxic products phosphoramide mustard and acrolein (Figure 7-12) (97). Phosphoramide mustard is probably the chief active species, whereas acrolein is an irritant that accumulates in the urine and may contribute to the hemorrhagic cystitis that often develops in patients treated with high doses of cyclophosphamide. The nitrosoureas not only give rise to carbonium ions that react with DNA, but also release isocyanates that form carbamoylated proteins (98).

Except for cyclophosphamide, which has a long half-life (mean about 6 hours), most alkylating agents disappear from the blood with half-lives of the order of minutes. Not only do they react with biomolecules, but also with water, and for this reason solutions should be used immediately. Metabolism is usually complete so that little or no unchanged drug can be found in the urine.

The structures of commonly used alkylating agents appear in Figures 7-12 and 7-13. Mitomycin is commonly listed among the antibiotics, but its mechanism of action involves the generation of active groups, such as carbonium ions, during an autoxidation process; alkylation and strand breakage result in treated DNA. Cis-diamminedichloroplatinum (II) is an unusual inorganic compound able to exchange its chloride ions for nucleophilic groups. In this way the drug can cross-link DNA strands (99) and thus function as an alkylating agent. The chief toxicity of this compound, renal tubular degeneration, can be prevented by inducing diuresis. Resistance to alkylating agents usually involves reduced uptake or increased levels of repair enzymes.

Bone marrow depression is the major toxicity of all the alkylating agents, and in addition, cyclophosphamide may cause hair loss (alopecia) and hemorrhagic cystitis, which requires high urine output for prevention; busulfan may cause minor pulmonary fibrosis. Early nausea and vomiting are produced by nitrogen mustard, cyclophosphamide, dacarbazine, and the nitrosoureas; dacarbazine may also have a flu-like effect.

Antimetabolites. This group of agents are analogs of naturally occurring metabolities that inhibit enzymatic pathways and are incorporated into macromolecules. The structures of some of these compounds appear in Figure 7-14. Except for hydroxyurea and methotrexate, the antimetabolites are analogs of purine and pyrimidine bases or nucleosides that require conver-

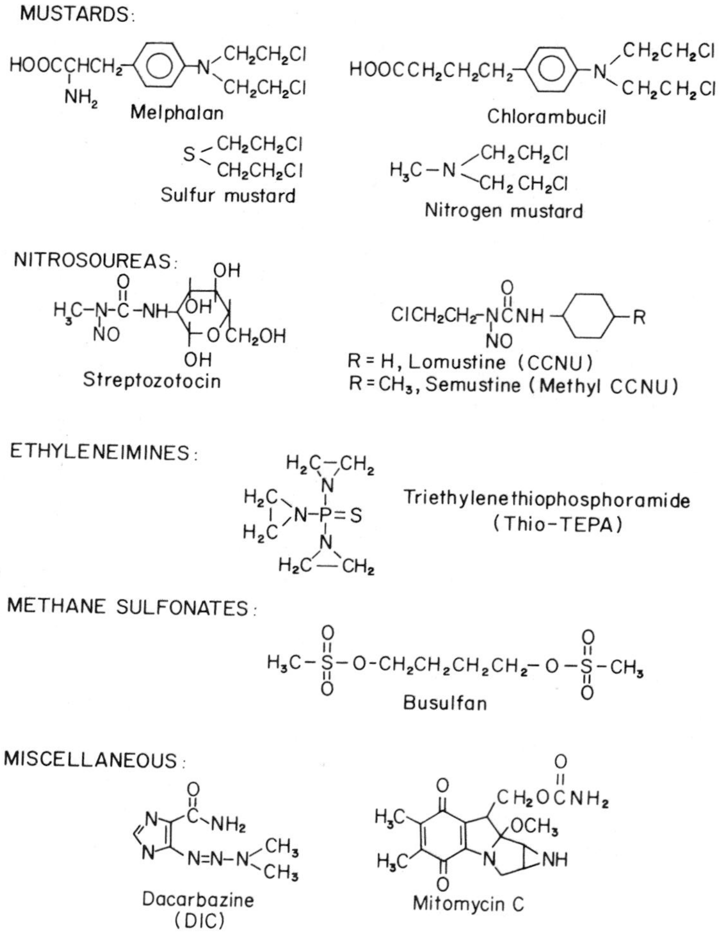

MUSTARDS:

$HOOCCH(NH_2)CH_2-C_6H_4-N(CH_2CH_2Cl)_2$
Melphalan

$HOOCCH_2CH_2CH_2-C_6H_4-N(CH_2CH_2Cl)_2$
Chlorambucil

$S(CH_2CH_2Cl)_2$
Sulfur mustard

$H_3C-N(CH_2CH_2Cl)_2$
Nitrogen mustard

NITROSOUREAS:

Streptozotocin

$ClCH_2CH_2-N(NO)C(=O)NH-C_6H_{10}-R$
R = H, Lomustine (CCNU)
R = CH_3, Semustine (Methyl CCNU)

ETHYLENEIMINES:

Triethylenethiophosphoramide
(Thio-TEPA)

METHANE SULFONATES:

$H_3C-SO_2-O-CH_2CH_2CH_2CH_2-O-SO_2-CH_3$
Busulfan

MISCELLANEOUS:

Dacarbazine
(DIC)

Mitomycin C

Figure 7-13 Alkylating agents.

sion to nucleotides to become active inhibitors. The principal sites of action of these compounds are indicated in Figure 7-15.

Methotrexate is a potent inhibitor of the enzyme dihydrofolate reductase, which synthesizes tetrahydrofolate needed for both thymidylate and purine biosynthesis. Thus, it stops DNA synthesis. The drug enters cells both by active transport and passive diffusion, and since the former process is frequently very limited, high doses of the antifolate have been widely used. The resulting high plasma levels serve to increase the rate of passive diffusion, ensuring the elevated intracellular concentrations needed for sustained inhibition of DNA synthesis. However, such levels are highly toxic to the bone marrow and other normal tissues, such as the mucosa, so that leukovorin or folinic acid, a tetrahydrofolate derivative, is administered after completion of the methotrexate infusion to supply needed reduced folate. It appears that bone marrow cells tend to recover their ability to synthesize DNA more rapidly than many tumors (100) and are thus better able to utilize the reduced folate. The very delayed portion of the methotrexate clearance curve is also modified, which lowers the retention time of the methotrexate. Studies of serum levels suggest that when they exceed 10^{-5}M at 24, 10^{-6}M at 48, and 10^{-7}M at 72 hours, severe toxicity may occur and intensive rescue is needed (101). Resistance to methotrexate is most commonly associated with a marked elevation in dihydrofolate reductase activity, directly ascribable to selective multiplication of the structural

Figure 7-14 Antimetabolites.

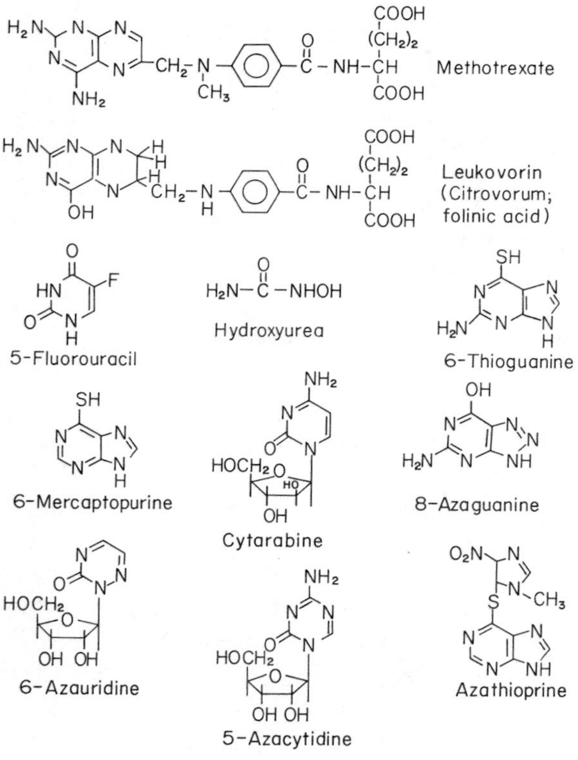

Methotrexate

Leukovorin (Citrovorum; folinic acid)

5-Fluorouracil

Hydroxyurea

6-Thioguanine

6-Mercaptopurine

Cytarabine

8-Azaguanine

6-Azauridine

5-Azacytidine

Azathioprine

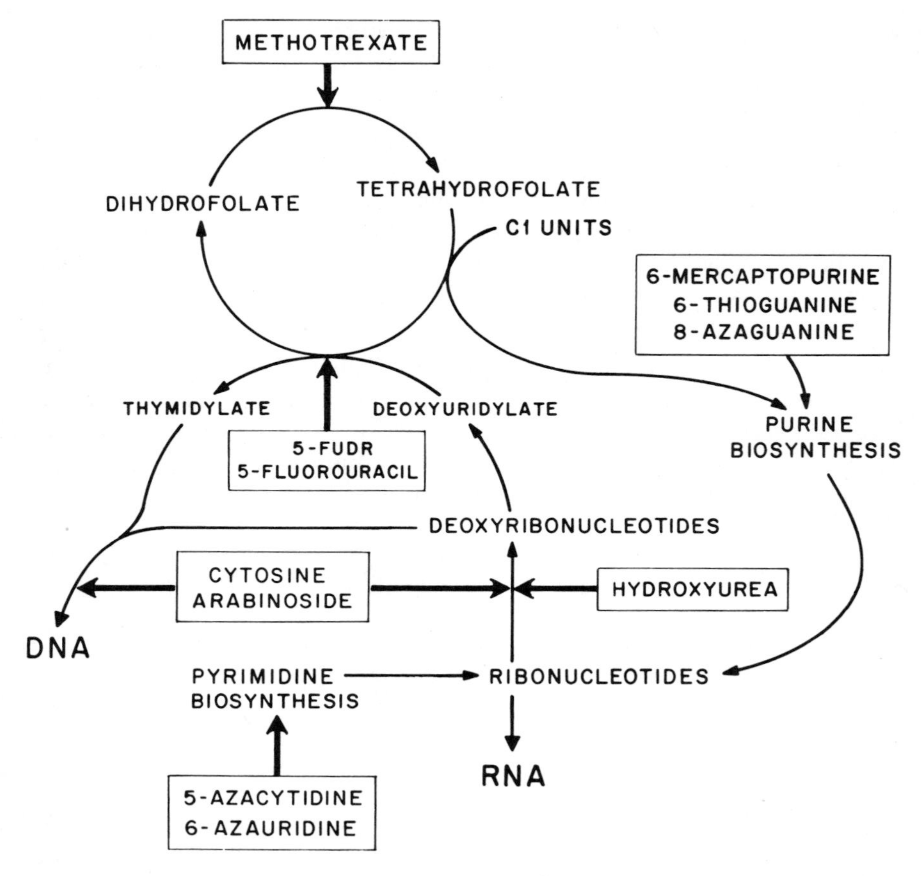

Figure 7-15 Principal sites of action of antimetabolites.

gene. For more information about this drug, the reader is referred to the review by Bertino (102).

The purine analogs *6-mercaptopurine and 6-thioguanine* are converted to their ribonucleotides; some 6-mercaptopurine is also metabolized to 6-methylmercaptopurine ribonucleotide and to the 6-thioguanine nucleotides. These nucleotides inhibit the first step on the pathway of purine biosynthesis, the formation of 5-phosphoribosylamine, as well as later steps in the interconversion of the various purine nucleotides. In addition, a certain amount of incorporation into nucleic acids occurs (103), which affects the function of these macromolecules (Figure 7-16). Bone marrow depression is the major toxic manifestation of these drugs, with a somewhat delayed leukopenia; evidence of liver damage has also been reported (104). Resistance to thiopurines takes the form of either reduced conversion to nucleotides or to an elevated intracellular level of alkaline phosphatase that degrades the nucleotides (105).

5-Fluorouracil in the form of 5-fluoro-2′-deoxyuridine 5′-monophosphate inhibits the formation of thymidylate. The nucleotide has a high affinity for thymidylate synthetase (106), but since it has a fluorine atom at the position where a methyl group is to be substituted, no methylation can occur. The deoxynucleoside of fluorouracil, 5-fluoro-2′-deoxyuridine (*FUDR*), is also occasionally used, but it has no clinical advantage over the free base. Toxicity takes the form of marrow depression, diarrhea, stomatitis, and ulceration of the gastrointestinal tract. Hair loss, dermatitis, and cerebellar damage seen as dizziness, slurred speech, and ataxia also occur occasionally.

Figure 7-16 Mechanisms for damage resulting from incorporation of analogs into nucleic acids.

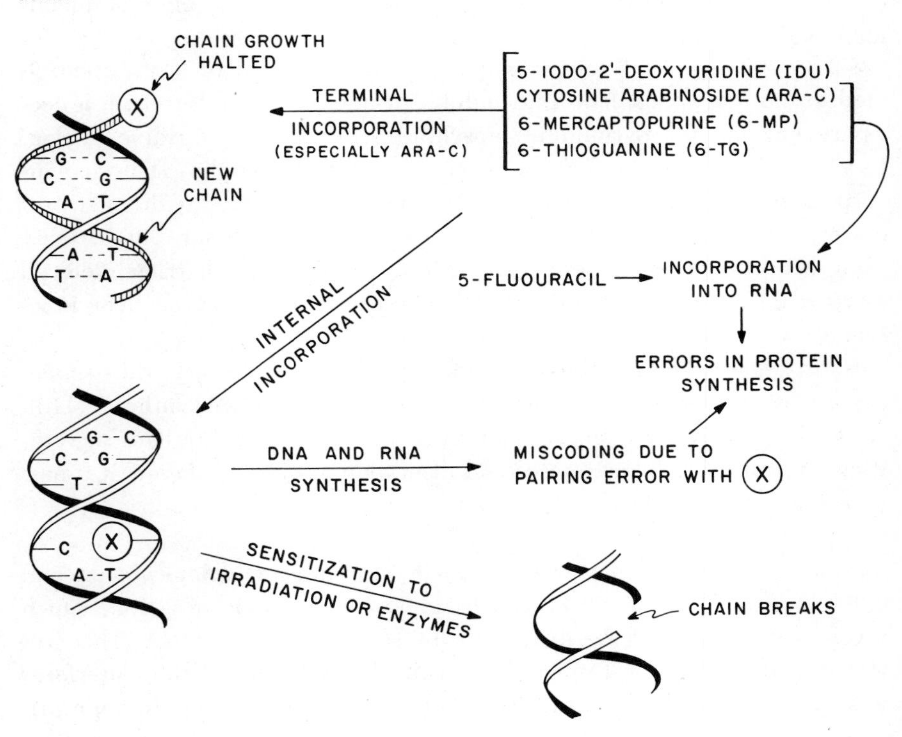

Since the drug is mainly metabolized by the liver, defective functioning of this organ will increase drug toxicity. A related halogenated pyrimidine is 5-iodo-2′-deoxyuridine, which is used as antiviral agent in treating herpes simplex infections of the eye. Further information on halogenated pyrimidines may be found in recent reviews (107,108).

Cytarabine (cytosine arabinoside) is converted metabolically to the triphosphate, which is the active nucleotide. A variety of mechanisms of action have been proposed (109). Although the most favored mechanism is inhibition of DNA polymerase, the nucleotide also inhibits the reduction of ribonucleotide diphosphates to deoxyribonucleotides and is incorporated into nucleic acids, where it may lead to termination of chain growth (110) or inhibition of initiation of chains (111). Resistance develops primarily through reduction in levels of deoxycytidine kinase, the enzyme that converts cytarabine to its monophosphate, but increase in cytidine deaminase, which converts cytarabine to the inactive uracil arabinoside, and a loss of affinity of DNA polymerase for the triphosphate, are other possibilities (109). Cytarabine is a potent myelosuppressive agent, which explains its use in leukemias, but it also causes gastrointestinal distress and oral inflammation and ulceration.

5-Azacytidine, like *6-azauridine*, is a compound that once phosphorylated to the monophosphate ester inhibits orotidylate decarboxylase, a necessary enzyme for pyrimidine biosynthesis. Unlike the uridine analog, however, 5-azacytidine also can be converted to the triphosphate and incorporated into RNA and DNA (112), where it interferes with such processes as the formation of ribosomal RNA from its precursor (90). Toxicity from this drug includes very severe nausea, vomiting and diarrhea, delayed marrow depression, and occasional hypotension and impaired liver function.

Hydroxyurea inhibits ribonucleoside diphosphate reductase, thus reducing the supply of deoxyribonucleotides needed for DNA synthesis (113). Toxicity is chiefly the result of bone marrow suppression, but nausea, vomiting, stomatitis, and gastrointestinal ulceration are also observed at times, as are dermatological side effects (90).

Antibiotics. The antibiotics *dactinomycin, Adriamycin, daunorubicin,* and *mithramycin* (Figure 7-17) have a basically similar mode of action, which involves interaction of the drug with the stacked bases of DNA. This creates a distortion or local unwinding of the DNA helix and thus interferes with the function of DNA and RNA polymerases, which require appropri-

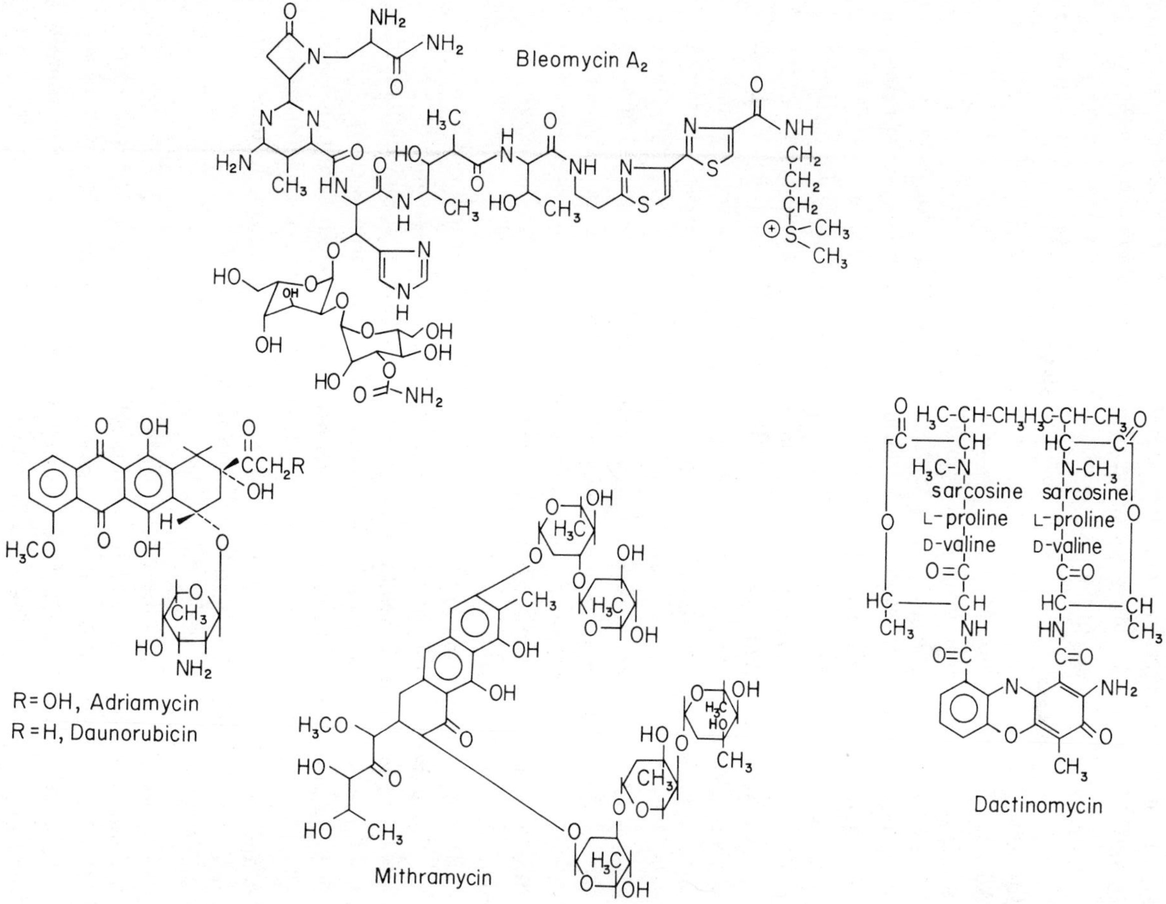

Bleomycin A_2

R = OH, Adriamycin
R = H, Daunorubicin

Mithramycin

Dactinomycin

Figure 7-17 Antitumor antibiotics.

ate orientation and separation of the strands for their activity. These interactions differ with the anticancer drug. Dactinomycin affects guanine bases, so that the planar rings of the chromophore intercalate between these bases with the polypeptides lying in the narrow groove of the helix (114). There they can obstruct the passage of RNA polymerase. On the other hand, Adriamycin and daunorubicin do not seem to affect these bases, and their amino sugar lies in the major groove; interaction between these drugs and DNA phosphate also occurs (115). Mithramycin is specific for guanine in a reversible and magnesium dependent interaction, but it does not appear to intercalate between the bases.

As regards toxicity, dactinomycin, which is mainly used for pediatric solid neoplasms, is myelosuppressive and causes severe nausea and vomiting, as well as frequent ulceration of the gastrointestinal tract, diarrhea, and occasional hair loss and acne. Adriamycin and daunorubicin may be myelosuppressive and also may produce nausea and diarrhea, but their chief limitation is cardiac toxicity of a type resembling congestive heart failure, which appears most commonly with a total dose in excess of about 500 mg/m^2. Mithramycin, once used for testicular cancers, has a variety of side effects, including hepatic and renal damage, marrow suppression, diarrhea, vomiting, and hemorrhage; it is now used in low, non-toxic doses to treat hypercalcemia.

Bleomycin is unusual in that it is a mixture with about half as bleomycin A_2, the active and less toxic form of the drug. This antibiotic interacts with DNA, releasing free bases to break strands, a reaction that may depend on the formation of an oxygen-labile complex (116). The drug is concentrated in lung and skin, where its chief toxicities are manifested. Oral mucositis, alopecia, edema and erythema of the hands and feet, sclerotic skin changes, and pulmonary toxicity manifested by dyspnea, cough, lung infiltrates, and even diffuse fibrosis have all been described.

Alkaloids. The alkaloids in current clinical use are the vinca alkaloids *vinblastine* and *vincristine* and the podophyllin derivatives *VM26* and *VP16-213* (Figure 7-18). Mitotic arrest in metaphase is the characteristic biological action of the *Vinca* alkaloids, which interact with tubulin, the subunit protein component of the microtubule system (117). By combining with this protein, which is in a state of dynamic equilibrium with microtubule-containing structures, the alkaloid drugs prevent its reassembly (polymerization) and thus, since dissociation is not affected, bring about the dissolution of those structures, including the mitotic spindle (118,119). This is

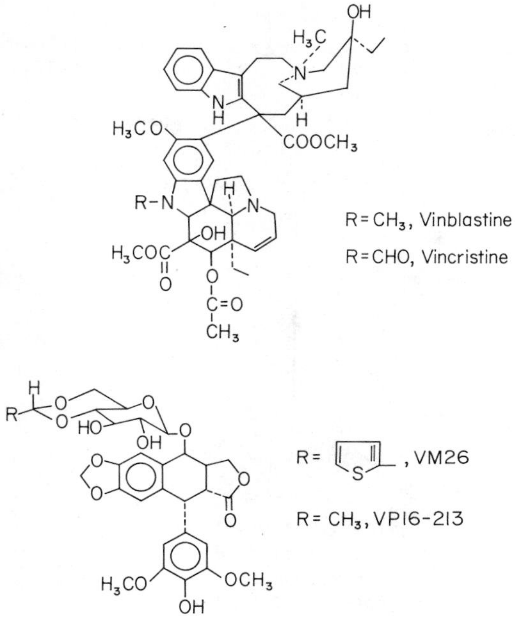

R = CH_3, Vinblastine
R = CHO, Vincristine

R = , VM26
R = CH_3, VP16-213

Figure 7-18 Clinically used plant alkaloids.

outlined in Figure 7-19, where it is evident that other structures containing microtubules, such as axons of nerve cells, as well as the aggregates of tubules involved in intracellular movements, will be affected, as will their functions. The latter include transport of neurotransmitter granules, secretion of many hormones, and phagocytosis. In addition to this microtubule action, the *Vinca* alkaloids can also inhibit biochemical pathways, including nucleic acid, protein, and lipid synthesis and carbohydrate metabolism, usually at somewhat higher levels of drug. These effects and other aspects of the pharmacology of the *Vinca* alkaloids have been reviewed recently (120). These two alkaloids show striking differences in their toxicities. Vinblastine is primarily myelosuppressive and only occasionally neurotoxic, whereas vincristine causes a severe neuropathy that includes loss of sensation in the extremities and loss of reflexes; it usually has no effect on the bone marrow. Hair loss is common with both drugs.

The epipodophyllotoxins VM26 and VP16-213 are derivatives of podophyllotoxin, which arrests mitosis, rather like vinblastine, except that it binds to a different site on the tubulin molecule, one for which colchicine

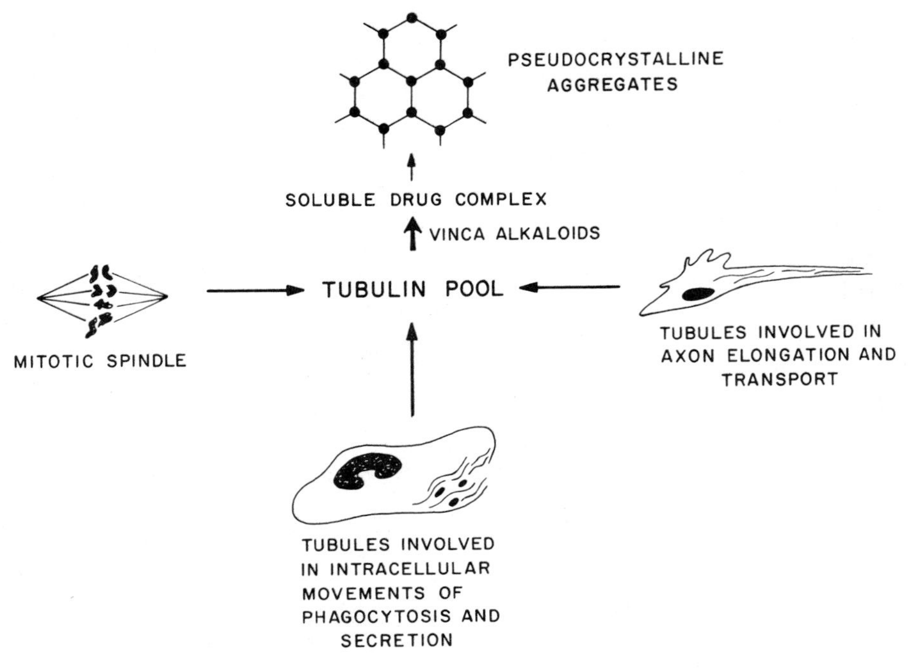

Figure 7-19 Action of the *Vinca* alkaloids on the microtubule system.

also has an affinity (117). Unlike the parent compound, however, VM26 and VP16-213 do not appear to cause dissolution of microtubules (121), and their main site of action on the cell cycle appears to be in G_2 phase; thus they reduce the mitotic index (122). Their mode of action is still unclear, although effects on electron transport (123) and nucleoside transport (121) have been described; DNA degradation also may occur. These alkaloids have nausea and vomiting, bone marrow suppression, and hair loss as their most frequent side effects. Chills, fevers, and anaphylactic reactions have also occurred.

Steroid hormones. A wide range of steroid hormones are used in cancer chemotherapy (Figure 7-20), but in general, this approach is largely empirical. In breast cancer, for example, estrogens may either inhibit or stimulate the growth of the tumor, and it is in the choice of therapy that the empirical element lies. If breast cancer makes its appearance 5 years or more after menopause, when circulating estrogen levels have fallen, it is unlikely to be stimulated by estrogens, whereas in a younger women, its growth may be estrogen dependent. Assay of hormone receptors has introduced one rational element to help in the choice of therapy. In general, all steroid hormones interact with receptors that occur intracellularly in the cytosol. These receptors transport the hormones into the nucleus in an active form where they modulate the activity of RNA polymerase through interacting at acceptor binding sites that are associated with DNA or at least chromatin (124). As a result, new specific messenger RNAs accumulate, but whether this results from induction, such as gene derepression, or from changes in the way nuclear RNA is processed, is not known. The messenger RNAs presumably code for new proteins, but these have been

Figure 7-20 Steroid hormones used in cancer therapy.

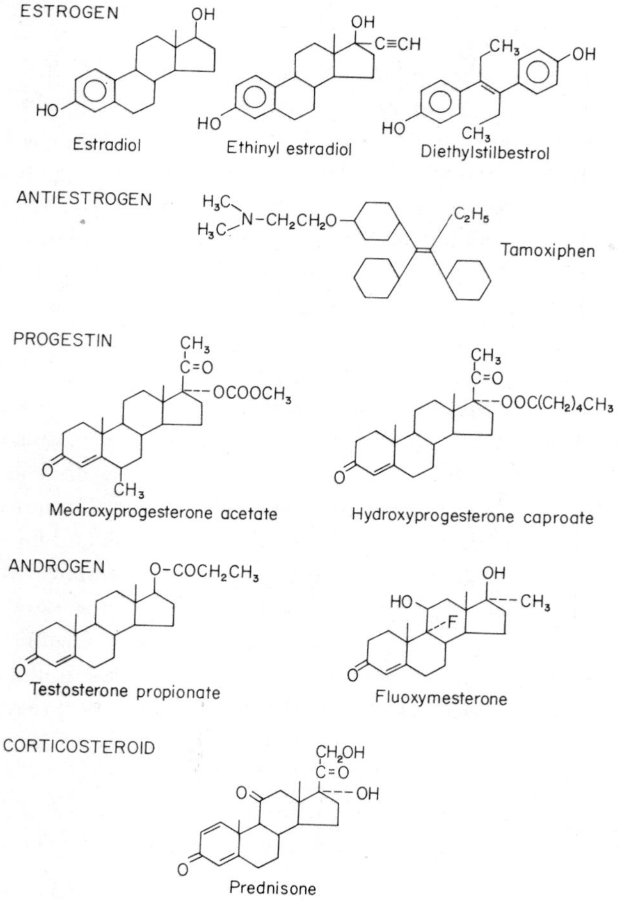

ESTROGEN

Estradiol

Ethinyl estradiol

Diethylstilbestrol

ANTIESTROGEN

Tamoxiphen

PROGESTIN

Medroxyprogesterone acetate

Hydroxyprogesterone caproate

ANDROGEN

Testosterone propionate

Fluoxymesterone

CORTICOSTEROID

Prednisone

identified in only a few cases (e.g., 125). The end result may be inhibition of growth, differentiation, stimulation of growth, or in the case of the corticosteroids and lymphoid tissues, cell kill.

These responses are keyed to the presence of appropriate receptors that are highly specific for different classes of steroids. Assay of hormone receptors involves homogenization and high-speed centrifuging of surgical specimens, incubation with radiolabeled steroid in the presence and absence of a physiologically potent non-labled steroid, and separation of the unbound and bound fractions. A correction must be made for nonspecific binding. The estrogen receptor has been studied most closely in view of the major clinical problem of breast cancer. In one study, 55 percent of patients having receptor responded to hormone manipulation as contrasted with only 8 percent of those without receptor (126). Such predictive reliability is of great value in delivering the most appropriate therapy at the earliest time, while avoiding non-beneficial treatment.

Major examples of therapeutic hormones are listed in Table 7-11, together with their most frequently encountered side effects. In considering these drugs, it should be noted that estrogens and androgens are in many respects mutually antagonistic. Thus, an androgen may suppress the growth of an estrogen-dependent tumor. Tamoxiphen, an antiestrogen, would in some respects act in the same antagonistic mode as androgens, but since it lacks the masculinizing effects of the latter, it can be used to avoid effects that can be very psychologically damaging to women.

Miscellaneous agents. A few clinically used drugs (Figure 7-21) do not fit any of the above classes. L-*Asparaginase* is an enzyme whose clinical use may be traced back to the ability of guinea pig serum to cause regression of rodent lymphomas. When L-asparaginase was identified as the active component, while other studies demonstrated that some tumor cells in culture have a requirement for L-asparagine, the basis was laid for rational use of the enzyme (90). Although there is a degree of selectivity with L-asparagine-dependent tumor cells, in which the supply of the needed nutrient is greatly reduced by the enzyme, the enzyme is far from innocuous. As a protein it can give rise to severe anaphylactic reactions in at least 25 percent of patients receiving it as part of a remission-induction regimen. Other side effects include liver damage and cerebral dysfunction. A review of this drug has appeared recently (127).

Mitotane, or *o,p'*-DDD, is an analog of the insecticide DDT used to treat cancer of the adrenal cortex because these compounds were originally

Table 7-11 Major uses and toxicity of steroids.

Drug	*Chief toxicity*	*Major use*
Estrogens		
Diethylstilbestrol* Ethinyl estradiol	Nausea, vomiting, fluid retention, hypercalcemia, thromboembolisms, uterine bleeding	Prostatic cancer, breast cancer in postmenopausal patients
Antiestrogens		
Tamoxiphen	Nausea, vomiting, hot flushes, transient leukopenia, vaginal bleeding, hypercalcemia	Breast cancer in postmenopausal patients
Progestins		
Medroxyprogesterone acetate Hydroxyprogesterone caproate † Megestrol acetate	Local pain, fluid retention, hypercalcemia	Endometrial cancer, renal cell cancer, breast cancer
Androgens		
Fluoxymesterone † Testosterone propionate Dromostanolone propionate	Masculinization, fluid retention	Breast cancer, 1 to 5 years postmenopausal
Testolactone	Hypercalcemia	Breast cancer, 1 to 5 years postmenopausal
Glucocorticoids		
Prednisone Prednisolone	Decalcification of bones Peptic ulcers, hypertension, impaired healing, increased risk of infection, fluid retention and fat accumulation	Acute and chronic lymphocytic leukemia, lymphomas, breast cancer

* Has produced vaginal carcinoma in offspring.
† Cholestatic jaundice has occurred.

found to cause atrophy of adrenal tissue (128); the mechanism is not understood.

Procarbazine is a hydrazine derivative known to produce chromosome breaks (129), although oxygen may be necessary for this to occur (130). The drug inhibits both RNA and DNA synthesis (131), but it is likely that some chemical breakdown product or metabolite is the active inhibitor. Major side effects are leukopenia and thrombocytopenia, but effects on the nervous system ranging from drowsiness to hallucinations and psychosis may occur, together with peripheral effects on sensation and reflexes, in up to

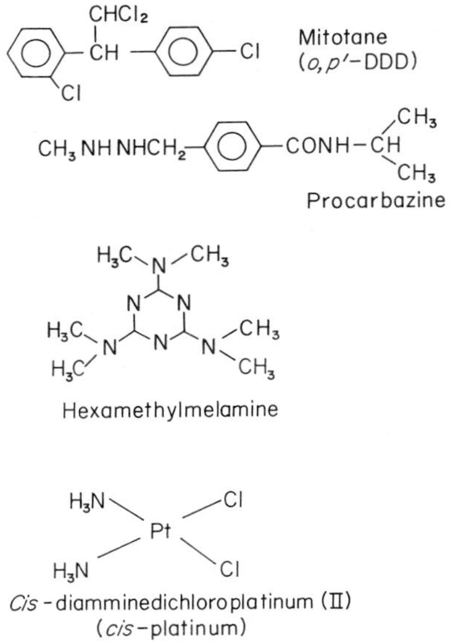

Mitotane (o,p'-DDD)

Procarbazine

Hexamethylmelamine

Cis-diamminedichloroplatinum (II)
(*cis*-platinum)

Figure 7-21 Miscellaneous anticancer drugs.

20 percent of patients. Since it also acts as a monomine oxidase inhibitor, interactions with sympathomimetic drugs, tricyclic antidepressants, and such tyramine-containing foods as cheese may occur; there is also an interaction with alcohol.

The choice of drugs

The choice of drugs for chemotherapy depends first upon whether the disease is generally responsive to drugs and second upon the particular spectrum of activity of individual compounds. Other factors that should be taken into account include pregnancy, because of the risk of teratogenetic effects on the fetus, the patient's tolerance of a particular medication, and compliance with the regimen. Table 7-12 lists the tumors that are generally responsive to chemotherapy, classified according to whether they are highly responsive, responsive (50 percent response rate); or moderately responsive (some increase in survival). The sensitive tumors listed account for less than 10 percent of all human cancers. In Table 7-13, the preferred drugs for treating many of these sensitive tumors are listed. The list is not comprehensive, and since all cancer treatment is to varying extents exper-

Table 7-12 Tumors most responsive to chemotherapy.

Response category	*Disease*
Highly responsive, with a large percentage achieving normal life expectancy	Burkitt's lymphoma Embryonal rhabdomyosarcoma Gestational choriocarcinoma Hodgkin's disease Wilms' tumor
Responsive with a 50% or greater response rate, prolonged survival and some apparent cures	Acute leukemia of childhood Ewing's sarcoma Histiocytic lymphoma Lymphocytic lymphoma Osteogenic sarcoma Testicular cancer
Moderately responsive with some increase in survival of responders	Adult acute leukemias Breast cancer Endometrial carcinoma Lung cancer (small cell) Multiple myeloma Neuroblastoma Ovarian carcinoma Prostatic carcinoma

Partially reproduced from Table 4-3, Ref. 90.

imental, it is subject to change. One point that emerges is the frequent use of combinations of drugs, and we shall now briefly consider the rationale for such combinations.

Combination therapy

In the earlier period of cancer chemotherapy, drugs were used sequentially. A patient would be treated with one agent until it was obvious that clinical resistance had developed, and then trial with a second drug would begin. The process was repeated as often as possible, but except for choriocarcinoma, few cures were achieved. Beginning with hematological malignancies, the trend toward using two or more drugs in combination gathered momentum, until it is now the most frequent approach in treatment. A major intent of this approach has been to avoid drug resistance and life-threatening side effects. For drugs with different mechanism of action, the probability of emergence of a resistant strain is the product of the probabilities of resistance to each component of the regimen. Although there is

Table 7-13 Drugs used in treating cancer (from the Medical Letter).

Disease	*Preferred drugs*	*Alternative drugs*
Hematological		
Acute lymphocytic leukemia	Induction: vincristine + prednisone	Daunorubicin, Adriamycin, cytarabine
	Intrathecal methotrexate ((or cranial irradiation)	L-asparaginase, cyclophophamide
	Maintenance: methotrexate + mercaptopurine	
Acute myelocytic leukemia	Adriamycin or daunorubicin + cytarabine	5-Azacytidine
	Cytarabine + thioguanine, vincristine + prednisone	
Chronic granulocytic leukemia	Busulfan	Hydroxyurea, dibromomannitol, mercaptopurine
Chronic lymphocytic leukemia	Chlorambucil or cyclophosphamide	Prednisone
Hodgkin's disease	Nitrogen mustard + vincristine + procarbazine + prednisone (MOPP)	Carmustine + cyclophosphamide + Vinblastine + procarbazine + prednisone (BCVPP)
		Adriamycin + bleomycin, vinblastine, dacarbazine (ABVD), hexamethylmelamine
Burkitt's tumor	Cyclophosphamide	Carmustine, methotrexate
Histiocytic lymphoma	Bleomycin + Adriamycin + cyclophosphamide + vincristine + prednisone (BACOP)	Lomustine, carmustine, Vinblastine
	Cyclophosphamide + Adriamycin + vincristine + prednisone (CHOP)	
Pediatric solid tumors		
Ewing's sarcoma	Cyclophosphamide + dactinomycin + vincristine	Adriamycin
Embryonal rhabdomyosarcoma	Cyclophosphamide + dactinomycin + vincristine	Adriamycin
Osteogenic sarcoma	High dose methotrexate + leukovorin, Adriamycin	Adriamycin + vincristine + cyclophosphamide + melphalan
Neuroblastoma	Cyclophosphamide or vincristine	Adriamycin

Retinoblastoma	Cyclophosphamide	
Wilms' tumor	Dactinomycin + vincristine	Adriamycin
Adult solid tumors		
Adrenocortical carcinoma	Mitotane	
Bladder	Adriamycin, thiotepa instilled in bladder	*Cis*-platinum, cyclophosphamide
Brain	Carmustine, lomustine	Procarbazine, Adriamycin, semustine
Breast	Cyclophosphamide + methotrexate + fluorouracil (CMF)	Adriamycin + cyclophosphamide
	Cyclophosphamide + methotrexate + fluorouracil + vincristine + prednisone (CMFOP)	
	Hormonal therapy depending on status	
Bronchogenic carcinoma (oat cell, small cell)	Cyclophosphamide + lomustine	Cyclophosphamide + Adriamycin VP 16-213
Cervix	Methotrexate	Bleomycin, *cis*-platinum, cyclophosphamide
Choriocarcinoma	Methotrexate	Dactinomycin, vinblastine, chlorambucil
Colon	Fluorouracil with or without semustine	Mitomycin, ftorafur
Endometrial carcinoma	Progestins	
Malignant insulinoma	Streptozotocin	
Malignant melanoma	Dacarbazine, semustine	Hydroxyurea
Ovary	Melphalan, cyclophosphamide	Hexamethylmelamine, *cis*-platinum, Thiotepa, chlorambucil, fluorouracil
Pancreas	Fluorouracil	Mitomycin, ftorafur
Prostate	Diethylstilbestrol	Cyclophosphamide, Adriamycin
Renal cell	Progestins	Testosterone, vinblastine, Adriamycin, Vincristine, cyclophosphamide
Sarcomas, miscellaneous	Adriamycin + dacarbazine	Dactinomycin, cyclophosphamide, vincristine
Stomach	Fluorouracil + semustine or lomustine	Mitomycin, Adriamycin
Testis	Vinblastine + bleomycin with or without *cis*-platinum	Dactinomycin + chlorambucil, mithramycin

little direct evidence that combination chemotherapy really does avoid the problem of resistance (132), there is no doubt of its greater success at both experimental (133) and clinical (134) levels. In selecting drugs for use in combination, three general criteria have been applied:

1. Drugs with activity against the specific tumor are used, unless a special pharmacological principle is involved, as in leukovorin rescue or the use of probenecid to reduce the elimination of methotrexate (132).
2. Agents with different mechanisms of action are the most appropriate choice. This may lessen the chance of emergence of resistance, but it also permits the oncologist to take advantage of different sites of biochemical action and cytokinetic intervention.
3. From the point of view of patient tolerance and safety it is best to minimize the overlap in toxicity. In this way it is possible to give the normal doses for single-drug usage, or close to those doses, without escalating a given side effect to intolerable intensity. The tumor, on the other hand, will be exposed to cumulative cytotoxic assaults.

The second of these factors merits a little expansion. From the biochemical point of view, when depletion of or damage to the end product of a series of reactions is the objective (Figure 7-22), three major types of combined intervention are possible. In sequential inhibition, successive steps along the pathway are blocked; in concurrent inhibition, alternate pathways may be blocked. The third type, complementary inhibition, may commonly occur in chemotherapy when an alkylating agent damages DNA the synthesis of which is also inhibited by antimetabolites. Cell cycle kinetic considerations enter the picture when, for example, *Vinca* alkaloids arrest cells in mitosis, a stage that is more susceptible to the action of alkylating agents (Table 7-6). For further consideration of combination chemotherapy, the reader is referred to several articles (132,133,135).

Finally, the use of different modalities in combination, when, for example, chemotherapy is initiated after surgery as adjuvant therapy for metastases, is becoming more widespread. This type of integrated approach means that it is not necessary to wait for recurrence of disease after surgery before resorting to radiation and chemotherapy; also, the small amount of tumor remaining after the operation should be more sensitive to these other modalities. Radiation, or on a few occasions chemotherapy, might be used to shrink a tumor that is difficult to remove in its entirety; this is sometimes done with Wilm's tumor.

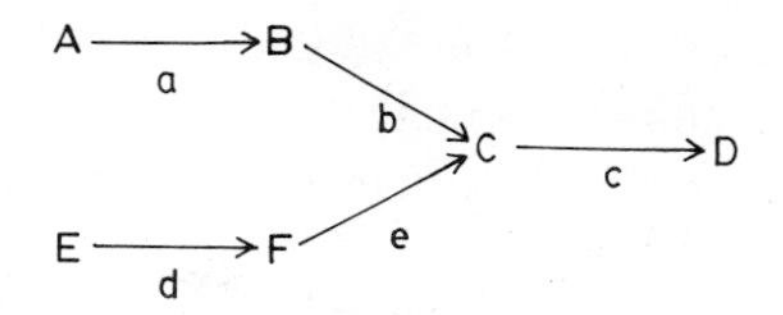

Figure 7-22 Diagram of possible biochemical interventions leading to enhanced cytotoxicity. Inhibition of steps a and c is sequential inhibition; blockade of a and d would be concurrent inhibition; inhibition of step a with damage or removal of the end product D is complementary inhibition.

IMMUNOTHERAPY

Attempts to vaccinate against cancer early in this century were unsuccessful, but the renewed interest in tumor immunology, which we documented in Chapter 6, led to new efforts at immunotherapy. Most tumors that have been examined show some antigenic activity, but unfortunately most patients with cancer are in an immunodepressed state, a state that tends to worsen as the disease progresses. Aspects of this situation were discussed in Chapter 6, and it is evident that tumor immunology is highly complex and attempts to manipulate it for therapeutic ends probably premature. Nevertheless, the concept has generated a lot of enthusiasm. Two approaches have been attempted: (1) efforts to increase specific immune response to the tumor and (2) efforts to increase immune capacity generally. Each of these two approaches may be further subdivided into active immunization with tumor cell preparations or general immunostimulants and passive immunization, in which such immunity is transferred by means of cells or sera from apparently immune individuals.

Specific immunization has been attempted in both experimental animals and humans with variable results (136,137), even when cells were pretreated with the enzyme neuramidase to expose more antigenic sites on their membranes (138). Nonspecific immunostimulation has relied upon the use of such bacterial agents as BCG (Bacille Calmette Guérin), a tuberculin preparation, and *Corynebacterium parvum* to stimulate general immune reactions. Although some success has been claimed in acute lymphoblastic leukemia (139), it is doubtful that the effect of the BCG could be separated from the action of the drug combination used, and in general, systemic BCG administration does not look promising. On the other hand, local administration of BCG, directly into melanoma lesions, has caused marked regression and complete disappearance (140), so this approach may have some limited application. The difference between the results of systemic and local BCG almost certainly reflects the necessity to sensitize local immune cell systems, which does not occur if the agent is injected into the peripheral circulation.

The present status of immunotherapy is uncertain, but enough is known to suggest that its future role may be an adjunctive one in which it is introduced after other modalities have been used to reduce tumor bulk to low levels. The possibility that tumor enhancement rather than tumor regression might be the result of immunotherapy cannot be passed over lightly; this, more than any other factor, urges caution.

CONCLUSION

At the present time about one-half of all newly contracted cancer may be cured. This depends upon three major treatment modalities—surgery, radiation, and chemotherapy—and upon a variety of techniques to obtain early diagnosis. After a trend toward ever more radical operations, surgeons now tend to carry out more circumscribed dissections in situations such as breast cancer, where there is a point of diminishing therapeutic returns and accelerating trauma to the patient. This has been accompanied by increased attention to reconstructive measures to improve the mental and physical well-being of those surviving cancer surgery. Radiation is also a highly curative modality for those diseases responsive to it. The use of higher energy radiation has meant that more effective, less toxic tumor doses can be used. Radiation protectors and sensitizers may further improve the therapeutic index. Although chemotherapy is effective in less than 10 percent of all human cancer, a number of formerly incurable conditions, such as acute lymphoblastic leukemia, are now among the most curable malignancies. This has been achieved by rational application of combination therapy that may often also involve other modalities in an integrated regimen. Immunotherapy is still in its infancy and much remains to be learned about tumor immunology before effective immunological intervention can occur, but this approach may eventually be crucial in increasing cure rates at low tumor loads (141). Interferon may help in this (142). As a final postscript to the subject of treatment, it is ironic that agents used to treat cancer, such as radiation and chemotherapy, can cause cancer (143). This is a finding that only became apparent as the success of these modalities began to show itself in increasing survivorship. Even with this possible side effect, the balance still remains strongly in favor of possible cure.

REFERENCES

1. A. M. Valsalva: *Deaure Humana Troatatus*, Bononrae: C. Pisarii, 1704.
2. F. LeDran: Memoire avec un precis de plusieurs observations sur le cancer. Mem. Acad. Roy. Chirur. *7:*224–310, 1757.
3. G. G. Morgagni: *The Seats and Causes of Diseases Investigated by Anatomy* (1769). London: Miller and Cadell (trans. B. Alexander, reprinted by Hafner, 1960, for New York Academy of Medicine).
4. B. Fisher: The changing role of surgery in the treatment of cancer. *In Cancer: A Comprehensive Treatise*, Vol. 6, F. F. Becker, ed., New York: Plenum Press, 1977, pp. 401–421.
5. W. S. Halsted: The results of radical operations for the cure of carcinoma of breast. Ann. Surg. *46:*1–19, 1907.
6. W. S. Handley: *Cancer of the Breast and Its Operative Treatment*. London: A. Murray, 1922.
7. R. T. Ashworth: A case of cancer in which cells similar to those in the tumours were seen in the blood after death. Aust. Med. J. *14:*146, 1869.

7A. T. C. Everson and W. H. Cole: *Sponanteous Regression of Cancer*. Philadelphia: W. B. Saunders, 1966.

8. I. Hellström, K. E. Hellström, and H. O. Sjögren: Serum mediated inhibition of cellular immunity to methylcholanthrene-induced murine sarcomas. Cell. Immunol. *1:*18–30, 1970.
9. G. A. Currie and C. Basham: Serum mediated inhibition of the immunological reactions of the patient to his own tumour: A possible role for circulating antigen. Br. J. Cancer *26:*427–438, 1972.
10. G. H. Heppner: *In vitro* studies of cell-mediated immunity following surgery in mice sensitized to syngeneic mammary tumors. Int. J. Cancer *9:*119–125, 1972.
11. A. B. Mikulska, C. Smith, and P. Alexander: Evidence for an immunological reaction of the host directed against its own actively growing primary tumor. J. Natl. Cancer Inst. *36:*29–35, 1966.
12. R. B. Whitney, J. G. Levy, and A. G. Smith: Influence of tumor size and surgical resection on cell mediated immunity in mice. J. Natl. Cancer Inst. *53:*111–116, 1974.
13. P. Alexander and J. G. Hall: The role of immunoblasts in lost resistance and immunotherapy of primary sarcomata. Adv. Cancer Res. *13:*1–37, 1970.
14. S. M. Watkins: The effects of surgery on lymphocyte transformation in patients with cancer. Clin. Exp. Immunol. *14:*69–76, 1973.
15. J. L. Odili and G. Taylor: Transience of immune responses to tumour antigens in man. Bri. Med. J. *4:*584–586, 1971.
16. R. D. Gershon and R. L. Carter: Factors controlling concomitant immunity in tumor bearing hamsters: Effects of prior splenectomy and tumor removal. J. Natl. Cancer Inst. *43:*533–543, 1969.
17. B. Fisher, N. Wolmark, J. Coyle, and E. A. Saffera; Effect of a growing tumor and its removal on the cytotoxicity of macrophages from cultured bone marrow cells. Cancer Res. *36:*2302–2305, 1976.
18. G. Poste and I. J. Fidler: The pathogenesis of cancer metastasis. Nature *283:*139–146, 1980.

19. W. D. DeWys: Studies correlating the growth rate of a tumor and its metastases and providing evidence for tumor related systemic growth retarding factors. Cancer Res. *32:*374–379, 1972.
20. L. Simpson-Herren, A. H. Sanford, and J. P. Holmquist: Cell population kinetics of transplanted and metastatic Lewis lung carcinoma. Cell Tissue Kinetics *7:*349–361, 1974.
21. F. M. Schabel, Jr.: Concepts for systemic treatment of micrometastases. Cancer *35:*15–24, 1975.
22. B. Fisher, E. Saffer, and E. R. Fisher: Studies concerning the regional lymph node in cancer. IV. Tumor inhibition of regional lymph node cells. Cancer *33:*631–636, 1974.
23. U. Veronesi: Curative surgery. *In Cancer Medicine.* J. F. Holland and E. Frei, III, eds. Philadelphia: Lea & Febiger, 1973, pp. 524–530.
24. G. F. Robbins and S. W. Berg: Bilateral primary breast cancer—a prospective clinicopathological study. Cancer *17:*1501–1527, 1964.
25. W. M. Kramer and B. F. Rush: Mammary duct proliferation in the elderly—A histopathologic study. Cancer *31:*130–137, 1973.
26. N. H. Slack, E. J. Bross, T. Nemoto, and B. Fisher: Experience with bilateral primary carcinoma of the breast in a cooperative study. Surg. Gynecol. Obstet. *136:*433–440, 1973.
27. F. M. Burnet: Immunologic aspects of malignant disease. Lancet *1:*1171–1174, 1967.
28. J. L. Hayward: The Guy's trial of treatments of early breast cancer. World J. Surg. *1:*314–316, 1977.
29. G. Crile, Jr., C. B. Esselstyn, Jr., R. H. Hermann, and S. O. Hoerr: Partial mastectomy for carcinoma of the breast. Surg. Gyn. Obst. *136:*929–933, 1973.
30. J. Bostwick, III, L. O. Vasconez, and M. J. Jurkiewicz: Breast reconstruction after a radical mastectomy. Plastic Reconstr. Surg. *61:*682–695, 1978.
31. L. R. Prosnitz and I. S. Goldenberg: Radiation therapy as primary treatment for early stage carcinoma of the breast. Cancer *35:*1587–1596, 1975.
32. T. V. Hubbard: Nonsimultaneous bilateral carcinoma of the breast. Surgery *34:*706–723, 1953.
33. W. W. Sutow and R. G. Martin: Bone and cartilaginous tumors. *In Cancer Medicine.* J. F. Holland and E. Frei, III, eds. Philadelphia: Lea & Febiger, 1973, pp. 1863–1879.
34. N. Jaffe, H. Watts, E. Fellows, and G. Vawter: Local en bloc resection for limb preservation. Cancer Treat. Rep. *62:*217–223, 1978.
35. F. R. Eilber, T. Grant, and D. L. Morton: Adjuvant therapy for osteosarcoma: Preoperative and postoperative treatment. Cancer Treat. Rep. *62:*213–216, 1978.
36. F. H. Kung and W. L. Nyhan: Wilms' tumor. *In Cancer Medicine.* J. F. Holland and E. Frei, III, eds. Philadelphia: Lea & Febiger, 1973, pp. 1881–1893.
37. C. E. Koop, W. B. Kiesewetter, and R. C. Horn: Neuroblastoma in childhood. Survival after major surgical insult to the tumor. Surgery *38:*272–1955.
38. R. Grattarola: La ovariectomia nel carcinoma mammorio. *In Atti Corso Oncologia Clinica.* Milan: C.E.A., 1971. Quoted in Ref. 39.
39. U. Veronesi: Noncurative surgery. *In Cancer Medicine.* J. F. Holland and E. Frei, III, eds. Philadelphia: Lea & Febiger, 1973, pp. 530–534.
40. K. M. Nelson and R. S. Bourke: Neurosurgical management of pain. *In Cancer Medicine.* J. F. Holland and E. Frei, III, eds. Philadelphia: Lea & Febiger, 1973, pp. 534–540.
41. L. V. Ackerman and J. A. Del Regato: *Cancer: Diagnosis, Treatment and Prognosis.* Saint Louis: C. V. Mosby Company, 1977.
42. American Cancer Society, Inc., sponsor: *Cancer Management.* Philadelphia: J. B. Lippincott, 1968.
43. W. Walters, ed.: *Lewis-Walters Practice of Surgery.* Hagerstown, Maryland: W. F. Prior, 1963 and updates.

44. J. F. Holland and E. Frei, III: *Cancer Medicine*. Philadelphia: Lea & Febiger, 1973.
45. J. T. Case: History of radiation therapy. *In Progress in Radiation Therapy*. F. Buschke, ed., New York: Grune and Stratton, 1958, pp. 1–18.
46. H. S. Kaplan: Present status of radiation therapy of cancer: An overview. *In Cancer: A Comprehensive Treatise*. Vol. 6. F. F. Becker, ed., New York: Plenum Press, 1977, pp. 3–38.
47. C. Regaud and R. Ferroux: Disordance des effets des rayons X, d'une part dans la peau, d'autre part dans le testicule, par le fractionne ment de la dose; diminution de l'efficacité dans le peau, maintien de l'efficacité dans la testicule. C. R. Soc. Biol. *97:*431–434, 1927.
48. C. Regaud, H. Coutard, and A. Hautant: Contribution au traitement des cancers endolarynges par les rayons-X. Xth Int. Congr. Otol. 19–22, 1922.
49. R. J. Shalek: Physics of radiation therapy. *In Cancer: A Comprehensive Treatise*. Vol. 6. F. F. Becker, ed., New York: Plenum Press, 1977, pp. 39–50.
50. E. J. Hall: High-LET radiations. *In Cancer: A Comprehensive Treatise*. Vol. 6. F. F. Becker, ed., New York: Plenum Press, 1977, pp. 281–315.
51. N. B. Strazhevskaya, ed.: *Molecular Radiobiology*, A. Mercado, translator. New York: John Wiley & Sons, 1975, pp. 6–51.
52. R. H. Thomlinson: Changes of oxygenation in tumours. *In Frontiers of Radiation Therapy and Oncology*. Vol. 3, G. Vaeth, ed. Basel: Karger, 1968, pp. 109–121.
53. J. Denekamp and J. F. Fowler: Cell proliferation kinetics and radiation therapy. *In Cancer: A Comprehensive Treatise*. Vol. 6. F. F. Becker, ed. New York: Plenum Press, 1977, pp. 101–137.
54. J. Denekamp: Changes in the rate of proliferation in normal tissues after irradiation. *In Radiation Research: Biomedical, Chemical and Physical Perspectives*. O. Nygaard, N. I. Adler, and W. K. Sinclair, eds. New York: Academic Press, 1975, pp. 810–825.
55. W. K. Sinclair: Cyclic X-ray responses in mammalian cells *in vitro*. Radiation Res. *44:*620–643, 1968.
56. M. M. Elkind and J. L. Redpath: Molecular and cellular biology of radiation lethality. *In Cancer: A Comprehensive Treatise*. Vol. 6. F. F. Becker, ed. New York: Plenum Press, 1977, pp. 51–99.
57. T. Alper: Cell death and its modification: The roles of primary lesions in membranes and DNA. *In Biophysical Aspects of Radiution Quality*. Vienna: I.A.E.A., 1971, pp. 171–184.
58. T. Alper: Observations relevant to the mechanism of RBE effects in the killing of cells. *In Biological Effects of Neutron Irradiation*. Vienna: I.A.E.A., 1974, pp. 133–147.
59. M. M. Elkind and C. Kamper: Two forms of repair of DNA in mammalian cells following irradiation. Biophys. J. *10:*237–245, 1970.
60. K. T. Wheeler and J. T. Lett: On the possibility that DNA repair is related to age in nondividing cells. Proc. Natl. Acad. Sci. U.S.A. *71:*1862–1865, 1974.
61. M. M. Elkind, C. Kamper, W. B. Moses, and H. Sutton-Gilbert: Sublethal-lethal radiation damage and repair in mammalian cells. Brookhaven Symp. Biol. *20:*134–160, 1967.
62. H. Deakin, M. G. Ord, and L. A. Stocken: Glucose-6-phosphate dehydrogenase activity and thiol content of thymus nuclei from control and x-irradiated rats. Biochem. J. *89:*296–304, 1963.
63. D. W. Van Bekkum: The effects of X-rays on phosphorylations *in vivo*. Biochim. Biophys. Acta *25:*487–493, 1957.
64. W. A. Creasey and L. A. Stocken: The effect of ionizing radiation on nuclear phosphorylation in the radiosensitive tissues of the rat. Biochem. J. *72:*519–523, 1959.
65. P. Todd: Metabolic changes induced by ionizing radiations. *In Antineoplastic and Immunosuppressive Agents*. I. A. C. Sartorelli and D. G. Johns, eds. Berlin: Springer-Verlag, 1974, pp. 474–488.
66. A. P. Casarett: *Radiation Biology*. Englewood Cliffs, N.J.: Prentice-Hall, 1968, p. 87.

67. J. F. Fowler and J. Denekamp: Radiation effects on normal tissues. *In Cancer: A Comprehensive Treatise*. Vol. 6. F. F. Becker, ed., New York: Plenum Press, 1977, pp. 139–180.
68. Proceedings of the National Cancer Institute Conference on the Delayed Consequences of Cancer Therapy: Proven and Potential Cancer. 37, Suppl. 2:999–1236, 1976.
69. F. Ellis: Dose, time and fractionation: A clinical hypothesis. Clin. Radiol. *20:*1–7, 1969.
70. J. Kirk, W. M. Gray, and E. R. Watson: Cumulative radiation effect. Part I: Fractionated treatment regimes. Clin. Radiol. *22:*145–155, 1971.
71. G. E. Adams: Hypoxic cell sensitizers for radiotherapy. *In Cancer: A Comprehensive Treatise*. F. F. Becker, ed., New York: Plenum Press, 1977, pp. 181–223.
72. S. Dische, A. J. Gray, G. E. Adams, I. R. Flockhart, J. L. Foster, G. D. Zanelli, R. Thomlinson, and L. M. Errington: Clinical testing of the radiosensitizer Ro-07-0582 (three papers). Clin. Radio. *27:*151–175, 1976.
73. M. G. Ormerod and P. Alexander: On the mechanism of radiation protection by cysteamine: An investigation by means of electron spin resonance. Radiation Res. *18:*495–509, 1963.
74. A. Locker and K. Flemming, eds.: Radioprotection. *Chemical Compounds—Biological Means*. Experientia Suppl. 27. Basel: Birkhäuser Verlag, 1977.
75. Lissauer: II. Zwei Fälle von Leucaemie. Berl. Klin. Wochenschr. *40:*403–404, 1865.
76. F. E. Adair and H. J. Bagg: Experimental and clinical studies on the treatment of cancer by dichloroethyl sulfide (mustard gas). Ann. Surgery *93:*190–199, 1931.
77. A. Gilman and F. S. Philips: The biological actions and therapeutic applications of β-chloroethyl amines and sulfides. Science *103:*409–415, 1946.
78. G. T. Beatson: On the treatment of inoperable cases of carcinoma of the mamma: Suggestions for a new method of treatment with illustrative cases. Lancet *2:*104–162, 1896.
79. C. Huggins and C. V. Hodges: Studies on prostatic cancer. I. The effect of castration, of estrogen and of androgen injection on serum phosphatases in metastatic carcinoma of the prostate. Cancer Res. *1:*293–297, 1941.
80. D. R. Seeger, D. B. Cosulich, J. M. Smith, and M. E. Hultquist: Analogs of pteroylglutamic acid. III. 4-amino derivatives. J. Am. Chem. Soc. *71:*1753–1758, 1949.
81. C. Heidelberger: Fluorinated pyrimidines. *In Progress in Nucleic Acid Research and Molecular Biology*. J. N. Davidson and W. E. Cohn, eds. New York: Academic Press, 1965, pp. 1–50.
82. G. B. Elion, E. Burgi, and G. H. Hitchings: Studies on condensed pyrimidine synthesis: IX. The synthesis of some 6-substituted purines. J. Am. Chem. Soc. *74:*411–414, 1952.
83. S. Farber, G. D'Angio, A. Evans, and A. Mitus: Clinical studies of actinomycin D with special reference to Wilms' tumor in children. Ann. N.Y. Acad. Sci. *89:*421–425, 1960.
84. R. L. Noble, C. T. Beer, and J. H. Cutts: Further biological activities of vincaleukoblastine—an alkaloid isolated from *Vinca rosea* (L.). *1:*347–348, 1958.
85. I. S. Johnson, J. G. Armstrong, M. Gorman, and J. P. Burnett, Jr.: The *Vinca* alkaloids: A new class of oncolytic agents. Cancer Res. *23:*1390–1427, 1963.
86. W. R. Bruce, B. E. Meeker, and F. A. Valeriote: Comparison of the sensitivity of normal hematopoietic and transplanted lymphoma colony-forming cells to chemotherapeutic agents administered *in vivo*. J. Natl. Cancer Inst. *37:*233–245, 1966.
87. H. E. Skipper: Cancer chemotherapy is many things: G. H. A. Clowes Memorial Lecture. Cancer Res. *31:*1173–1180, 1971.
88. D. A. Karnofsky: Problems and pitfalls in the evaluation of anticancer drugs. Cancer *18:*1517–1528, 1965.
89. E. M. Hersh, J. P. Whitecar, K. B. McCredie, G. P. Bodey, and E. J. Freireich: Chemotherapy, immunocompetence, immunosuppression and prognosis in acute leukemia. New Eng. J. Med. *285:*1211–1216, 1971.

90. W. B. Pratt and R. W. Ruddon: *The Anticancer Drugs*. New York, Oxford: Oxford University Press, 1979.
91. W. A. Creasey: *Drug Disposition in Humans: The Basis of Clinical Pharmacology*. New York, Oxford University Press, 1979.
92. G. P. Wheeler: Alkylating agents, *In Cancer Medicine*. J. F. Holland and E. Frei, III, eds. Philadelphia: Lea & Febiger, 1973, pp. 791–806.
93. D. B. Ludlum: Molecular biology of alkylation: An overview. *In Handbook of Experimental Pharmacology*. Vol. 38, pt. II. Heidelberg: Springer-Verlag, 1975, pp. 6–17.
94. W. A. Creasey: Biologic effects of cancer chemotherapeutic agents. Comprehensive Therapy *1:*31–39, 1975.
95. D. R. Krieg: Ethyl methanesulfonate-induced reversion of bacteriophage T_4 r II mutants. Genetics *48:*561–580, 1963.
96. J. J. Roberts, T. P. Brent, and A. R. Crathorn: The mechanism of the cytotoxic action of alkylating agents on mammalian cells. *In The Interaction of Drugs and Subcellular Components in Animal Cells*. P. M. Campbell, ed. London: Churchill, 1968, pp. 5–27.
97. T. A. Connors, P. J. Cox, P. B. Farmer, A. B. Foster, and M. Jarman: Some studies of the active intermediates formed in the microsomal metabolism of cyclophosphamide and isophosphamide. Biochem. Pharmacol. *23:*115–129, 1974.
98. C. J. Cheng, S. Fujimura, D. Grunberger, and I. B. Weinstein: Interaction of 1-(2-chloroethyl)-3-cyclohexyl-1-nitrosourea (NSC 79037) with nucleic acids and proteins *in vivo* and *in vitro*. Cancer Res. *32:*22–27, 1972.
99. J. J. Roberts and J. M. Pascoe: Cross-linking of complementary strands of DNA in mammalian cells by antitumor platinum compounds. Nature *235:*282–284, 1972.
100. M. Tattersall, N. Jaffe, and E. Frei, III: The pharmacology of methotrexate rescue studies. *In Pharmacological Basis of Cancer Chemotherapy*. Baltimore: Williams & Wilkins, 1975, pp. 105–107.
101. N. Nirenberg, C. Mosende, B. M. Mehta, A. L. Gisolfi, and G. Rosen: High-dose methotrexate with citrovorum factor rescue: Predictive value of serum methotrexate concentrations and corrective measures to avert toxicity. Cancer Treat. Rep. *61:*779–783, 1977.
102. J. R. Bertino: Folate antagonists. *In Antineoplastic and Immunosuppressive Agents*. Part II, A. C. Sartorelli and D. G. Johns, eds. Berlin: Springer-Verlag, 1975, pp. 468–483.
103. G. A. LePage and J. P. Whitecar: Pharmacology of 6-thioguanine in man. Cancer Res. *31:*1627–1631, 1971.
104. J. Shorey, S. Schenker W. N. Suki, and B. Combes: Hepatotoxicity of mercaptopurine. Arch. Int. Med. *122:*54–58, 1968.
105. M. Rosman, M. H. Lee, W. A. Creasey, and A. C. Sartorelli: Mechanisms of resistance to 6-thiopurines in human leukemia. Cancer Res. *34:*1952–1956, 1974.
106. D. V. Santi, C. S. McHenry, and H. Sommer: Mechanism of interaction of thymidylate synthetase with 5-fluorodeoxyuridylate. Biochemistry *13:*471–480, 1974.
107. C. Heidelberger: Fluorinated pyrimidines and their nucleosides. *In Antineoplastic and Immunosuppressive Agents*, Part II. A. C. Sartorelli and D. G. Johns, eds. Berlin: Springer-Verlag, 1975, pp. 193–231.
108. W. H. Prusoff, M. S. Chen, P. H. Fischer, T. S. Lin, and G. T. Shiau: 5-lodo-2′-deoxyuridine. *In Antibiotics V*, Part 2. F. E. Hahn, ed. Berlin: Springer-Verlag, 1979, pp. 236–261.
109. W. A. Creasey: Arabinosylcytosine. *In Antineoplastic and Immunosuppressive Agents*, Part II. A. C. Sartorelli and D. G. Johns, eds. Berlin: Springer-Verlag, 1975, pp. 232–256.
110. R. L. Momparler: Kinetic and template studies with 1-β-D-arabinofuranosylcytosine 5′-

triphosphate and mammalian deoxyribonucleic acid polymerase. Mol. Pharmacol. *8:*362–370, 1972.

111. A. Friedland: Inhibition of deoxyribonucleic acid chain initiation: A new mode of action for 1-β-D-arabinofuranosylcytosine in human lymphoblasts. Biochemistry *16:*5308–5312, 1977.
112. L. H. Li, E. J. Olin, H. H. Buskirk, and L. M. Reineke: Cytotoxicity and mode of action of 5-azacytidine on L1210 leukemia. Cancer Res. *30:*2760–2769, 1970.
113. I. H. Krakoff, N. C. Brown, and P. Reichard: Inhibition of ribonucleoside diphosphate reductase by hydroxyurea. Cancer Res. *28:*1559–1565, 1968.
114. H. M. Sobell and S. C. Jain: Stereochemistry of actinomycin binding to DNA. II. Detailed molecular model of actinomycin-DNA complex and its implications. J. Mol. Biol. *68:*21–34, 1972.
115. W. J. Pigram, W. Fuller, and L. D. Hamilton: Stereochemistry of intercalation: Interaction of daunomycin with DNA. Nature New Biol. *235:*17–19, 1972.
116. E. A. Sausville, J. Peisach, and S. B. Horwitz: A role for ferrous ion and oxygen in the degradation of DNA by bleomycin. Biochem. Biophys. Res. Commun. *73:*814–822, 1976.
117. L. Wilson, K. A. Anderson, and D. Chin: Nonstoichiometric poisoning of microtubule polymerization: A model for the mechanism of action of the vinca alkaloids, podophyllotoxin and colchicine. *In Cold Spring Harbor Conference on Cell Proliferation. III. Cell Motility.* R. Goldman, T. Pollard and J. Rosenbaum, eds. New York: Cold Spring Harbor Laboratory, 1976, pp. 1051–1064.
118. R. L. Margolis and L. Wilson: Opposite end assembly and disasembly of microtubules at steady state *in vitro.* Cell *13:*1–8, 1978.
119. S. E. Malawista, H. Sato, and K. G. Bensch: Vinblastine and griseofulvin reversibly disrupt the living mitotic spindle. Science *160:*770–772, 1968.
120. W. A. Creasey: The vinca alkaloids. *In Antibiotics V,* Part 2. F. E. Hahn, ed. Berlin: Springer-Verlag, 1979, pp. 414–438.
121. J. D. Loike and S. B. Horwitz: Effects of podophyllotoxin and VP 16-213 on microtubule assembly *in vitro* and nucleoside transport in HeLa cells. Biochemistry *15:*5435–5443, 1976.
122. A. Krishan, K. Paika, and E. Frei, III: Cytofluorometric studies on the action of podophyllotoxin and epipodophyllotoxins (VM 26, VP 16-213) on the cell cycle traverse of human lymphoblasts. J. Cell Biol. *66:*521–530, 1975.
123. M. Gosalvez, J. Perez-Garcia, and M. Lopez: Inhibition of NADH-linked respiration with the anti-cancer agent 4′-demethyl-epipodophyllotoxin thenylidene glucoside (VM 26). Europ. J. Cancer *8:*471–473, 1972.
124. J. R. Pasqualini, ed.: *Receptors and Mechanisms of Action of Steroid Hormones.* New York: Marcel Dekker, Part 1, 1976; Part II, 1977.
125. M. H. Mackman, B. Dvorkin, and A. White: Evidence for induction by cortisol *in vitro* of a protein inhibitor of transport and phosphorylation processes in rat thymocytes. Proc. Natl. Acad. Sci. U.S.A. *68:*1269–1273, 1971.
126. W. L. McGuire, P. P. Carbone, M. E. Sears, and G. C. Escher: Estrogen receptors in human breast cancer: An overview. *In Estrogen Receptors in Human Breast Cancer.* W. L. McGuire, P. P. Carbone, and E. P. Vollmer, eds. New York: Raven Press, 1975, pp. 1–7.
127. M. K. Patterson, Jr.: L-Asparaginase: Basic aspects; and H. F. Oettgen: L-Asparaginase: Current status of clinical evaluation. *In Antineoplastic and Immunosuppressive Agents,* Part II. A. C. Sartorelli and D. G. Johns, eds. Berlin-Heidelberg-New York: Springer-Verlag, 1975, pp. 695–722; 723–746.

128. O. Vilar and W. W. Tullner: Effects of o,p'-DDD on histology and 17-hydroxycorticosteroid output of the dog adrenal cortex. Endocrinology *65:*80–86, 1959.
129. A. Rutishauser and W. Bolag: Cytological investigations with a new class of cytotoxic agents: Methylhydrazine derivatives. Experientia *19:*131–132, 1963.
130. K. Bernies, M. Kofler, W. Bolag, A. Kaiser, and A. Langemann: The degradation of deoxyribonucleic acid by new tumor inhibiting compounds: The intermediate formation of hydrogen peroxide. Experientia *19:*132–133, 1963.
131. A. C. Sartorelli and S. Tsunamura: Studies on the biochemical mode of action of a cytotoxic methylhydrazine derivative, N-isopropyl-α-(2-methylhydrazine)-*p*-toluamide. Mol. Pharmacol. *2:*275–283, 1966.
132. W. A. Creasey: Pharmacological considerations in combination chemotherapy. Pharmacol. Ther. A. *1:*307–325, 1977.
133. A. Goldin, J. M. Venditti, and N. Mantel: Combination chemotherapy: Basic considerations. *In Antineoplastic and Immunosuppressive Agents,* Part I. A. C. Sartorelli and D. G. Johns, eds. Berlin: Springer-Verlag, 1974, pp. 411–448.
134. V. T. DeVita, R. C. Young, and G. P. Canellos: Combination versus single agent chemotherapy: A review of the basis for selection of drug treatment of cancer. Cancer *35:*98–110, 1975.
135. A. C. Sartorelli and W. A. Creasey: Combination chemotherapy. *In Cancer Medicine.* J. F. Holland and E. Frei III, eds. Philadelphia: Lea & Febiger, 1973, pp. 707–717.
136. H. F. Oettgen and K. E. Hellstrom: Tumor immunology. *In Cancer Medicine.* J. F. Holland and E. Frei, III, eds. Philadelphia: Lea & Febiger, 1973, pp. 951–990.
137. E. M. Hersh, G. M. Mavligit, and J. U. Gutterman: Immunotherapy as related to lung cancer. Seminars in Oncol. *1:*273–278, 1974.
138. R. L. Simmons, A. Rios, G. Lundgren, P. K. Ray, C. F. McKhann, and G. Haywood: Immunospecific regression of methylcholanthrene-fibrosarcomas using neuroaminidase. Surgery *70:*38–46, 1971.
139. G. Mathe, J. L. Amiel, L. Schwartzenberg, M. Schneider, A. Cattan, J. R. Schlumberger, M. Hayat, and F. DeVassal: Demonstration de l'efficacite de l'immunotherapie active dans la leukemie aigue lymphoblastique humaine. Rev. Franc. d'et Clin. Biol. *13:*454–1968.
140. D. L. Morton, F. R. Eilber, R. A. Malmgren, and W. C. Wood: Immunological factors which influence response to immunotherapy in malignant melanoma. Surgery *68:*158–164, 1970.
141. E. M. Hersch, G. M. Mavligit, J. U. Gutterman, and S. P. Richman: Immunotherapy of human cancer. *In Cancer: A Comprehensive Treatise.* Vol. 6. F. F. Becker, ed. New York: Plenum Press, 1977, pp. 425–532.
142. B. R. Blum: Interferons and the immune system. Nature *284:*593–595, 1980.
143. S. M. Sieber and R. H. Adamson: The clastogenic, mutagenic, teratogenic and carcinogenic effects of various antineoplastic agents. *In Pharmacological Basis of Cancer Chemotherapy.* Baltimore: Williams & Wilkins, 1975, pp. 401–468.

8. Unproven and dietary treatments for cancer

Unorthodox treatments for disease have always existed, but at one time the distinction between what was accepted and what was not was purely arbitrary. As medicine came to emphasize its rational aspects, many of its original practices were abandoned in favor of approaches based on scientific knowledge, while traditional and unorthodox treatments were looked on with suspicion. In this way the distinction between official medical practice and the unorthodox became quite definitive. Many of these unorthodox approaches originated in folk medicine, whereas others were devised by individuals, who often acted with a strong profit motive. Some of these remedies ultimately proved their worth and became medically accepted, but most remained at the fringe, their fate decided by public fads and fancies and the changing prevalence of various diseases. Cancer, because of its severity, has always received more than its share of unorthodox remedies and will undoubtedly continue to do so, as long as so many malignancies are not curable. Such treatments extend from bizarre electrical apparatus, through herbs and chemicals, to dietary regimens. We shall briefly review some of the more important examples of these, and point out where there is rational basis for their use.

LAETRILE

Many popular remedies have been proposed as cancer cures, but none has achieved the widespread publicity or become as controversial as laetrile.

Its proponents argue that it is a natural, harmless nutrient—vitamin B_{17}—that is lacking in a normal modern diet, and is capable of benefiting or even curing many cancer patients (1). To its opponents it is not merely worthless, but actually dangerous. The success of its proponents in gaining a measure of legal approval, in the face of opposition from such bodies as the FDA (2), reflects to some extent a contemporary protest against what is perceived by many as the overzealous paternalism of government, coupled with entrenched self-interest on the part of the pharmaceutical industry and the medical profession. However, there is undoubtedly another component, the strong conviction, or wishful thinking of many patients and their families that laetrile can be beneficial in the treatment of cancer.

Laetrile is a cyanogenic glycoside present in a wide variety of plants. These include bitter almonds, the kernels and seeds of apricots, apples, cherries, nectarines, peaches, pears and plums, broad beans, chick peas, blackberries, cranberries, strawberries, alfalfa, barley, oats, brown rice, and bamboo shoots (3). Although it was originally thought to be a glucuronide, laetrile is now considered identical to amygdalin (L-mandelonitrile-β-D-glucosido-6-β-D-glycoside), which has been known since 1845 (4). Laetrile preparations have generally been found to contain no more than 70 or 80 percent of amygdalin, and often much less (5). It has been proposed that laetrile acts by releasing hydrogen cyanide, which accounts for 6% of its weight, as a result of β-glucuronidase or β-glucosidase action; the intermediate mandelonitrile may also be toxic (Figure 8-1). Cyanide ion is toxic for both malignant and normal cells, but the latter are assumed to be protected by rhodanese (thiosulfate-cyanide sulfurtransferase), an enzyme that converts cyanide to the harmless thiocyanate, thus providing selective lethality for cancer cells (6). There is, however, some controversy regarding the reality of the claimed distribution pattern of these enzymes. Tumors do not have less rhodanese than normal tissues, nor uniformly, more glucuronidase, and β-glucosidase is present at trace levels in most animal tissue (7,8). Since the major component of laetrile amygdalin is a glucoside not a glucuronide, formation of cyanide by endogenous β-glucosidase could not be extensive, a conclusion that is in accord with the very limited data on the metabolism of laetrile given to patients intravenously (9). Thus, the rationale for laetrile use is weakened significantly. As a result, other mechanisms have been proposed, such as that cyanide groups interact with the cell membrane to increase its permeability to cations, which tends to increase the pH of the intracellular milieu (3).

In discussions of the possible toxicity of laetrile, it is the release of cya-

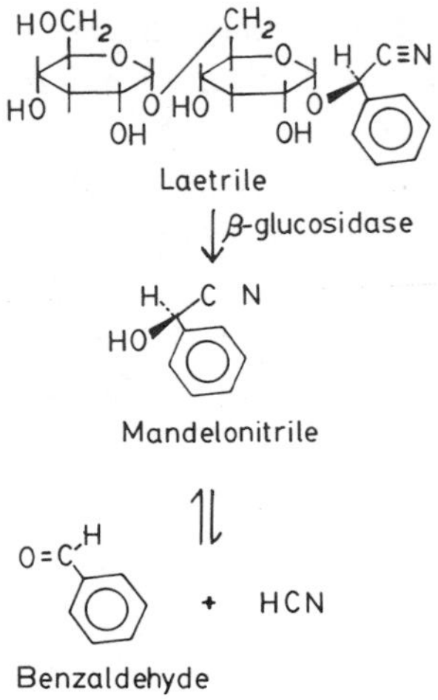

Laetrile

β-glucosidase

Mandelonitrile

Benzaldehyde + HCN

Figure 8-1 Postulated products of laetrile metabolism.

nide that has given rise to most concern. In a study carried out in dogs, ingestion of laetrile together with sweet almond paste, which contains β-glucosidase, led to neurological impairment and to behavioral, cardiovascular, and respiratory changes characteristic of cyanide intoxication. Six out of ten dogs died after receiving laetrile at the therapeutic dosage level (10). There are a number of reports in the literature of fatal poisoning from laetrile ingestion (e.g., Ref. 11), and the recorded symptoms are clearly those associated with cyanide poisoning and are compatible with blood cyanide in excess of 2 μg/ml (12). The oral route is most likely to cause release of cyanide, because the intestinal mucosa has some glucosidase activity, foods containing the enzyme may be present, and the intestinal flora also contain the enzyme. Finally, it should be remembered that poisoning from eating pits and seeds containing cyanogenic glycosides is well documented around the world. Thus, it can hardly be claimed that laetrile is without risk of toxicity, and this risk may be greatly enhanced by the manner of administration and the foods ingested. There is also the added complication that extraction and purification without adequate quality control may lead to extensive hydrolysis by endogenous enzymes in the plant.

There is little evidence of laetrile's efficacy against experimental tumors in animals, and most of this has appeared in publications other than scientific journals (3). A report from the Sloan-Kettering Institute included only two experiments by Kanematsu Sugiura that showed activity against tumor metastases. The somewhat confusing situation surrounding this report, including the use of the highly refractory CD_8F, spontaneous mouse mammary carcinoma in its original host, have been described (13), but this did not negate the strongly negative tenor of the report. Southern Research Institute also failed to document any activity of laetrile alone, or combined with β-glucosidase, in rodents bearing Ridgeway osteogenic sarcoma, Lewis lung carcinoma, and P388 leukemia (14). The leukemia and sarcoma are generally considered to be sensitive tumors that respond to most clinically effective drugs. In another study, at Arthur D. Little, Inc., laetrile, with or without β-glucosidase, was inactive against leukemia L1210, P388 lymphocytic leukemia, B16 melanoma, and Walker 256 carcinosarcoma (15). With isolated Ehrlich ascites carcinoma cells, laetrile has been reported both to affect (16), and to be without any effect (17) on, respiration.

Clinical evidence for the efficacy of laetrile consists for the most part of testimonials and anecdotal or inadequately documented material that does not meet the usual criteria for scientific study (18,19). This is unfortunate, because many of those directly involved are without a doubt sincere in their convictions, even if others would appear to be unscrupulous. The completion of the NIH-sponsored studies may clarify the problem. A consistent theme in the available material is that patients may experience marked relief of pain (20). This could be a placebo effect (see Chapter 9), reflecting subjective effects of merely taking medication, or it could be an effect of the laetrile. Such subjective effects would be less noticeable in experimental animals with tumors, but their confirmation in the clinic might provide a rational basis for the palliative use of the compound. This once more underscores the need for adequately designed trials, even if special exemption from the usual requirements for preclinical efficacy is necessary. However, it should be borne in mind that, realistically, even totally negative findings would not lead to early abandonment of an agent with such an ardent following.

There would appear to be no justification for claims of a conspiracy to suppress laetrile. The compound has been known for more than 130 years, and there were traditional uses for apricot pits and apricot oil to treat tumors in sixth-century China and seventeenth-century England, respectively (21). Many other natural products with similar reputations as cancer cures have been investigated, some have been given clinical trials, and a few have earned their place as accepted active drugs, but none of them would have been pursued further if their preclinical data had been as negative as those of laetrile. Lastly, from the point of view of the pharmaceutical industry, antitumor drugs are not profitable items because research and development are so costly. In this context, it is known that a search for tumor-inhibitory activity, which is guided by folklore and traditional use of plants for treating cancer, is twice as likely as random screening to disclose plants with scientifically demonstrable activity (22). Thus, attention to folklore makes good economic sense.

OTHER UNPROVEN AND FOLK REMEDIES

Plant products are very prominent among unproven remedies. The reviews by Hartwell (23) list about 3,000 plants that have been used historically to treat cancer. One particularly ancient remedy is garlic (*Allium sativum*), which was described in the Ebers papyrus, compiled about 1550 B.C., as an external application to treat skin indurations that may have been skin cancers (24). Later, Hippocrates, and then the Indian physicians of the fifth century (A.D.), recommended eating garlic for uterine and abdominal tumors (23). It appears that an antibacterial and antitumor agent allicin (allylthiosulfinicallylester) is formed enzymatically within the plant, and this is the active agent (25). Only a limited clinical study was attempted, with negative results.

The sap of the bloodroot *Sanguinaria canadensis* (L.) (Papaveraceae), was first used by Indians of the Great Lakes region and then by later European settlers in America, and also as a folk remedy in Russia, to treat warts, polyps, and skin cancers (23,26,27). Sanguinarine and chelerythrine (Figure 8-2) are the alkaloids in the plant that are active against Ehrlich carcinoma and sarcoma 37 in mice (23,28). A paste containing the sap was employed clinically in the nineteenth century, and its use was revived in some studies undertaken with superficial tumors of the nose and external ear in the early 1960's (21).

The rhizomes of the May apple *Podophyllum peltatum* (L.) were used by Indians in Maine to treat cancer (23), and later became the treatment of choice for condylomata acuminata—venereal warts (29). The active agent, the lignan podophyllotoxin, has served as a starting point for a number of synthetic derivatives discussed earlier in this book (p. 204). This is a good example of a folk remedy becoming an accepted medicinal agent. Other folk remedies have been less successful. For example, sassafras tea, derived from *Sassafras albidum*, had a reputation as a cancer cure in Virginia, but the presence of the carcinogen safrole (Figure 8-2) makes its use question-

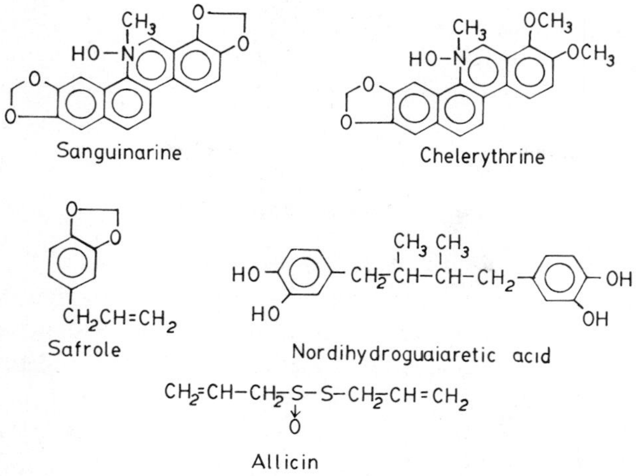

Sanguinarine

Chelerythrine

Safrole

Nordihydroguaiaretic acid

$CH_2{=}CH{-}CH_2{-}S(\rightarrow O){-}S{-}CH_2{-}CH{=}CH_2$

Allicin

Figure 8-2 Components identified in plants that have been used against cancer.

able, to say the least (21). Another Indian remedy that failed in clinical trials is Chaparral tea (30). This is made by steeping the leaves of the creosote bush *Larrea divaricata* Cav. in hot water. The active agent in the extract is nordihydroguaiaretic acid (Figure 8-2), which is an inhibitor of respiration and of the growth of tumor cells *in vitro*, but was unfortunately found to be ineffective in animals, and in a larger clinical trial, although it appeared promising in a small initial group of patients.

Those wishing to follow up specific unproven remedies might find the long series of articles in *CA/A Cancer Journal for Clinicians* a useful source of references. Typical examples would be the Hubbard E-Meter and Electrometer (31), a battery-operated galvanometer device; M/P virus, a live lymphocytopenic virus derived from Ehrlich carcinoma cells (32); sera and vaccines, such as the Bonifacio anticancer goat serum, based on the idea that goats are resistant to cancer (33); the Livingston vaccine, with its premise that cancer is a disease caused by microorganisms of the pleuropneumonia-like (PPLO) type (34); plant materials, such as Ferguson plant products (35), obtained from the Jivaro Indians of South America, presumably on the basis that what shrinks heads may shrink tumors; simple compounds like hydrazine sulfate (36), which at least is cheap; and complex regimens such as Issels combination therapy (37), which involves surgery, dietary modification, enzymes for the digestive tract, vaccines to induce fever, desensitization transfusions, and psychotherapy. There is no proof of efficacy for any of these remedies. As therapeutic approaches to cancer become more successful, it is hoped that worthy elements from the "fringe" will be incorporated into orthodox treatment and the rest will die out.

DIETARY REGIMENS AND VITAMIN THERAPY

In an earlier chapter we discussed the dietary problems of the cancer patient. Some of these problems, which reflect the interaction between the tumor and the host, include such factors as physical obstruction and psychological changes, whereas others result from the side effects of therapy. However, there is another dimension to these problems. There is a widespread concept, of recent origin, that cancer results from a breakdown in the normal defense system of the body as a result of an improper diet combined with the effects of pollution and food additives; it is thus believed that this situation can be remedied by nutritional programs. Some of the latter programs have essentially no rational basis. Examples of these are the grape diet (38), which dates back to 1556, and prescribes eating only grapes to facilitate elimination of wastes that cause disease; the Chase dietary methods (39), with a similar concept of the origin of cancer, to be corrected in this case by fasting, bed rest, and then a diet of raw fruits, salads, and large amounts of fruit juices; and the Gerson diet (40), a complex regimen with an initial 6-week diet of fresh fruit, vegetables, and oatmeal, followed by the consumption of milk protein products, vitamins A and D, brewer's yeast, defatted bile, liver, calcium phosphate, Lugol's solution (as a source of iodine), and blended vegetables, with regular enemas, and no salt, spices, alcohol, or tobacco or aluminum utensils.

Other dietary programs are more rational, demanding the avoidance of processed food and "junk" foods, consumption of as many raw items as possible, large amounts of dietary fiber, and vitamin and mineral supplements at levels greatly in excess of those officially regarded as adequate (3). As we have seen earlier, lack of dietary fiber, with the resultant diminished stool bulk and diminished intestinal mobility and increased transit time through the digestive tract, does appear to be associated with an increased incidence of bowel cancer (p. 152). Most processed and "junk" foods are already looked on by nutritionists as being low in important dietary components and high in calories. Thus, apart from their megavitamin content, such diets are merely rational programs in good nutrition. The elevated vitamin and mineral supplements are usually justified on the basis of older reports linking low blood vitamin levels or low vitamin intake with increased death rates (41) and on indications of depleted stores and increased demand for vitamins in cancer patients. Irrespective of whether such claims are really justified, this popular movement toward what has been termed "supernutrition" has coincided with a new awareness within established medical circles of the importance of diet in the overall management of the cancer patient. This is typified by such approaches as hyperalimentation, which was discussed earlier. We shall first review what is known of the role of dietary factors in cancer and then, on this basis, discuss the dietary modes that have been recommended.

Vitamin A

Vitamin A and other retinoid derivatives are the dietary components that most clearly show a relationship to cancer (42). Norwegian (43) and British (44) reports noted an association between low intake or low blood levels of vitamin A and lung cancer; about 15 percent of the population in the United States has blood or liver concentrations of the vitamin below the acceptable normal limits of 0.2 μ/ml and 40 μg/g, respectively (45). In all such studies, it can be argued, however, that the deficiency state is a consequence rather than a cause of the disease. More direct evidence is available from studies in animals. For example, increasing dietary supplements of vitamin A led to a decrease in the incidence of oral cancers induced in hamsters by application of carcinogens (46). In the same species, the prophylactic use of vitamin A lowered the incidence of lung cancer due to inhaled benzo(α)pyrene from 30 to less than 2 percent (47). Similarly impressive was the 76 percent reduction in the incidence of skin tumors in carcinogen-treated mice given vitamin A (48). Maugh has reviewed many similar findings reported at a conference held in Bethesda, Maryland in 1974 (49).

Vitamin A plays a role in the induction and control of cellular differentiation in normal epithelia. Deficiency of vitamin A seems to potentiate the conversion of glandular to squamous epithelium, the so-called squamous metaplasia, with its increased risk of cancer. It is also known that vitamin A is required for the formation of fucose-containing membrane glycopeptides and glycolipid intermediates (50), which may account for its anticancer activity. The type of epithelial metaplasia induced by carcinogens resembles that seen in vitamin A deficiency and may be antagonized by the vitamin (51). Alternatively, it is known that vitamin A and the retinoids act as antioxidants (they are highly unsaturated) to prevent the oxidative metabolism of such carcinogens as benzo(α)pyrene to their active hydroxylated derivatives (52). However, neither of these two mechanisms provides a satisfactory explanation for the marked potentiation of the antitumor action of the alkylating agent BCNU by vitamin A (53), so some other action must be responsible. Officially recommended daily intakes of vitamin A are 4,000 to 5,000 IU for adults, 2,000 to 3,000 IU for children aged from one to ten years and 1,400 to 2,000 IU for infants. In megavitamin therapy, 25,000 to 35,000 IU are generally given, although daily doses of emulsified vitamin A that are 100 times greater have been used for cancer (3). A major caution to the use of very high doses of vitamin A is its toxicity, which includes anorexia, vomiting, dry itchy skin, irritability, headache, elevated intracranial pressure, inflammation of oral tissues, liver damage, and bone abnormalities. The bulk of the vitamin is stored in the liver and in the blood binding occurs with a specific carrier protein. Clinical trials now underway have used 13-*cis*-retinoic acid rather than vitamin A, since this synthetic derivative is not stored in the liver, is bound nonspecifically by serum albumin, and may be less toxic. Finally, it should be mentioned that not all the data regarding vitamin A are favorable. Some experiments have suggested that high levels of the vitamin actually may enhance induction of cancers by polycyclic hydrocarbons (54).

Vitamin C

A role for ascorbic acid in preventing or treating cancer is more problematical than that for vitamin A. Blood concentrations of ascorbic acid appear to be lower in patients with cancer than with other chronic diseases (55); they are also lower in cigarette smokers, who are more susceptible to lung cancer than non-smokers (56). Like vitamin E, ascorbic acid functions as an antioxidant and this is manifested in a number of ways. It inhibits the formation of carcinogenic N-nitroso compounds from nitrite and various amines and heterocyclics (57). Initiation of skin tumors in rodents by benzo[α]-pyrene is reduced by ascorbic acid, apparently by preventing *in vivo* activation or by increasing the detoxification rate of a reactive intermediate (58). In addition to this antioxidant action, since ascorbic acid enhances lymphocyte blastogenesis induced by phytohemagglutinin, and since lymphocyte reactivity is associated with better prognosis, there could be an immunological role for vitamin C in cancer (59). In a large clinical study, doses of ascorbic acid of the order of 10 g per day were found to give a threefold increase in the life-span of "untreatable" cancer patients (60). This dosage is enormous compared with the recommended dose of 60 mg, and has raised the question of predisposition to kidney stones. There are also problems in the matching of each vitamin C-treated patient with ten controls, and formal randomization was not used; thus, the study is open to objections. The reported prolongation of survival has been attributed to inhibition of hyaluronidase by ascorbic acid, which would reduce the infiltrative spread of malignment tumors (61), rather than to its antioxidant or immunostimulant properties. Another interesting clinical finding is complete or partial regression of rectal polyps in five of seven patients treated with ascorbic acid (62). However, preliminary results of a double-blind, randomized study of 128 patients with advanced cancer did not show any difference between the control and vitamin C-treated (10 g per day) group (63). Thus, although some data suggest a role for vitamin C in cancer prevention and therapy, there are also negative findings, which point up the need for more research to resolve the issue.

Vitamin E

As an antioxidant, vitamin E (α-tocopherol) would be expected to have some of the same actions as ascorbic acid. Indeed, in experiments in which tumors were induced in mice with 7,12-dimethyl benz[α]anthracene (DMBA), and promoted with croton oil or resin, it was found that vitamin E was almost twice as effective as ascorbic acid in preventing tumor development. The best time to give the vitamin was at days 2 to 21, when peroxidation was at a peak (64). In another experiment, ultraviolet-induced skin cancers were prevented by vitamin E: at the same time, the amount of cholesterol alpha-oxide, suspected of being carcinogenic, was reduced (65). On the other hand, vitamin E was not effective in reducing benzo[α]pyrene-induced cancers in rats, although the synthetic antioxidants butylated hydroxyanisole, butylated hydroxytoluene, and ethoxyquin were very effective (66,67). Since there may be a possible increased risk of cancer from diets high in polyunsaturated fats (68), several studies were undertaken in rodents. Here, polyunsaturated fats seem to increase the incidence of tumors produced by carcinogens, perhaps because of the formation of reactive lipoperoxides that can damage membranes and biopolymers; antioxidants such as vitamin E could prevent the propagation of peroxide radicals and the resultant biological damage (64,69,70).

Selenium

Dietary selenium is one of the more recent concerns regarding cancer. In surveys undertaken more than a decade ago, Shamberger and his colleagues found an inverse relationship between blood levels of selenium and cancer death rate (71). These data are reproduced in Table 8-1, and although they permit a linear regression line to be drawn, the negative correlation coefficient of 0.434 reflects the marked scatter. In other studies, the frequency of breast cancer was found to fall by 28 percent as selenium levels in local crops rose from 0.03 to 0.26 ppm (72). Schrauzer compared dietary intake of selenium in New Zealand, the United States, and Venezuela, which were 56, 167 and 220 μg per day, respectively, with the mortality from various cancers, and found that colorectal, lung, pancreatic, bladder, breast, and prostate cancer followed an inverse relation to selenium intake. This was not true of stomach, liver, thyroid, uterine, esophageal, and head and neck cancer (73). Asian diets, with their low levels of polyunsaturated fats and high selenium contents, have also been invoked

Table 8-1 Relation between blood levels of selenium and human cancer death rate—1962–1966.

City	*Blood selenium* (*μg/100 ml*)	*Cancer deaths per* 100,000
Rapid City, SD	25.6	94
Cheyenne, WY	23.4	104
Spokane, WA	23.0	179
Fargo, ND	21.7	142
Little Rock, AR	20.1	176
Phoenix, AZ	19.7	126
Meridian, MS	19.5	125
Missoula, MT	19.4	174
El Paso, TX	19.2	119
Jacksonville, FL	18.8	199
Red Bluff, CA	18.2	176
Geneva, NY	18.2	172
Billings, MT	18.0	138
Montpelier, VT	18.0	164
Lubbock, TX	17.8	115
Lafayette, LA	17.6	145
Canandaigua, NY	17.6	168
Muncie, IN	15.8	169
Lima, OH	15.7	188

Data derived from R. J. Shamberger and C. E. Willis (71).

to help explain the lower breast cancer incidence among Asian women (74). As with vitamin E, dietary selenium, and selenium applied to the skin close to the site of application of carcinogenic hydrocarbons, reduced the incidence of cancer in mice (75,76). When C3H mice, which are highly susceptible to spontaneous mammary carcinomas, received selenium in their drinking water, there was an eightfold reduction in the incidence of tumors (77). It is possible that this effect of selenium results from its participation in the glutathione peroxidase enzyme system, which may play a role in preventing the peroxidation of lipids (74). However, there does not appear to be a correlation between selenium intake and the blood levels of glutathione peroxidase activity (73), which would argue against involvement of this enzyme. Another role that selenium, together with vitamin E, could play, is to stimulate the immune response, an effect that has been seen in rabbits (78). Thus, at present, although selenium appears to be an important dietary component from the point of view of reducing the incidence of some forms of cancer, nothing definitive can yet be said about its mechanism of action.

CONCLUSION

Unconventional treatments for cancer have varied from completely worthless gadgetry to products of natural origin and diets that may have, at least in part, a rational basis. There is an obvious need for more study of some of the postulated treatments that fall into the latter category, since positive results of preliminary or poorly designed experiments are frequently highly publicized, and "cures" are rapidly marketed to an eager public. This is hardly the way to establish the true worth of a treatment or preventive modality. Naturally, this demands some restraint on the part of those enthusiastically pushing their product and a degree of open-mindedness on the part of those engaged in experimental and clinical oncology.

From this brief survey it is possible to conclude that laetrile appears most unlikely to be an active anticancer drug. A few of the plants, such as garlic and bloodroot, might prove to be worth further study, along with other materials that have been found to be positive in preclinical screens. There would appear to be a basis for the use of some vitamins and selenium, especially in view of the frequently unfavorable nutritional status of many patients with cancer. However, there is really no justification for megavitamin therapy at present. This could change if some role for such large doses were demonstrated. For example, should it be discovered that the large endogenous production of nitrite does indeed generate nitrosamines that produce cancer in humans, large doses of vitamins C and E might be very effective antidotes.

REFERENCES

1. E. T. Krebs, Jr.: The nitrilosides (vitamins B-17): Their nature, occurrence and metabolic significance: Antineoplastic vitamin B-17. J. Appl. Nutr. *22:*75–86, 1970.
2. B. J. Culliton and W. K. Waterfall: Apricot pits and cancer. Br. Med. J. *1:*802–803, 1979.
3. R. A. Passwater: *Cancer and Its Nutritional Therapies.* New Canaan, Conn.: Keats Publishing, Inc., 1978.
4. H. M. Summa: Amygdalin, a physiologically active therapeutic agent in cancer. Krebsgeschehen *4:*110–118, 1972. Abstracted in Excerpta Med., Cancer *24:*2098, 1973.
5. J. P. Davignon, L. A. Trissel, L. M. Kleinman, and J. Cradock: Pharmaceutical assessment of amygdalin (Laetrile) products. Cancer Treat. Rep. *62:*99–104, 1978.
6. E. T. Krebs, Jr., and N. R. Bouziane: Nitrilosides (Laetriles). Their rationale and clinical utilization in human cancer. *In The Laetriles-Nitrilosides in the Prevention and Control of Cancer.* Montreal: The McNaughton Foundation.
7. E. M. Gal, F. Fung, and D. M. Greenberg: Studies on the biological action of malononitriles II. Distribution of rhodanese (transulfurase) in the tissues of normal and tumor-bearing animals and the effects of malononitriles theron. Cancer Res. *12:*574–579, 1952.
8. J. Conchie, J. Findley and G. A. Levy: Mammalian glycosidases-distribution in the body. Biochem. J. *71:*318–325, 1959.
9. M. M. Ames, J. S. Kovach, and K. P. Flora: Initial pharmacologic studies of amygdalin (Laetrile) in man. Res. Comm. Chem. Pathol. Pharmacol. *22:*175–185, 1978.
10. E. S. Schmidt, G. W. Newton, S. M. Sanders, J. P. Lewis, and E. E. Conn: Laetrile toxicity studies in dogs. J. Am. Med. Ass. *239:*943–947, 1978.
11. L. Sadoff, K. Fuchs, and J. Hollander: Rapid death associated with laetrile ingestion. J. Am. Med. Ass. *239:*1532, 1978.
12. J. A. Ortega and J. E. Creek: Acute cyanide poisoning following administration of Laetrile enemas. J. Pediatr. *93:*1059, 1978.
13. N. Wade: Laetrile at Sloan-Kettering: a question of ambiguity. Science *198:*1231–1234, 1977.
14. W. R. Laster, Jr., and F. M. Schabel, Jr.: Experimental studies of the anti-tumor activity of amygdalin MF (NSC-15780) alone and in combination with β-glucosidase (NSC-128056). Cancer Chemother. Rep. *59:*951–965, 1975.
15. I. Wodinsky and J. K. Swiniarski: Antitumor activity of amygdalin MF (NSC-15780) as a single agent with β-glucosidase (NSC-128056) on a spectrum of transplantable rodent tumors. Cancer Chemother. Rep. *59:*939–950, 1975.
16. D. Burk, A. R. L. McNaughton, and M. Von Ardenne: Hyperthermy of cancer cells with amygdalin-glycosidase, and synergistic action of derived cyanide and benzaldehyde. Panminerva Med. *13:*520–522, 1971.
17. L. Levi, W. N. French, I. J. Bickis, and I. W. D. Henderson: Laetrile: a study of its physicochemical properties. Canad. Med. Ass. J. *92:*1057–1061, 1965.
18. J. A. Richardson and P. Griffen: *Laetrile Case Histories.* Toronto, New York, London: Bantam Books, 1977.
19. J. W. Yarbro: Laetrile 'case histories'—A review and critique. Missouri Med. *76:*195–202, 1979.

20. J. A. Morrone: Chemotherapy of inoperable cancer, preliminary reports of 10 cases treated with laetrile. Exp. Med. Surg. *20:*299–308, 1962.
21. W. H. Lewis and M. P. F. Elvin-Lewis: *Medical Botany.* New York: John Wiley and Sons, 1977.
22. R. W. Spjut and R. E. Perdue, Jr.: Plant folklore: A tool for predicting sources of antitumor activity? Cancer Treatment Rep. *60:*979–985, 1976.
23. J. L. Hartwell: Plants used against cancer: A survey. Lloydia *30:*379–436, 1967; *ibid 31:*71–170, 1968; Cancer Chemother. Rep. 19–24, 1960.
24. B. Ebbell: *The Papyrus Ebers. The Greatest Egyptian Medical Document.* London: Oxford University Press, 1937.
25. A. S. Weisberger and J. Pansky: Tumor-inhibiting effects derived from an active principle of garlic (*Allium sativum*). Science *126:*1112–1114, 1957.
26. J. W. Fell: *A Treatise on Cancer and its Treatment.* London: J. Churchill, 1857.
27. A. Osol and G. E. Farrar, Jr.: *The Dispensatory of the United States of America,* ed. 24, Philadelphia: Lippincott, 1947, p. 1928.
28. O. Stickl: Chemotherapeutische Versuche gegen das Übertraghore Mäusecarcinom. Virchow's Arch. Pathol. Anat. *270:*801–867, 1929.
29. I. W. Kaplan: Condylomata acuminata. New Orleans Med. Surg. J. *94:*388, 1942.
30. Unproven methods of cancer management: Chaparral tea. CA-Cancer J. Clin. *20:*112–113, 1970.
31. Hubbard E-Meter and Hubbard Electrometer. CA-Cancer J. Clin. *16:*214–215, 1966.
32. M-P Virus. CA-Cancer J. Clin. *21:*186–189, 1971.
33. Bonifacio anticancer goat serum. CA-Cancer J. Clin. *21:*43–45, 1971.
34. Livingston vaccine. CA-Cancer J. Clin. *18:*46–47, 1968.
35. Ferguson plant products. CA-Cancer J. Clin. *22:*113–117, 1972.
36. Hydrazine sulfate. CA-Cancer J. Clin. *26:*108–110, 1976.
37. Issels combination therapy. CA-Cancer J. Clin. *22:*188–191, 1972.
38. Grape diet. CA-Cancer J. Clin. *24:*144–146, 1974.
39. Chase dietary methods. CA-Cancer J. Clin. *19:*125–126, 1969.
40. Gerson diet. CA-Cancer J. Clin. *23:*314–317, 1973.
41. H. D. Chope and L. Breslow: Nutritional status of the aging. Am. J. Public Health *46:*61–67, 1956.
42. Vitamin A and cancer prophylaxis. Br. Med. J. *2:*2–3, 1976.
43. E. Bjelke: Dietary vitamin A and human lung cancer. Int. J. Cancer *15:*561–565, 1975.
44. A. Sakula: Vitamin A and lung cancer. Br. Med. J. *2:*298, 1976.
45. O. A. Roels: Vitamin A physiology. J. Am. Med. Ass. *214:*1097–1102, 1970.
46. N. H. Rowe and R. J. Gorlin: Effect of vitamin A deficiency upon experimental oral carcinogensis. J. Dental Res. *38:*72–83, 1959.
47. U. Saffioti: Experimental cancer of the lung: Inhibition by vitamin A of the induction of tracheobronchial squamous metaplasia and squamous cell tumors. Cancer *20:*857–864, 1967.
48. R. J. Shamberger: Inhibitory effect of vitamin A on carcinogenesis. J. Natl. Cancer Inst. *47:*667–673, 1971.
49. T. H. Maugh: Vitamin A: Potential protection from carcinogens. Science *186:*1198, 1974.
50. L. DeLuca, M. Schumacher, and G. Wolf: Biosynthesis of a fucose-containing glycolipid from rat small intestine in normal and vitamin A-deficient conditions. J. Biol. Chem. *245:*4551–4558, 1970.
51. C. C. Harris, M. B. Sporn, D. G. Kauffman, J. M. Smith, F. E. Jackson, and U. Saffioti: Histogenesis of squamous metaplasia in the hamster tracheal epithelium caused by vitamin A deficiency or benzo[α]pyrene-ferric oxide. J. Natl. Cancer Inst. *48:*743–761, 1972.
52. D. Hill and T. W. Shih: Vitamin A compounds and analogs as inhibitors of mixed-function

oxidases that metabolize carcinogenic polycyclic hydrocarbons and other compounds. Cancer Res. *34:*564–570, 1974.

53. M. H. Cohen and P. P. Carbone: Enhancement of the antitumor effects of 1,3-*bis* (2-chloroethyl)-1-nitrosourea and cyclophosphamide by vitamin A. J. Natl. Cancer Inst. *48:*921–926, 1972.
54. D. M. Smith, A. E. Rogers, and P. M. Newberne: Vitamin A and benzo(α)-pyrene carcinogenesis in the respiratory tract of hamsters fed a semi-synthetic diet. Cancer Res. *35:*1485–1488, 1975.
55. O. Bodansky, F. Wroblewski, and B. Markardt: Concentration of ascorbic acid in plasma and white cells of patients with cancer and non-cancerous chronic disease. Cancer Res. *11:*238, 1951.
56. O. Pelletier: Vitamin C status of cigarette smokers and non-smokers. Am. J. Clin. Nutrition *23:*520–524, 1970.
57. S. S. Mirvish, L. Wallcave, M. Eagen, and P. Shufik: Ascorbate-nitrite reaction: Possible means of blocking the formation of carcinogenic N-nitroso compounds. Science *177:*65–68, 1972.
58. T. J. Slaga and W. M. Bracken: The effects of antioxidants on skin tumor initiation and aryl hydrocarbon hydroxylase. Cancer Res. *37:*1631–1635, 1977.
59. R. H. Yonemoto, P. B. Chretien, and T. F. Fehniger: Enhanced lymphocyte blastogenesis by oral ascorbic acid. Proc. Am. Ass. Cancer Res. and ASCO *17:*288, 1976.
60. E. Cameron and L. Pauling: Supplemental ascorbate in the supportive treatment of cancer: Prolongation of survival times in terminal human cancer. Proc. Natl. Acad. Sci. U.S.A. *73:*3685–3689, 1976.
61. E. Cameron and L. Pauling: Ascorbic acid and glucosaminoglyans. Oncology *27:*181–192, 1973.
62. J. J. DeCosse, M. B. Adams, J. F. Kuzma, P. LoGerfo, and R. E. Condon: Effect of ascorbic acid on rectal polyps of patients with familial polyposis. Surgery *78:*608–612, 1975.
63. E. T. Creagan, C. G. Moertel, A. J. Schutt, and M. J. O'Connell: Vitamin C (ascorbic acid) therapy of preterminal cancer patients. Proc. Am. Ass. Cancer Res. and ASCO *20:*355, 1979.
64. R. J. Shamberger: Increase of peroxidation in carcinogenesis. J. Natl. Cancer Inst. *48:*1491–1497, 1972.
65. W. B. Lo and H. S. Black: Inhibition of carcinogen formation in skin irradiated with ultraviolet light. Nature *246:*489–491, 1973.
66. S. S. Epstein, S. Joshi, J. Andrea, J. Forsyth, and N. Mantel: The null effect of antioxidants on the carcinogenicity of 3,4,9,10-dibenzpyrene to mice. Life Sci. *6:*225–233, 1967.
67. L. W. Wattenberg: Inhibition of carcinogenic and toxic effects of polycyclic hydrocarbons by phenolic antioxidants and ethoxyquin. J. Natl. Cancer Inst. *48:*1425–1430, 1972.
68. M. L. Pierce and S. Dayton: Incidence of cancer in men on a diet high in polyunsaturated fat. Lancet *1:*464–467, 1971.
69. Y. V. Arkhipenko, S. K. Dobrina, V. E. Kagan, Y. P. Kozlov, N. K. Nadirov, V. A. Pisarev, V. B. Ritov, and R. Kh. Khafizov: Stabilizing effect of vitamin E on biological membranes during lipid peroxidation. Biokhimiya *42:*1525–1531, 1977; in CA *87:*166420h, 1977.
70. S. W. Rothman and S. A. Broitman: Fecal bacterial β-glucuronidase, dietary fat and rat colonic tumors. Abst. Ann. Meeting Am. Soc. Microbiol. 1977, p. 24.
71. R. J. Shamberger and C. E. Willis: Selenium distribution and human cancer mortality. Crit. Rev. Clin. Lab. Sci. *2:*211–221, 1971.
72. R. J. Shamberger and D. V. Frost: Possible protective effect of selenium against human cancer. Canad. Med. Ass. J. *100:*682, 1969.

73. G. N. Schrauzer and D. A. White: Selenium in human nutrition: Dietary intakes and effects of supplementation. Bioinorg. Chem. *8:*303–318, 1978.
74. C. S. Wilson and N. L. Petrakis: Selenium as a protective against breast cancer in non-western diets. Fed. Proc. *35:*578, 1976.
75. R. J. Shamberger and G. Rudolph: Protection against cocarcinogenesis by antioxidants. Experientia *22:*116, 1966.
76. R. J. Shamberger: Relationship of selenium to cancer. I. Inhibitory effect of selenium on carcinogenesis. J. Natl. Cancer Inst. *44:*931–936, 1970.
77. G. N. Schrauzer and D. Ishmael: Effects of selenium and of arsenic on the genesis of spontaneous mammary tumors in inbred C3H mice. Annals Clin. Lab. Sci. *4:*441–447, 1974.
78. T. F. Berenshtein: Effect of selenium and vitamin E on antibody formation in rabbits, Zdravookhr. Beloruss. *18:*34–36, 1972; *in* Chem. Abstr. *78:*24162, 1973.

9. The cancer research endeavor

an experiment—
brief view of reality
condensed to a point.

Cancer research is a multifaceted effort supported by very extensive private and governmental funding. A dramatic illustration of this is the graph in Figure 9-1 showing the growth of expenditures by the National Cancer Institute in the United States; corresponding institutions in other countries have made proportionate investments in cancer research. Although organized national efforts to support research into the causes and treatment of cancer have been in effect for most of this century, the bulk of the total expenditures to date have been made during the period of escalating funding that followed World War II. During this era, the successes achieved against infectious diseases encouraged hope that cancer, too, could be cured, given sufficient financial commitment. Unfortunately, despite these major efforts, overall progress in reducing cancer mortality has been disappointingly slow, as we showed in Table 1-1. In only a few relatively rare forms of childhood cancers, the leukemias and the lymphomas, has progress been spectacular. Cure rates for solid tumors in general have improved slowly, due to the combined effects of earlier diagnosis, improvements in the equipment and capabilities of radiotherapy, and refinements in surgery. Chemotherapy, which has been a major factor in the improved outlook for patients with soft tissue cancers, has had minimal impact on

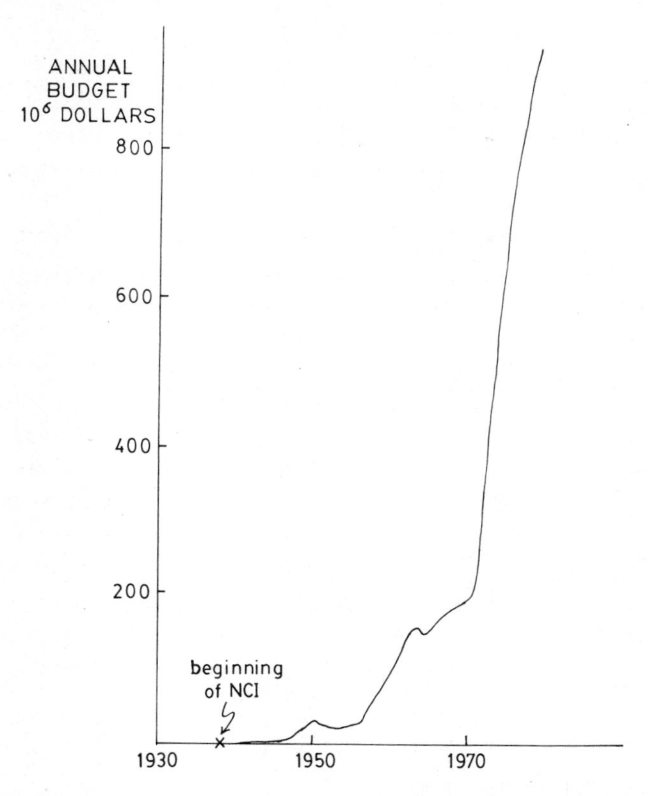

Figure 9-1 Expenditures of the National Cancer Institute since its inception in 1937.

solid tumors. For some cancers, cure rates have changed little over the past 30 years, while death rates from lung cancer have soared.

Thus, if we measure the success of cancer research solely in terms of curing human cancer, the total picture is not altogether reassuring, despite a number of undeniable bright spots. However, the element of basic research must also be figured in, and here progress has been phenomenal. Whereas much basic research involves direct study of human or animal cancer cells, and of the mechanisms of action of drugs or other modalities used in treatment, other endeavors supported as cancer research may appear to have tenuous links, or even no connections at all, to cancer. However, no one can deny that research into molecular biology, using bacteria or viruses, for example, has made major contributions that have helped our understanding of cancer cells and how they function. Thus it is impossible to draw a line that clearly demarcates basic research allied to oncology from totally unrelated studies.

Since the major obstacle to the cure of cancer is its systemic spread by infiltration and metastasis, it is not surprising that the major effort in both research and funding has gone into those areas related to systemic or wide-field therapy—chemotherapy, immunotherapy, and radiation. Comparatively little public funding has gone into surgery, although surgeons have contributed extensively to the other well-supported modalities, notably chemotherapy, through carrying out procedures needed for organ perfusions or intraventricular administration of drugs, for example. Prevention has been an especially neglected area.

In this brief consideration of cancer research, we will discuss some elements of basic and clinical research. Studies on the etiology and growth of cancer have already been reviewed in earlier chapters, so the stress here will be on treatment. Two areas that will be dealt with in more detail, because of the high level of effort committed to them, are drug development and clinical trials. Concerning the latter, we will discuss ethical problems because of the frequency with which they arise. Finally, we shall give some indication of research approaches that seem promising in the light of current knowledge and of other areas where there is need of more information.

DRUG DEVELOPMENT

There are three major sources of new drugs: synthetic compounds; naturally occurring compounds; and traditional folklore remedies. The latter two sources essentially involve the same type of activity, but as was stressed in Chapter 8, folkloric remedies are a much better source of active drugs than random samples of the plant population. Chemical synthesis of new drugs may take the form of devising entirely new structures that appear to have the potential to act as antimetabolites, or of modifying preexisting drug structure to accomplish specific goals, such as increasing binding to target enzymes, slowing down the rate of metabolism and excretion, or modifying the patterns of absorption and distribution. Screening for naturally occurring agents has been focused chiefly on the higher plants and fungi, from which a variety of alkaloids and antibiotics have been derived. The overall process of drug development is outlined in Figure 9-2, and we shall use this as the framework for our discussion.

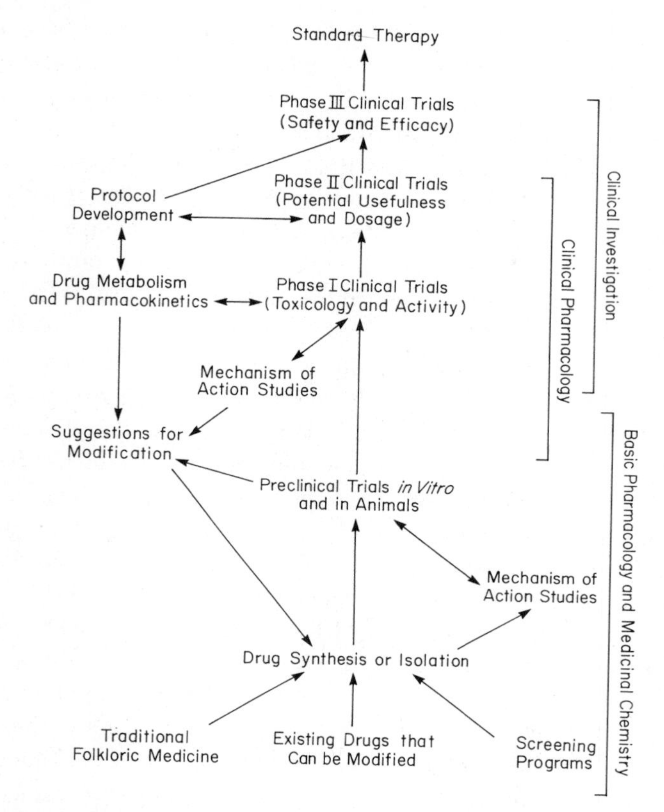

Figure 9-2 Chart showing the elements of drug development and clinical trials.

Screening

Traditionally, potential anticancer drugs have been screened for activity against several transplantable mouse tumors. Although still bearing the nomenclature of the originally isolated tumor, many of these experimental cancer systems are now rather undifferentiated cell lines with very high growth rates and have little in common with the major human cancers. The chief of these tumors is L1210 mouse leukemia, an extremely fast-growing line, with a doubling time of only about 12 hours, carried as ascites cells in the peritoneal cavity. Other commonly used tumors in the older screen were sarcoma 180 and Ehrlich carcinoma, both usually in the ascites form, but also carried as solid tumors, adenocarcinoma 755, and Walker 256 carcinosarcoma, a rat tumor. Most of these tumors are very responsive to drugs or radiation. A particular advantage of ascites tumors is the ease with which responses may be evaluated. This is done simply by determining the increase in survival that occurs as a result of treatment. Untreated mice bearing ascites tumors tend to die within a relatively brief time span, which is characteristic for each tumor, and for all such tumors usually lies between 7 and 18 days after inoculation. As a result of such reproducibility, increases in survival may be determined in a relatively short time with a high degree of confidence. In contrast, animals bearing solid tumors may survive for months, and the rather irregular growth rates must be assayed by frequent measurements with calipers and final excision and weighing.

Although in general the responses to drugs by ascites tumors have been fairly good indicators of how human leukemias and lymphomas will respond, correlation with the effects on solid human tumors has been poor. This has led to modification of the screening procedure. Since ascites tumors are useful in identifying *potentially* active agents, a prescreening step using the P388 mouse leukemia has been introduced. The P388 leukemia has been found to be a better predictor of clinical activity for both natural and synthetic compounds than the L1210. Occasionally, such cell culture systems as the human KB and HeLa cells have been used for initial screening rather than the P388 leukemia. In the next step, the potentially active agents are tested against a number of signal tumors, namely, mouse colon, breast, lung, B16 melanoma, and L1210 leukemia, and occasionally xenografts of human colon, breast, and lung cancers, that is, human tumors growing in immunodeficient nude mice or other immune sanctuary. This wide spectrum helps to provide a more reliable guide to the potential usefulness of a new agent. For further discussion of screening the reader is referred to other reviews (1,2).

Toxicology

The legal requirement that there be evidence of both efficacy and safety, if a drug is to be approved, carries with it the need to evaluate the preclinical toxicity before the drug is administered to humans. Such evaluation should include, in addition to small rodents, dogs or some other larger mammals and non-human primates. Hitherto, parameters of acute toxicity have been the ones examined. These include suppression of bone marrow function, neurological damage, gastrointestinal damage, hepatic and renal damage, weight loss, and lethality. Effects on immune function should probably also be determined routinely, because of the importance of immunity in tumor control. The survival of many patients on intensive chemotherapy regimens also means that attention should be paid to the long-term effects of drugs. This would include developmental abnormalities, behavioral changes or evidence of impaired nerve function, and various fibroses and other chronic tissue changes. At present, no effort is being made to evaluate such long-term effects on a routine basis. Thus from animal toxicology, certain expectations regarding likely tolerated dosage levels, and most probable toxic symptoms, will be generated for the clinical trials that represent the next stage of development.

Mechanism of action studies

These primarily biochemical studies are less necessary as part of the drug development pathway than they are as indicators of appropriate ways to work a drug into combination chemotherapy regimens. As we stressed in the last chapter, varied mechanisms of action and choice of appropriate sites to be inhibited are important factors in devising effective drug combinations. Another useful application of mechanism studies is that it may frequently be possible to use the knowledge obtained to develop tests predictive of tumor response. The best known example of this is the determination of estrogen receptors, but a variety of other biochemical tests have been developed for different drugs (3).

CLINICAL TRIALS

Design

Clinical trials are conventionally based on the Phase I, II, and III scheme outlined in Figure 9-2. In Phase I trials, small numbers of patients (often fewer than 30) receive drug on an escalating dosage basis in order to determine a tolerable dose range and the types of toxicity encountered. Frequently, a modified Fibonacci series is used to set the dosage escalation, for example 0.5, 1.0, 1.5, 2.5, 4.0, and 6.5 mg/m^2. It appears that dosage based on body surface area is more reliable and has a greater comparability with dosages in other species than does dosage based on body weight, but knowledge of preclinical pharmacokinetics helps in assessing appropriate dosage (4). About three patients would be studied at each dose level and escalation would continue until there were signs of significant toxicity. At this stage, the clinical pharmacology of the drug would be studied to elucidate its pharmacokinetics. Phase II studies are intended to evaluate primarily the activity of the drug against tumors. Increasingly, Phase I and II studies are being performed conjointly to expedite the development process. Much of the pharmacological and toxicological data uncovered during Phase I–II trials may be used as feedback at earlier stages of drug development, especially if they indicate how the drug may be modified or administered differently to enhance antitumor action. Phase III trials are undertaken when it is certain that a drug has activity against a tumor; they are intended to establish the value of the agent by comparing it with currently used regimens. By present protocol, the new agent is very likely to be added to a preexisting regimen or substituted for another drug, for comparison, which would thus also be an evaluation of the agent as a component of a combination.

In setting up trials in which two forms of therapy are to be compared, several factors should be considered. First, the study populations should be matched on the basis of age, sex, and stage of disease. Second, if the protocol entails sequential treatments, it is important that one therapeutic approach not always be done first, for as the cancer progresses the chance of response will decrease. A *crossover design*, in which the order the different treatments are given is alternated, will compensate for this change in disease status. To eliminate other biases, such as physician prejudice in assigning patients to a group or evaluating response to a "favorite" treatment, which is our third consideration, randomization of patient entry and blind studies are used. In a *blind study*, the nature of the treatment is concealed from the patient; in a *double-blind study* the clinician also does not know: the medication used is coded. A fourth consideration is the use of placebos. *Placebo*, a Latin word meaning "I shall please," is applied to a pharmacologically inert substance, such as lactose, given to a patient group to control for the effect of simply taking medication. This may be an important factor in the action of psychoactive drugs or analgesics, in which the so-called placebo effect may involve actual physiological changes such as the action of enkephalins at opiate receptors (5). In the case of cancer, subjective improvement may well occur, but objective improvement seems unlikely, so the placebo effect hardly needs to be allowed for. A much more powerful argument against using placebos in a study of cancer treatment is that in such a serious disease it is certainly unethical to deny any group of patients the most effective known medication. Thus, the typical Phase III study involves new medication versus the established, most-effective regimen, if there is one. Finally, the fifth consideration concerns numbers of patients. No study that involves discomfort, or even minor hazard to patients, should be undertaken if there is doubt that it can answer the questions being asked. Two factors need to be taken into account: experimental design and statistical considerations. In terms of experimental design, it is clear that the groups should be set up in such a way as to give an unequivocal answer by avoiding changing too many variables, by providing standard criteria for evaluation, and by eliminating patients whose physiological status may lead to aberrant responses. Statistical input into protocol design should ensure that sufficient patients enter the study to enable a defined percentage difference in response to be established and that the results are not obscured by the poor distribution of particular subgroupings of the population.

In many cases, especially with such rare diseases as Wilms' tumor, it is impossible for any one institution to accumulate a sufficient number of patients within a reasonable time (usually 2 years) to make statistically significant conclusions. For this reason, cooperative clinical trials were introduced, in which a number of institutions adhere to a common protocol, with centralized evaluation and data management. The Cooperative Group Program of the National Cancer Institute is now nationwide, with both geographical and disease-oriented groups, including association with a European group, so as to be in a position to evaluate new therapies expeditiously and to provide uniform treatment (6).

Institutional review boards and the ethics of treating cancer

In any kind of medical treatment, the understanding and cooperation of the patient is vitally necessary if compliance with instructions and effective therapeutic management are to take place. This presupposes a degree of forthrightness on the part of the clinician in explaining the disease and the therapy. This is doubly important when experimental procedures or agents are to be used, for lack of compliance would make the whole study worthless. To ensure that such communication exists, Institutional Review Boards have been set up in all institutions that carry on clinical research. The role of such Boards, which may include clinicians, other local or outside experts, and lay persons, is to act as advocates for the patients, trying to balance the gains to be made from the research against the hazards and discomforts inflicted on the patients as a result of experimental procedures. In the case of cancer therapy, which in some measure is always to be viewed as experimental, the hazards are often major because of the narrow therapeutic margins of the modalities used. Since the disease is so often fatal, however, the ratio of risk to benefit may still be low enough to justify a particular treatment protocol.

In general, the Review Board in its deliberations requires a written protocol explaining the background and nature of the study, why it is being done, what it hopes to achieve, what kinds of patients are to participate and what kinds are to be excluded, and details of procedures and treatments used. A patient consent form must also be submitted. Clinicians are expected to explain the study orally to their patients and to answer any questions they may have, as well as to present the consent form for their consideration and signature. This form should, in layman's language, outline the procedures, benefits, and risks and alert the patient to his or her rights to have any further questions answered, to withdraw from the study without jeopardizing future treatment, and to receive compensation for injury if any is available. Such a written form does not afford protection against legal action, but by adhering to the approved protocol, the investigator at least has the backing of the institution, although it is questionable whether institutional malpractice insurance specifically covers research.

Institutional Review Boards are constantly caught up in arguments about ethical aspects of research with cancer patients, and a few observations are in order here.

Firstly, although full disclosure is the better way, and is mandated by law if treatment under a research protocol carries any risk, a good case can be made that such disclosure makes studies involving placebos or randomization difficult or impossible to carry out. Patients may justifiably be unwilling to sign up for a study in which they may be among those that do not receive effective treatment. Even if the currently most effective therapy is being compared with the same therapy plus an added new component, patients may seek out the newer treatment, especially if it has been publicized in a magazine or newspaper report. Thus, there is unlikely to be sufficient number of patients to complete such studies. In these circumstances, the investigator may be tempted to resort to some limited deception in terms of downplaying the randomization or stating that the drug "may be effective in treating . . ." when in fact only some of the patients will receive this medication. It is best to avoid any such form of deception in the interests of patient accrual, and instead to modify experimental designs so as to eliminate placebos, for example (7).

Secondly, although it is recognized that the Cooperative Group Program has done much to upgrade the treatment of cancer on a national basis, concerns are often expressed that patients may be assigned to standard protocols without proper consideration of their individual needs. This is a legitimate concern even at the biological level where variation in response and toxicity is to be expected, and some flexibility in treatment should thus be required. Although dose modification schemes are frequently included in protocols to deal with this problem, individual changes in the scheduled treatment can lead to invalidation of patient entries by the Group's central office. Since too many such invalidations may lead to loss of funding or group membership, there is obviously a degree of pressure to conform, which might not always be in the patient's best interests.

Thirdly, the whole concept of consent may be cast in doubt if one considers a scenario in which a patient, or worse a pediatric patient with a distraught family, newly informed of the diagnosis of cancer, is asked to sign a rather complex form outlining the method of treatment and its possible side effects. Under such stressful conditions, many might sign without really reading or comprehending the document. It is already known that in such circumstances patients have poor recall of the contents of consent forms (8), and this renders the whole process suspect. Thus, a common practice is to obtain preliminary informal consent at the time of initial discussion of treatment options, and written consent at a later date when the initial psychological reaction has passed.

Fourthly, the increasing legislative attention to human experimentation may be reaching the point of harming rather than protecting patients. Written discussion of rare side effects and complications and disclaimers of institutional compensation do not engender patient confidence in the investigator, and really undermine patient care. Some of the absurdities that arise from undue attention to the wording of consent forms have been pointed out by others, for example, Levine: "I want to treat you with drug X which should (may reasonably be expected to) stop your bleeding. There are no alternatives. If it does not work, you are likely to bleed to death. . . . You are free to decline drug X without prejudicing your rights or future care." (9). Such a written paragraph can in no way reassure a patient about the care he or she is to receive, and it certainly cannot benefit medical research. In all the undue emphasis on written documentation of informed consent, what is being neglected is the process of obtaining consent through the compassionate attitude and willingness of the physician to explain the study, and this neglect is truly unethical (10).

Fifthly, a major concern is how to evaluate risks when one is dealing with patients with a fatal disease. For example, a therapeutic regimen may include an element of outpatient treatment, with the patient taking the medication at home. This may introduce a certain risk through forgetting, deliberately omitting, or overdosing with the drug, a risk not as pronounced when all the therapy is carried out in the hospital, yet the patient may prefer to be at home, and other patients may benefit through the hospital bed space made available. Here there is a three-way balance between individual risk, individual preference, and societal benefit (11). In other cases, particularly in Phase I trials, individual patients may derive no benefit from the study, the main purpose of which is to determine tolerated dosages and clinical pharmacology, which is likely to benefit medical knowledge and ultimately perhaps other patients. Few would consider that such studies should be forbidden because they do not benefit the individual.

Regulation by the Food and Drug Administration

The Food and Drug Administration (FDA) exercises control over clinical trials of new drugs or new combinations of drugs, specifically those shipped in interstate commerce. Before a drug can be administered to humans, an Investigational New Drug (IND) exemption must be filed with the FDA. This includes a detailed report of the properties and preclinical pharmacology and toxicology of the agent, as well as a description of the proposed study—all in all a bulky document. This must be followed up by reports, particularly of adverse reactions. When sufficient data on the drug's safety and efficacy are available, a New Drug Application (NDA) must be filled. On approval, the drug may be marketed for the specific indications for which evidence is provided in the NDA. Use for other purposes is not authorized, and would require filing new IND and NDA applications. The overall process is a long one, taking up to 3 years from the filing of an NDA to approval, although 6 months is the statutory requirement. Thus, FDA processing makes a significant contribution to the time span of the as much as 7 to 10 years required to develop a new drug. This order of delay has been compared with that in Britain, for example, where new drugs appear to be developed more expeditiously, and for a wider range of indications, and suggestions have been made for improving the situation in the United States (12). Among the measures proposed are reduction in the amount of FDA surveillance of Phase I–II trials, which have a good safety record, speeding up the review process at the FDA, perhaps through the use of consultants and/or increased numbers of reviewing officers, and abandoning Phase III trials in favor of a more intensive postmarketing surveillance, as was done in the case of L-Dopa, the anti-parkinsonian drug. In the case of anticancer therapy, abandonment of Phase III trials might not be such a good idea because of the toxicity of these agents and because cancer chemotherapy is always in large measure experimental, with no truly standard effective treatment. The other suggestions, however, are entirely applicable to cancer therapy.

RECENT AREAS OF RESEARCH ACTIVITY IN THERAPEUTICS

It is now appropriate to turn to some of the more recent areas of basic research activity strongly relevant to cancer therapy.

Biological modulators of growth

Apart from hormonal therapy and stimulation of the immune system, which represent biological mechanisms for modulating cellular proliferation, a number of other systems currently under intensive study modulate growth.

Interferons. The interferons, a group of rather species-specific glycoproteins of molecular weights 20,000 to 120,000 or more, are released by cells infected with viruses and then help to prevent viral infection of other cells. They appear to act by causing production of a repressor polypeptide, which interacts with RNA to prevent synthesis of viral nucleic acids and proteins (13). A variety of bacterial and protozoal products and synthetic polymers, such as poly (IC), and tilorone, can also induce interferon release (14). These glycoproteins seem to have a very wide spectrum of activity, being able to inhibit the proliferation of bacteria, fungi, and protozoa, in addition to viruses (13), and exerting various effects on the immune system ranging from augmentation of cell-mediated cytotoxicity (13) to suppression of the antibody response to sheep red cells (15) and of acute inflammatory responses (16). However, it is the reported inhibition of the growth of cancer cells *in vitro* (17,18) and a large number of findings of prolonged life-span of mice bearing virally induced and non-virally induced transplantable tumors (e.g., Refs. 19,20) that have focused attention on interferon. This has naturally led to clinical trials using such interferon inducers as tilorone (21) and poly (IC) (22), but the results have been disappointing. Attempts to use recombinant DNA techniques to induce bacterial synthesis of interferon are promising, since the availability of large enough amounts of purified human interferons is essential for proper evaluation of the material as anticancer therapy. This is an area that needs intensive exploration and the progress that is being made in elucidating the gene sequence of human interferons (23) will help in this.

Whereas the antiviral action of interferons appears to reside in the induction of intracellular mediators that repress RNA function (24), the mechanism for antitumor effects may be more complex. Although, in general, antiviral and antitumor activity are coordinated (25), suggesting a close relationship between them, there is evidence that antitumor effects may have, at least in part, an immunological basis. Thus interferon appears to be a primary regulator of natural killer (NK) cells, the non-B, non-T lymphocytes that attack transformed cells, both in mice (26) and in humans, in whom leukocyte interferon induces the appearance of NK cells (27). It is of interest that in tissue culture lines of Burkitt's lymphoma, resting cells are more sensitive to interferon than are cells in mitotic cycle (28). This suggests the value of combining chemotherapy, with its primary effect on proliferating cells, with interferon, thus attacking a larger proportion of the tumor cell population. Some studies in mice do suggest that the combination may be synergistic (29), but it is clear that in order to take advantage of the differential effects of the two modalities, more attention to cell cycle kinetics is needed.

Chalones. The chalones (30), tissue-specific inhibitors of mitosis, reduce not only the proliferation of normal epithelial cells, melanocytes, fibroblasts, granulocytes, and lymphocytes, but also the growth of tumor cell lines derived from these cell types. Chalones are glycoproteins, most of which have molecular weights in the range of 30,000 to 50,000 daltons. In general they appear to act by arresting cells in cycle at the G_1 phase, but the mechanism of action is not known. Attallah has suggested a primarily cell-surface action of these agents, with intracellular cyclic AMP as the modulator (31). The chalone is normally part of the cell membrane, from which it may be removed by injury, proteolytic enzymes, or serum mitogenic factor (which stimulates mitosis), for example. Since the chalone is considered to modulate the activity of adenyl cyclase, loss of chalone may lower intracellular cyclic AMP levels. A relation between cyclic AMP levels and cellular proliferation, in which resting cells have greater cyclic AMP content, has been known for a long time (32–34); in contrast, cyclic GMP levels rise markedly in proportion to the degree of cellular division (35).

The chalones seem to be produced, or released, in large amounts by some tumors that have been examined (31), yet tumors in general appear to have a lower endogenous content and to be less responsive to the factor than normal cells (36,37). It is tempting to speculate that this could be part of the mechanism that maintains tumor cells in a permanently immature state. Secretion of proteases and other degradative enzymes at the tumor cell surface, leading to chalone release or to the weaker binding of chalone, could explain why the lower levels of this factor have been found. The converse of this is that chalones, or perhaps modified fragments containing active groupings, could add a potential new chemotherapeutic modality. Differential sensitivity might enable chalone-responsive normal cells to be kept in a resting phase, while the less sensitive tumor cells continue to divide and thus remain responsive to cytotoxic chemotherapy.

Maturation factors. The possible therapeutic role for chalones leads us into a new area of cancer treatment. Cancer therapy today is based on the concepts of excision for surgery, and cytotoxicity for radiation, chemotherapy, and immunotherapy, but are these the only approaches? If, as we indicated in earlier chapters, the major defect in cancer cells is that maturation is anomalous or incomplete, would it not be possible in some way to stimulate the differentiation of tumor cells, rather than attempt to kill them, given the narrow margin of selectivity between malignant and normal cells? Studies with tumor cell lines growing in culture have provided a number of examples of temporary or occasionally permanent conversion of malignant cells to cells having characteristics of normal lines, by the action of various agents. These agents include such plant lectins as concanavalin A (38,39); the anticancer drug Adriamycin (40); colony-stimulating factor, which may cause mouse myeloid leukemia to differentiate into mature macrophages and granulocytes (40); nerve growth factor, which causes some neuroblastoma lines to differentiate (41); beef thymus extracts (42); and cyclic AMP (43). Spontaneous maturation and regression of tumor also occurs, particularly with neuroblastoma (44), which suggests the operation or reinforcement of innate control factors. Thus there is sufficient preliminary information to suggest that maturation therapy is a practical possibility in systemic treatment of cancer. Clearly, much more information on the substances having this ability, and on mechanisms for ensuring the permanence of the transformation, is needed before the approach can be applied.

Newer approaches in the design and delivery of chemotherapy

As a result of the information gathered from thirty years of experience with drugs, it is possible to point out a number of approaches that need to be studied if the success of chemotherapy is to be enhanced (45). These include designs that avoid the potential for metabolism to carcinogenic derivatives, perhaps by metabolic stabilization, avoidance of immunosuppression, tailoring of drugs for greater affinity for isozymes characteristic of cancer cells, targeting of drugs for bioactivation at specific sites, and utilization of endocytosis for selective delivery of drugs. This latter has been developed more fully and deserves further discussion.

Selective endocytosis. The concept that cancer cells are more dependent upon external supplies of metabolites, and that such uptake processes as endocytosis are more active than in normal cells, is longstanding (46–48). Thus, tumor cells should take up more of a drug that is bound to a complex material the cell can pinocytose. Several approaches have been used. We know that DNA complexes readily with such drugs as daunorubicin and its congener Adriamycin and that the products are taken up by cells where lysosomal action releases the free drug intracellularly (49,50). Since a major problem with these antibiotics is cardiotoxicity, and since myocardial cells do not appear to undertake pinocytosis, this approach, outlined in Figure 9-3, has the potential for reducing the cardiac damage that limits the use of these drugs. In other cases, drugs may be encased in lipids to form vesicles known as liposomes. Reports of enhanced responses to such liposomes, as compared with the free drug, have been published for actinomycin D (51), cytosine arabinoside (52), BCNU, and nitrogen mustard (53). It is possible that additional specificity might be obtained by incorporating antibodies (54) or lectin receptors (55) into the drug-liposome complex. Non-liposomal complexes of anti-ferritin immunoglobulin with radioiodine have also been used with favorable results as a radiotherapeutic approach to liver cancer (55A). On the other hand, it is also possible that in many cases the affinity of the antibody or lectin for cell surface receptors may prevent access of the complex to the internal milieu of the cell. In the case of non-liposomal conjugates of daunorubicin with concanavalin A (56), and of the aziridine alkylating agent Trenimon with a tumor-specific immunoglobulin fraction (IgG) (57), there is evidence of enhanced antitumor activity. However, neither of these observations can be taken to indicate that entry of the drugs into the cells is enhanced. Both Trenimon, through al-

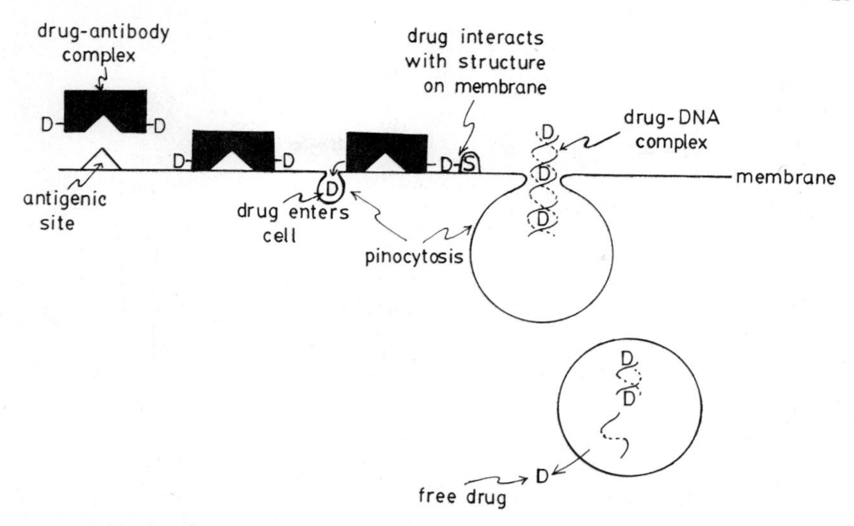

Figure 9-3 Schematic illustration of the principles of selective endocytosis.

kylation, and daunorubicin, through lipid peroxidation (58), could damage the cell by attacking membrane components in the vicinity of the receptors to which they are attached.

Non-traditional sites of drug action. The site of action of most drugs in current use involves the synthesis and function of nucleic acids or the activities of the mitotic apparatus. In other words, their target is cell division. This leaves large areas of intermediary metabolism that might be susceptible to the antimetabolite approach. Among more recent agents that have different sites of action are anguidine and bruceantin, which are inhibitors of protein synthesis; 4-hydroxy-4-androstene-3, 17-dione, an inhibitor of estrogen synthesis that might obviate the need for surgical ablation of all sites at which this synthesis occurs; and tilorone, the inducer of interferon. One other new agent, N-(phosphonacetyl)-L-aspartate (PALA), inhibits pyrimidine synthesis, but at the very first step, aspartate transcarbamylase (59); thus it does not fit in with the typical nucleoside analogs. It is particularly promising in that preclinical screens showed marked activity against solid tumors. The structures of these compounds appear in Figure 9-4.

Glycolysis. Warburg's postulate that tumor cells differ from normal cells in having an increased capacity for glycolysis, even in the presence of oxy-

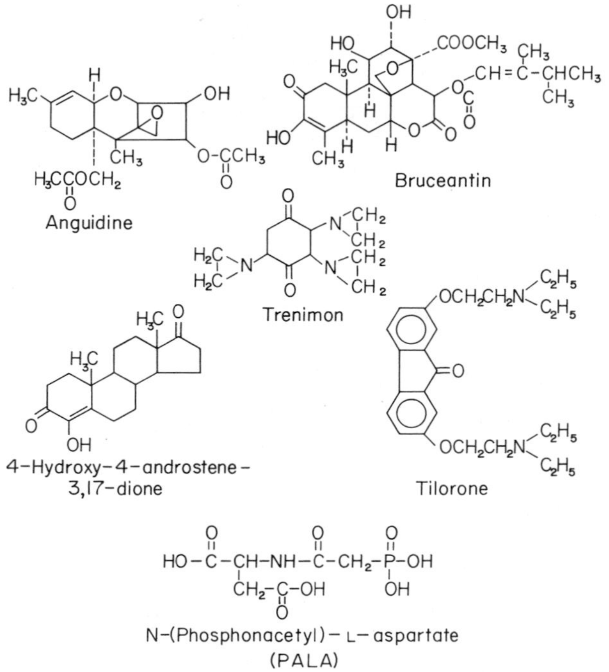

Anguidine

Bruceantin

Trenimon

4-Hydroxy-4-androstene-3,17-dione

Tilorone

N-(Phosphonacetyl)-L-aspartate (PALA)

Figure 9-4 Structures of some newer anticancer drugs with novel sites of action.

gen, led to continuing interest in possible inhibitors of this metabolic pathway, but selective cytotoxicity with such potential agents as pyridine nucleotide analogs (60) has not been achieved. Perhaps further consideration of this metabolic area is needed. In most cells, oxygen inhibits glycolysis, with a shift to respiration that is a more economical mechanism for the synthesis of ATP; this is known as the Pasteur effect. The mechanisms involved in this shift include allosteric inhibition of phosphofructokinase by ATP, produced by mitochondrial respiration, and release of this inhibition by increased levels of fructose 6-phosphate and 1,6-diphosphate, which activate hexokinase (through reduced glucose 6-phosphate) and pyruvate kinase, respectively (61) (Figure 9-5). More detailed examination (62) indicates that in both tumor and proliferating cells the levels of all the intermediates of the pentose phosphate pathway are increased, especially phosphoribosyl pyrophosphate (P-ribosyl-PP), which is required for nucleotide synthesis. The additional aerobic glycolysis is needed for this synthetic pathway and does not reflect non-existence of the Pasteur effect. Furthermore, there is a possible blockade of the M_2 form of pyruvate kinase due to phosphorylation of the protein, and this may be non-reversible in cancer cells and reversible in normal proliferating cells. It is interesting that the net changes in proliferating cells are lowered NADPH/NADP ratios, reduced regeneration of glutathione, and increased phosphoribosylpyrophosphate levels. These changes undoubtedly facilitate conversion of antimetabolites to their nucleotides and may increase sensitivity to radiation through lowered thiol content and lack of reducing power. Advantage could be taken of the glycolytic pathway by introducing synthetic substrates that may be converted to analogs of fructose diphosphate or phosphoribosyl pyrophosphate; these analogs would have the potential to inhibit the protein kinase that blocks the M_2 form of pyruvate kinase (62). Alternatively, analogs of P′, P^4-di (adenosine-5′-) tetraphosphate ($A_{P4}A$), which also inhibits the protein kinase, might be a useful approach, provided the synthesis of such a charged molecule is engineered to occur intracellularly (63).

Figure 9-5 Outline of cellular glycolysis showing the interrelationships with respiration and nucleotide formation. Broken arrows represent modulation of enzyme activities; (⊕) stimulation and (⊖) inhibition. In proliferating cells as well as cancer cells, the activities of the pathways denoted by heavy arrows are greatly elevated.

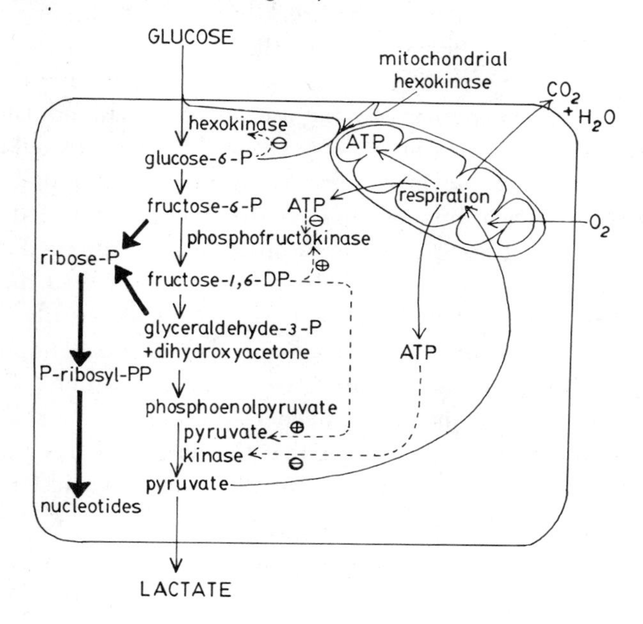

CONCLUSION

I have briefly considered some aspects of cancer research that bear most directly on treatment. In doing so, I realize that many lines of study have been omitted. Among these are such procedures as bone marrow transplantation, which has been established as a viable treatment for aplastic anemia when a compatible donor of marrow is available. The record for treating leukemia by this approach has been less satisfactory, although some notable successes have been achieved (64). Also it is clearly not feasible to review a vast array of basic research connected with cancer, including recombinant DNA work. It is not impossible that such a technique could ultimately be of practical value, but much development is needed first.

Therefore, in this chapter the main outlines of drug development and clinical trials have been given, together with brief consideration of a few potentially promising leads. It is in the nature of the research process that new leads and insights may change a given field totally; the helical DNA model in biochemistry and plate tectonics in geology are good examples of this. The same is undoubtedly true of cancer research.

My own personal view is that, although it is necessary to refine existing therapeutic modalities so as to extract the greatest possible improvement in survival they can offer, no major breakthrough is to be expected from this approach. It is much more likely that a major advance will come through an ability to intervene in the process of metastasis more effectively than can be done now, perhaps by the use of biological modulators of cell growth and differentiation. Current conventional treatment would probably still be necessary for removing or destroying major tumor bulk, but prevention of recurrence would depend on the new modality. At the same time, it is urgent that great attention be paid to prevention. If we look at the major diseases of former times, the greatest advances in their control came not from medical treatment of those who had already contracted them, but rather from preventive medicine that included improved personal and social hygiene, altered life-styles, and vaccinations. Changes in our modern life-styles might also be needed to bring about a similar reduction in cancer, with the added bonus that the forms of cancer most likely to be reduced, such as lung cancer, are the ones now most resistant to treatment.

REFERENCES

1. F. M. Schabel, Jr., D. P. Griswold, Jr., W. R. Laster, Jr., T. H. Corbett, and H. H. Lloyd: Quantitative evaluation of anticancer agent activity in experimental animals. Pharmacol. Ther. A *1*:411–435, 1977.
2. J. M. Venditti: Relevance of transplantable animal-tumor systems to the selection of new agents for clinical trial. *In Pharmacological Basis of Cancer Chemotherapy.* Baltimore: Williams & Wilkins, 1975, pp. 245–270.
3. T. C. Hall, D. Kessel, D. W. Roberts, A. Nahas, and B. Hacker: Prediction of clinical response to cancer therapy. *In Pharmacological Basis of Cancer Therapy.* Baltimore: Williams & Wilkins, 1975, pp. 281–296.
4. A. M. Guarino and D. J. Prieur: Increasing the reliability of extrapolation of preclinical toxicologic data of antineoplastic agents. *In Pharmacoloical Basis of Cancer Therapy.* Baltimore: Williams & Wilkins, 1975, pp. 351–381.
5. J. D. Levine, N. C. Gordon, R. T. Jones, and H. L. Fields: The narcotic antagonist naloxone enhances clinical pain. Nature *272*:826–827, 1978.
6. National Cancer Program: *1979 Director's Report and Annual Plan for FY 1981–1985.* NIH Publication, 80–2214.
7. F. A. Saber and R. D. Reece: The use of placebo and deception. IRB *1*:4–6, June/July 1979, The Hastings Center, Hastings-on-Hudson, N.Y.
8. B. J. Kennedy and A. Lillehaugen: Patient recall of informed consent. Med. Pediatr. Oncol. *7*:173–178, 1979.
9. R. J. Levine: The Senate's proposed statutory definition of "Voluntary and informed consent." IRB *2*:8–10, 1980.
10. E. F. Loftus and J. F. Fries: Informed consent may be hazardous to health. Science *204*:11, 1979.
11. R. M. Veatch: Risk-taking in cancer chemotherapy. IRB *1*:4–6, 1979.
12. W. Wardell: R_x: More regulation or better therapies. Regulation *3*:25–33, 1979.
13. S. E. Grossberg: The interferons and their inducers: Molecular and therapeutic considerations. New Eng. J. Med. *287*:13–19; 122–128, 1972.
14. E. M. Hersh, G. M. Mavligit, J. U. Gutterman, and S. P. Richman: Immunotherapy of human cancer. *In Cancer: A Comprehensive Treatise,* Vol. 6. F. F. Becker, ed., New York: Plenum Press, 1977, pp. 425–532.
15. B. R. Brodeur and T. C. Marigan: Suppressive effect of interferon on the humoral immune response to sheep red blood cells in mice. J. Immunol. *113*:1319–1325, 1974.
16. M. Koltai and E. Mecs: Inhibition of the acute inflammatory response by interferon inducers. Nature *242*:525–526, 1973.
17. I. Gresser, D. Brouty-Boyé, M. T. Thomas, and A. Macieira-Coelho: Interferon in cell division. I. Inhibition of the multiplication of mouse L-1210 leukemia cells *in vitro* by interferon preparations. Proc. Natl. Acad. Sci. U.S.A. *66*:1052–1058, 1970.
18. W. E. Stewart, I. Gresser, M. G. Tovey, M. T. Bandu, and S. LeGoff: Identification of the cell multiplication inhibitory factors in interferon preparations as interferons. Nature *262*:300–302, 1976.
19. E. F. Wheelock and R. P. B. Larke: Efficacy of interferon in the treatment of mice with established Friend virus leukemia. Proc. Soc. Exp. Biol. Med. *127*:230–238, 1968.
20. I. Gresser: Antitumor effects of interferon. *In Cancer: A Comprehensive Treatise,* Vol. 5. F. F. Becker, ed., New York: Plenum Press, 1977, pp. 521–571.
21. W. Regelson: Clinical immunoadjuvant studies with tilorone, DEAA fluorene (RMI 11,002 DA), and *Corynebacterium parvum* and some observations on the role of host resistance and herpes-like lesions in tumor growth. Ann. N.Y. Acad. Sci. *277*:269–287, 1976.

22. O. R. McIntyre, K. Rai, O. Glidewell, and J. F. Holland: Polyriboinosinic: polyribocytidylic acid as an adjunct to remission maintenance therapy in acute myelogenous leukemia. *In Immunotherapy of Cancer: Present Status of Trials in Man.* W. Terry and D. Windhorst, eds., New York: Raven Press, 1978, pp. 423–430.
23. M. Houghton: Human interferon gene sequences. Nature *285:*536, 1980.
24. P. J. Farrell, G. C. Sen, M. F. Dubois, L. Ratner, E. Slattery, and P. Lengyel: Interferon action: Two distinct pathways for inhibition of protein synthesis by double-stranded RNA. Proc. Natl. Acad. Sci. U.S.A. *75:*5893–5897, 1978.
25. A. Adams, H. Strander, and K. Cantell: Sensitivity of the Epstein-Barr virus transformed human cell lines to interferon. J. Gen. Virol. *28:*207–217, 1975.
26. R. M. Welsh and R. M. Zinkernagel: Heterospecific cytotoxic cell activity induced during the first three days of acute lymphoblastic choriomeningitis virus infection in mice. Nature *268:*646–648, 1977.
27. J. R. Huddlestone, T. C. Merigan, Jr., and M. B. A. Oldstone: Induction and kinetics of natural killer cells in humans following interferon therapy. Nature *282:*417–419, 1979.
28. J. S. Horoszewicz, S. S. Leong, and W. A. Carter: Noncycling tumor cells are sensitive targets for the antiproliferative activity of human interferon. Science *206:*1091–1093, 1979.
29. M. A. Chirigos and J. W. Pearson: Cure of murine leukemia with drug and interferon treatment. J. Natl. Cancer Inst. *51:*1367–1368, 1973.
30. J. C. Houck and A. M. Attallah: Chalones (specific and endogenous mitotic inhibitors) and cancer. *In Cancer: A Comprehensive Treatise.* Vol. 3. F. F. Becker, ed., New York: Plenum Press, 1975, pp. 287–326.
31. A. M. Attallah: Chalones and cancer. Clin. Proc. Children's Hosp. Natl. Med. Ctr. *31:*215–222, 1975.
32. J. R. Sheppard: Difference in the cyclic adenosine 3′,5′-monophosphate levels in normal and transformed cells. Nature New Biol. *236:*14–16, 1972.
33. O. H. Iverson: The regulation of cell numbers in epidermis. Acta Pathol. Microbiol. Scand. Suppl. *148:*91–96, 1961.
34. J. J. Vorhees, E. A. Duell, and W. H. Kelsey: Dibutyryl cyclic AMP inhibition of epidermal cell division. Arch. Dermatol. *105:*384–386, 1972.
35. M. Abou-Sabé, ed.: *Cyclic Nucleotides and the Regulation of Cell Growth.* Stroudsburg, Pennsylvania: Dowden, Hutchison and Ross, 1976.
36. W. S. Bullough and E. B. Lawrence: Control of mitosis in rabbit V x 2 epidermal tumours by means of the epidermal chalone. Eur. J. Cancer *4:*587–594, 1968.
37. T. Rytömaa and K. Kiviniemi: Control of DNA duplication in rat chloroleukemia by means of the granulocyte chalone. Eur. J. Cancer *4:*595–606, 1968.
38. M. J. Karnovsky and E. R. Unanue: Mapping and migration of lymphocyte surface macromolecules. Fed. Proc. *32:*55–59, 1973.
39. R. J. Mannino, K. Ballmer, and M. M. Burger: Growth inhibition of transformed cells with succinylated concanavalin A. Science *201:*824–826, 1978.
40. L. Sachs: Control of normal cell differentiation and the phenotypic reversion of malignancy in myeloid leukemia. Nature *274:*535–539, 1978.
41. L. F. Sinks: Neuroblastoma. *In Cancer Medicine.* J. F. Holland and E. Frei, III, eds., Philadelphia: Lea & Febiger, 1973, pp. 1893–1900.
42. E. O. Rijke and R. E. Ballieux: Is thymus-derived lymphocyte inhibitor a polyamine? Nature *274:*804–805, 1978.
43. K. N. Prasad and S. Kumar: Expression of differentiated functions in neuroblastoma cell culture. *In The Cell Cycle in Malignancy and Immunity.* J. C. Hampton, ed. Technical Information Center ERDA, 1975, pp. 132–155.

44. J. B. Beckwith and R. F. Martin: Observations on the histopathology of neuroblastomas. J. Pediatr. Surg. *3:*106–110, 1968.
45. E. J. Ariëns: Drug design and cancer. *In Pharmacological Basis of Cancer Chemotherapy.* Baltimore: Williams & Wilkins, 1975, pp. 127–152.
46. T. Ghose, R. C. Nairn, and J. E. Fothergill: Uptake of proteins by malignant cells. Nature *196:*1108–1109, 1962.
47. J. Whang-Peng, S. Perry, and T. Knutsen: Maturation and phagocytosis by chronic myelogenous leukemia cells *in vitro.* A preliminary report. J. Natl. Cancer Inst. *38:*969–977, 1967.
48. C. H. Sutton and N. H. Becker: Lysosomes and pinocytosis in human and experimental brain tumors. Ann. N.Y. Acad. Sci. *159:*497–508, 1969.
49. A. Trouet, D. Deprez-de Campeneere and C. De Duve: Chemotherapy through lysosomes with a DNA-daunorubicin complex. Nature New Biol. *239:*110–112, 1972.
50. D. W. Henry: Adriamycin (NSC-123127) and its analogs. Cancer Chemother. Rep. Part 2, *4:*5–9, 1974.
51. G. Gregoriadis and E. D. Nerrunjun: Treatment of tumour-bearing mice with liposome-entrapped actinomycin D prolongs their survival. Res. Commun. Chem. Pathol. Pharmacol. *10:*351–362, 1975.
52. E. Mayhew, D. Papahadjopoulous, Y. M. Rustum, and C. Dave: Inhibition of tumor cell growth *in vitro* and *in vivo* by 1-β-D-arabinofuranosyl-cytosine entrapped within phospholipid vesicles. Cancer Res. *36:*4406–4411, 1976.
53. R. J. Rutman, C. A. Ritter, N. G. Avadhani, and J. Hansel: Liposomal potentiation of the antitumor activity of alkylating agents. Cancer Treat. Rep. *60:*617–618, 1976.
54. G. Gregoriadis and E. D. Nerrunjun: Homing of liposomes to target cells. Biochem. Biophys. Res. Commun. *65:*537–544, 1975.
55. R. L. Juliano and D. Stamp: Lectin-mediated attachment of glycoprotein-bearing liposomes to cells. Nature *261:*235–238, 1976.
55A. S. Order: Treatment found for liver cancer. Science News *118:*229, 1980.
56. T. Kitao and K. Hattori: Concanavalin A as a carrier of daunomycin. Nature *265:*81–82, 1977.
57. J. H. Linford, G. Froese, I. Berczi, and L. G. Israels: An alkylating agent-globulin conjugate with both alkylating and antibody activity. J. Natl. Cancer Inst. *52:*1665–1667, 1974.
58. W. B. Pratt and R. W. Ruddon: *The Anticancer Drugs.* New York, Oxford: Oxford University Press, 1979, p. 168.
59. K. D. Collins and G. R. Stark: Aspartate transcarbamylase. Interaction with the transition state analog N-(phosphonacetyl)-L-aspartate. J. Biol. Chem. *246:*6599–6605, 1971.
60. L. S. Dietrich: Cytotoxic analogs of pyridine nucleotide coenzymes. *In Antineoplastic and Immunosuppressive Agents II.* A. C. Sartorelli and D. G. Johns, eds. Berlin-Heidelberg-New York: Springer-Verlag, 1975, pp. 539–543, 891–892.
61. G. A. Tejwani: Th role of phosphofructokinase in the Pasteur effect. Trends Biochem. Sci. *3:*30–33, 1978.
62. E. Eigenbrodt and H. Glossmann: Glycolysis—one of the keys to cancer? Trends Pharmacol. Sci. *1:*240–245, 1980.
63. B. R. G. Williams, R. R. Golgher, R. E. Brown, C. S. Gilbert, and I. M. Kerr: Natural occurrence of 2-5A in interferon-treated EMC virus-infected L cells. Nature *282:*582–586, 1979.
64. G. W. Santos: Bone marrow transplantation. Adv. Int. Med. *24:*157–182, 1979.

Index